Toll-Like Receptors in Diseases of the Lung

Edited by

Catherine M. Greene

Respiratory Research Division
Department of Medicine
Royal College of Surgeons in Ireland
Ireland

CONTENTS

FOREWORD

The lung is the largest surface area of the body in contact with the external environment and it is constantly exposed to a wide array of microbes and particles. As a result the body's immune system evolved a series of systems which enables it to distinguish potentially harmful agents from those which are innocuous. Two of the major systems are the adaptive and innate immune responses. The innate system is fast responding and recognizes a wide variety of potentially noxious stimuli coming into the lungs. In the majority of cases these may be microbial products, however on occasion the innate immune system can also respond to host-derived danger signals not normally encountered in the healthy lung. A key component of this response is the germ-line encoded pattern recognition receptor family of Toll-like receptors. TLRs regulate the lung's response to potential pathogens or other environmental hazards and communicate closely with the adaptive immune response to orchestrate effective resolution of infection and a return to homeostasis. Our understanding of the role of TLRs in infectious, environmental and genetic lung diseases has advanced greatly over the last fifteen years. In this book experts from around the world offer their insights into the mechanisms of TLR-mediated responses in a number of common but serious diseases of the lung, and explore how our growing knowledge of the mode of action of TLRs can be exploited for therapeutic use.

Noel G. McElvaney
Consultant Respiratory Physician, Beaumont Hospital, Dublin Ireland
Professor of Medicine, Royal College of Surgeons in Ireland
Ireland

PREFACE

Since the discovery of the mammalian Toll-like receptors in the 1990s, we have seen advances in our understanding of the basic biology, genetics and function of this family of proteins at a rate rarely paralleled. It is hoped that this book will provide the reader with a comprehensive review of what is now known regarding the roles of TLRs in maintaining pulmonary health and will outline why TLRs are so important in orchestrating the host's innate immune response during a variety of common and often life threatening pulmonary diseases. Topics that are covered in the ten chapters include the expression, function and activation of TLRs during bacterial, viral and fungal infection of the airways – concentrating on global diseases such as pneumonia and tuberculosis; the role of TLRs in the pathogenesis of important genetic and environmental pulmonary disorders such as cystic fibrosis, COPD and asthma; and TLR biology in the context of transplantation. Each chapter highlights recent advances in the area, explores the usefulness and current status of TLR-directed therapies and all are written by leading experts in the field.

Catherine M. Greene
Respiratory Research Division
Department of Medicine
Royal College of Surgeons in Ireland
Ireland

List of Contributors

Gillina Bezemer

Division of Pharmacology, Utrecht Institute for Pharmaceutical Sciences, Faculty of Science, Utrecht University, Utrecht, The Netherlands.

Sanjay H. Chotirmall

Respiratory Research - Dept. Medicine, Royal College of Surgeons in Ireland, Education and Research Centre, Beaumont Hospital, Dublin 9, Ireland; Email: schotirmall@rcsi.ie

Catherine A. Coughlan

Respiratory Research - Dept. Medicine, Royal College of Surgeons in Ireland, Education and Research Centre, Beaumont Hospital, Dublin 9, Ireland; Email: catherinecoughlan@rcsi.ie

Gert Folkerts

Division of Pharmacology, Utrecht Institute for Pharmaceutical Sciences, Faculty of Science, Utrecht University, Utrecht, The Netherlands; Email: G.Folkerts@uu.nl

J. Garssen

Division of Pharmacology, Utrecht Institute for Pharmaceutical Sciences, Faculty of Science, Utrecht University, Utrecht, The Netherlands and Danone Research - Centre for Specialised Nutrition, Wageningen, The Netherlands.

Niki A. Georgiou

Division of Pharmacology & Pathophysiology, Department of Pharmaceutical Sciences, Faulty of Science, Utrecht University, Utrecht, The Netherlands, and Danone Research Centre for Specialised Nutrition, Bosrandweg 20, 6704 PH Wageningen, The Netherlands.

Catherine M. Greene

Respiratory Research - Dept. Medicine, RCSI Education and Research Centre, Beaumont Hospital, Dublin 9, Ireland; Email: cmgreene@rcsi.ie

Markus O. Henke

Philipps-University Marburg, Department of Pulmonary Medicine, Baldingerstraße 1, 35043 Marburg, Germany; Email: markus.henke@staff.uni-marburg.de

Toshihiro Ito

Department of Pathology, University of Michigan Medical School, Ann Arbor, Michigan 48109, USA.

Gerrit John

Comprehensive Pneumology Center, Institute of Lung Biology and Disease, Helmholtz Zentrum München, Ingolstädter Landstraße 1, 85764 Neuherberg, Germany; Tel: +49-89-31873795; E-mail: gerrit.john@helmholtz-muenchen.de

Sebastian Johnston

Department of Respiratory Medicine, National Heart & Lung Institute, Imperial College London W2 1PG, London UK Tel: +44 20 7594 3764 Fax: +44 20 7262 8913; Email: s.johnston@imperial.ac.uk

Shaf Keshavjee

The Latner Thoracic Surgery Research Laboratories, Toronto General Research Institute, University Health Network, Department of Surgery, Faculty of Medicine, University of Toronto, Canada

Sylvia Knapp

Center for Molecular Medicine & Department of Medicine 1, Division of Infectious Diseases and Tropical Medicine, Medical University Vienna, Waehringer Guertel 18-20, Vienna, 1090, Austria; Tel: +43-1-40400-5139; E-mail: sylvia.knapp@meduniwien.ac.at

Aletta D. Kraneveld

Division of Pharmacology, Utrecht Institute for Pharmaceutical Sciences, Faculty of Science, Utrecht University, PO box 80082, 3508 TB Utrecht, The Netherlands. Tel: +31302534509; E-mail: A.D.Kraneveld@uu.nl

Steven L. Kunkel

Department of Pathology, University of Michigan Medical School, Ann Arbor, Michigan 48109, USA; E-mail: slkunkel@umich.edu

Mingyao Liu

Faculty of Medicine, University of Toronto, 101 College Street, Toronto Medical Discovery Tower, Room 2-814,Toronto, Ontario, M5G 1L7 Canada; Tel: 416-581-7500; E-mail: mingyao.liu@utoronto.ca

Valerie Quesniaux

University of Orleans and CNRS UMR6218 Molecular Immunology and Embryology, 3B rue de la Ferollerie, 45071 Orleans Cedex 2, France; E-mail: quesniaux@cnrs-orleans.fr

Emer P. Reeves

Department of Medicine, Royal College of Surgeons in Ireland, Education and Research Centre, Beaumont Hospital, Dublin 9, Ireland; Tel: 353-1-8093877; E-mail: emerreeves@rcsi.ie

Siel Sagar

Division of Pharmacology & Pathophysiology, Department of Pharmaceutical Sciences, Faulty of Science, Utrecht University, Utrecht, The Netherlands, and Danone Research Centre for Specialised Nutrition, Bosrandweg 20, 6704 PH Wageningen, The Netherlands

Stephanie Traub

Department of Respiratory Medicine, National Heart & Lung Institute, Imperial College London W2 1PG, London UK; Email: s.traub@imperial.ac.uk

Jeroen van Bergenhenegouwen

Danone Research – Centre for Specialised Nutrition, Wageningen, The Netherlands and Division of Pharmacology, Utrecht Institute for Pharmaceutical Sciences, Faculty of Science, Utrecht University, Utrecht, The Netherlands

Jonathan C. Yeung

The Latner Thoracic Surgery Research Laboratories, Toronto General Research Institute, University Health Network, Department of Surgery, Faculty of Medicine, University of Toronto, Canada

CHAPTER 1

The Toll-like Receptor Family

Catherine M. Greene[*]

Respiratory Research Division, Department of Medicine, Royal College of Surgeons in Ireland

Abstract: Toll-like receptors (TLRs) comprise a major family of pattern-recognition receptors (PRRs) that fulfill a key role in recognizing, discriminating and responding appropriately to microbial infection. Although expressed principally by macrophages and dendritic cells, TLRs expression is widespread and includes, but is not limited to cells of myeloid and lymphoid origin. Activation of TLRs by their cognate ligands can lead to induction of proinflammatory cytokine and antimicrobial peptide expression or up regulation of type 1 interferons. Whilst central to innate immunity, TLRs can additionally communicate with the adaptive immune response *via* modulation of cell-adhesion and co-stimulatory molecules to induce longer term immunity. Interestingly a selection of non-microbial endogenous factors can also activate certain TLRs, with dysregulation of these events having potentially deleterious consequences. Since the first report of human TLR4 by Medzhitov and Janeway in 1997 [1] there has been huge progress in elucidating the fundamental processes controlling the biology of the TLR family.

Keywords: TLRs, PAMPs, DAMPs, MyD88-dependent, TRIF-dependent signaling.

1. INNATE AND ADAPTIVE IMMUNITY

Innate immunity represents the first line of defense against invading micro-organisms. It provides a rapid but short-lived reaction. In contrast, the adaptive immune response is activated more slowly but provides longer-lasting antigen-specific responses that involve antibody and cell-mediated immunity. Antigen receptors are important in the adaptive immune response and can provide customized specificity to individual antigens *via* somatic recombination of the genes encoding variable regions of these receptors. Originally thought to be non-discriminatory, the innate immune system is in fact highly specific. This attribute is due to PRRs, a collection of germ-line encoded receptors central to the innate immune system. PRRs have broad specificities for conserved, invariant structures of microbes. TLRs are a subclass of PRRs that can detect particular molecular patterns and have unique properties that are shared by members of the TLR family.

2. WHAT DO TLRs DO?

The function of dendritic cells and macrophages is to ingest pathogens, release cytokines and activate antigen-specific T- and B-cell clones. The first step in this process is the recognition of invading microbes by these phagocytic cells, largely *via* the engagement of TLRs with specific structures present on the microbes; two co-incidental events rapidly ensue (Fig. **1**). (i) Intracellular signaling pathways are activated that can lead to transcriptional induction of antimicrobial defenses including antimicrobial peptide, pro-inflammatory or antiviral cytokine expression. IL-1β, TNF and IL-6, for example, co-ordinate local and systemic inflammatory responses, activate the endothelium to induce vasodilation enabling leucocyte recruitment, local coagulation occurs to prevent microbial dissemination, and acute phase proteins are produced which, in turn, can activate complement and opsonize pathogens for phagocytosis. Type 1 interferons bind to interferon receptors and induce the expression of genes with anti-viral and anti-tumor effects. (ii) The expression of a subset of cell surface receptors (*e.g.* B7, CD80) is concomitantly induced which, in conjunction with MHC class II molecules displaying antigen, can engage with CD28 and the T cell receptor (TCR), respectively, on naïve T cells. This stimulates the adaptive immune response and in turn leads to maturation of T cell subtypes, further lymphocyte-specific cytokine expression (*e.g.* IL-12 and IL-23 stimulate the production of Th1 and Th17 cells, respectively) and initiation of B cell expansion and antibody production.

***Address correspondence to Catherine M. Greene:** Respiratory Research - Dept. Medicine, RCSI Education and Research Centre, Beaumont Hospital, Dublin 9, Ireland. E-mail: cmgreene@rcsi.ie

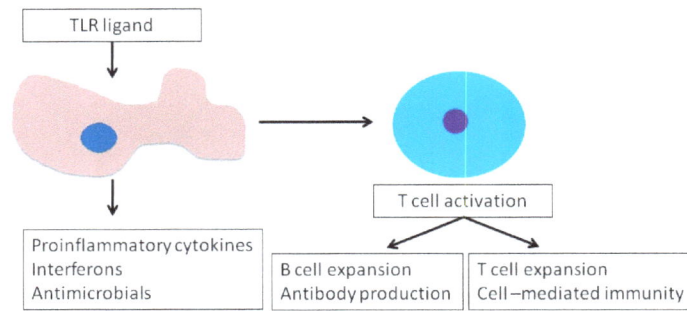

Figure 1: Effects of TLR activation.

3. DISCOVERY OF TLRs

TLRs were first identified in the fruit fly *Drosophila melanogaster*. Initially *Drosophila* or dToll was described as a protein with an important a role in regulating dorsal-ventral axis formation during fly embryogenesis [2]. Subsequently dToll was found to have a role in antimicrobial defense in the adult fly [3]. It was not until 1997 that the first human Toll-like receptor was cloned and characterized [1]. This receptor became known as TLR4 and was first described as a type I transmembrane protein with an extracellular domain consisting of leucine-rich repeats (LRR) and a cytoplasmic domain homologous to the cytoplasmic domain of the human IL-1 type 1 receptor (IL-1RI). Both dToll and IL-1R1 signal *via* evolutionarily conserved signaling pathways leading to activation of the transcription factor Dorsal or its mammalian homologue NFκB, respectively [4]. This finding provided functional confirmation of the earlier report that both dToll and IL-1R1 share sequence similarity in their intracellular domains [5]. TLR4's identity as the mammalian LPS receptor came soon after from studies on the LPS hypo-responsive mouse strain C3H/HeJ [6]. These mice can withstand challenge with lethal doses of LPS due an inactivating Pro712His mutation in TLR4.

It is now known that there are 13 members of the mammalian TLR family, TLR1-13. To date 10 functional TLRs have been identified in humans; 12 exist in mice. TLRs 1-9 are conserved in both species, in the mouse TLR10 is non-functional due to a retroviral insertion and TLRs 11-13 have been lost from the human genome.

4. STRUCTURE & CELLULAR LOCALISATION

TLRs belong to a larger family of proteins called the IL-1 receptor (IL-1R)/TLR superfamily. All are type 1 integral membrane glycoproteins. Members of this family share sequence similarity in their intracellular domains but have either leucine-rich repeat motifs or immunoglobulin-like domains in their ectodomains. The TLR subfamily has LRRs; these mediate the recognition of TLR ligands. Recently, there has been progress in the elucidation of the crystal structures of several TLR ectodomains with their ligands [7-10]. For most TLRs the initial step in signal transduction involves dimerization of two receptor chains following binding of a specific ligand. TLR7, TLR8 and TLR9, however can be present in the cell as a preformed but inactive dimer, with ligand binding causing a reorientation of the TIR domains to allow signal transduction to occur [11]. Unlike the other TLRs, TLR4 forms a complex together with the GPI-anchored protein CD14 and a protein called MD2 that resides in the outer leaflet of the cell membrane [12]. This process is unique among the TLR family however TLR2 may also utilize CD14 and/or MD2 in certain circumstances [13].

The intracellular signaling domain of TLRs carries a functional signature motif known as the TIR (Toll/interleukin-1 receptor) domain. This cytosolic domain is a conserved region of approximately 200 amino acids [14] that is essential for signaling. TIR-TIR interactions between TLRs and specific intracellular adaptor proteins transduce the message that ligand activation has occurred.

Depending on their cellular localization TLRS can be divided into two subgroups. TLRs that are expressed on the cell surface include TLR1, TLR2, TLR4, TLR5, TLR6 and TLR11, whereas TLR3, TLR7, TLR8 and TLR9 are expressed in intracellular vesicles such as the endoplasmic reticulum (ER) and endolysosomes. TLR7 and TLR9 are sequestered in the ER in unstimulated cells and their trafficking to endolysosomes is regulated *via* UNC93B1 [15, 16]. Two other ER proteins also regulate TLR trafficking to the plasma membrane or endolysosomes: PRAT4 and gp96 [17-19]. Unlike the other TLRs, TLR9 has been shown to require proteolytic cleavage within the endolysosome by proteases such as the cysteinyl cathepsins B, L, S, H and K or asparaginyl endopeptidase in order to become functional [20-24].

5. TLR LIGANDS

TLR ligands include structures expressed by bacteria, fungi, protozoans and viruses. These tend to be essential invariant motifs not expressed by eukaryotes and have been designated the acronym PAMPs, denoting pathogen-associated molecular patterns, however this is a misnomer in that PAMPs are not only expressed by pathogens but also by non-pathogenic microbial species. Host-derived factors can also activate TLRs and these so-called danger or damage-associated molecular patterns (DAMPs) represent factors not normally encountered in healthy tissue due to mislocalization, protease-mediated damage or as a result of infectious or sterile insults [13].

6. PAMPs AND DAMPs

6.1. PAMPs

TLR1, TLR2 and TLR6

These TLRs arose from an evolutionary gene duplication event and are very similar in their primary sequences [25]. Homo- or heterodimerization between TLR2 and either TLR1 or TLR6 allows the recognition of a wide array of ligands [26]. For example, together TLR2 and TLR1 recognize triacylated lipopeptides whilst TLR2-TLR6 heterodimers recognize diacylated lipopeptides. Amongst TLR2 agonists, bacterial lipoproteins are the most potent [27, 28]. Microbial lipids, acylated sugars and proteins, unmodified protein complexes, and some polysaccharides also act as TLR2 agonists [29, 30]. Examples of these include zwitterionic polysaccharides from Group B *Streptococcus* [31], type 2b heat-labile enterotoxin from enteropathogenic *Escherichia coli* [32] and porin B from pathogenic *Neisseriae* sp. [33]. In addition to TLR1 and TLR6, other co-receptors such as CD36 [34] and dectin-1 can co-operate with TLR2 in the recognition of certain PAMPs *e.g.* β-glucan [35].

TLR3

TLR3 recognizes viral double-stranded RNA (dsRNA), certain small interfering RNAs and polyriboinosinic-polyribocytidylic acid (poly I:C), a synthetic analog of dsRNA [36, 37]. Genomic dsRNA from reovirus and dsRNA produced during the replication of ssRNA viruses including West Nile virus and respiratory syncytial virus has also been reported to activate TLR3. In addition, polyriboadenylic-polyribouridylic acid (poly A:U) is an agonist of both TLR3 and TLR7 [38].

TLR4

TLR4 is the key receptor involved in the recognition of bacterial lipopolysaccharide (LPS) and is important to the host response when combating against Gram-negative bacterial infections [6, 39-42]. TLR4 can also recognize other microbial agonists including mannans from *Saccharomyces*, *Candida* and *Cryptococcus* species, protozoan glycophspholipidinositols, pneumolysin [43], Hsp60 from *Chlamydia pneumoniae,* flavolipin, murine retroviruses and fusion protein from respiratory syncytial virus (RSV) [44-47]. The plant-derived products taxol and paclitaxel can also bind to TLR4 [48, 49].

TLR5

The TLR5 receptor recognizes flagellin, a principal protein component of bacterial flagella expressed on gram-negative bacteria [50, 51].

TLR7 and TLR8

TLR7 and 8 are found in endosomes of monocytes and macrophages. Both of these receptors recognize guanosine- and uridine-rich viral single-stranded RNA [52, 53]. TLR7 can recognize ssRNA derived from vesicular stomatitis virus and influenza A virus, synthetic poly(U) RNA, some siRNAs and the imidazoquinoline derivatives imiquimod and resiquimod (R-848). TLR8 is phylogentetically most similar to TLR7. In humans TLR8 is activated by viral ssRNA and imidazoquinolines.

TLR9

TLR9 acts as a receptor for unmethylated 2'- deoxyribo (cytodine-phosphate-guanosine) (CpG) motifs in bacteria and DNA viruses [54]. These motifs commonly occur in bacterial and viral DNA, whereas in vertebrate DNA they are rarer and are usually in a methylated form. The *Plasmodium falciparum* haemoglobin digestion product hemozoin is also directly recognized by TLR9 [55].

TLR10-TLR13

Human TLR10 is an orphan member of the TLR family [56]. In mice TLR11 responds to a surface-exposed factor on uropathogenic *E. coli* and protozoan profilin [57, 58] however full length TLR11 expression in humans is prevented due to a stop codon mutation. TLR12 and TLR13 are expressed in mice but not in humans. TLR13 is located intracellularly in murine macrophages and dendritic cells in the spleen and can respond to vesicular stomatitis virus.

6.2. DAMPs

It is increasingly clear that TLRs respond not only to PAMPs but also to self-antigens to trigger inflammatory responses. The endogenous molecules responsible are produced mainly as a result of cell death or injury, or by tumor cells, and have been coined DAMPs for danger/damage-associated molecular patterns [13]. The major DAMPs that have been identified include protease-generated degradation products of the extracellular matrix (biglycan, versican, hyaluronic acid, fibronectin extradomain A), high mobility group box 1 proteins, heat-shock proteins, amyloid-β, surfactant protein A, oxidized low density lipoproteins and phospholipids, immune complexes, LL-37, and self chromatin-DNA and ribonucleoprotein-RNA complexes and neutrophil elastase. TLR2, TLR4 and TLR6 have been implicated in the responses to most of these signals with the occasional involvement of co-receptors such as CD36. TLR7 and TLR9 also recognize and respond to self nucleic acids that are complexed to autoantibodies, HMGB1 or LL-37 and are delivered to endosomes *via* FcγRIIa or RAGE, for example.

7. TLR SIGNALING PATHWAYS

A family of TIR domain-containing adaptor protein exists that is responsible for mediating intracellular signaling by TLRs. These are MyD88, TIRAP (also called Mal), TRIF (or TICAM-1), TRAM (or TICAM-2) and SARM. Activating functions have been assigned to MyD88, TIRAP, TRIF [59, 60] and TRAM whilst SARM acts as a negative regulator of TRIF-dependent TLR signaling. All TLRs with the exception of TLR3 signal *via* MyD88 with TIRAP being utilized by TLR2 and TLR4 to engage with MyD88. TLR3 and TLR4 can utilize TRIF, either directly (for TLR3) or *via* TRAM (in the case of TLR4) (Fig. **2**). In addition to SARM a selection of endogenous and microbial inhibitors have been identified that can interfere with TLR signaling *via* a variety of mechanisms (reviewed in [61]).

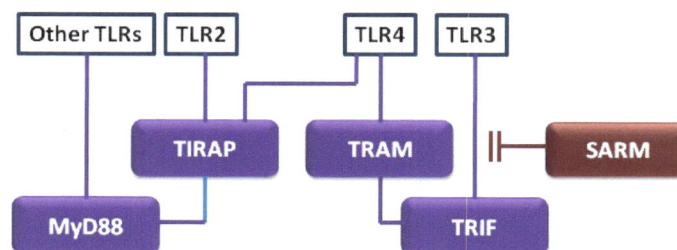

Figure 2: TLR adaptor proteins.

7.1. MyD88-Dependent

Signaling *via* MyD88 leads to activation of the transcription factor NFκB and the mitogen-activated protein kinases (MAPKs) to induce proinflammatory cytokine expression [62, 63] (Fig. **3**). Following association of the TIR domain of MyD88 with TIRAP or a TLR, an intracellular signaling cascade is activated involving the sequential activation of IL-1 receptor-associated kinase 4 (IRAK4), IRAK1 and IRAK2, and the E3 ubiquitin ligase TRAF6. Lysine63-linked ubiquitination of TRAF6 and IRAK1 occurs *via* the ubiquitin-conjugating enzymes Ubc13 and Uev1. In turn the regulatory proteins TAB2 and TAB3 bind and activate TAK1, the kinase responsible for activation of the IKK complex *via* phosphorylation of IKKβ. IκB proteins are phosphorylated, ubiquitinated and degraded by the proteosome, revealing nuclear localization sequences on NFκB that allow it to translocate into the nucleus, bind to NFκB consensus sequences in NFκB–regulated genes and induce their expression. TAK1 also phosphorylates the MAPKs ERK1, ERK2, p38 and JNK which can induce AP1 activation and influence translation. IRF5 activation by TRAF6 also leads to induction of proinflammatory cytokine genes, whilst IRF7 can also be activated by TRAF6 *via* TRAF3 leading to type I interferon induction.

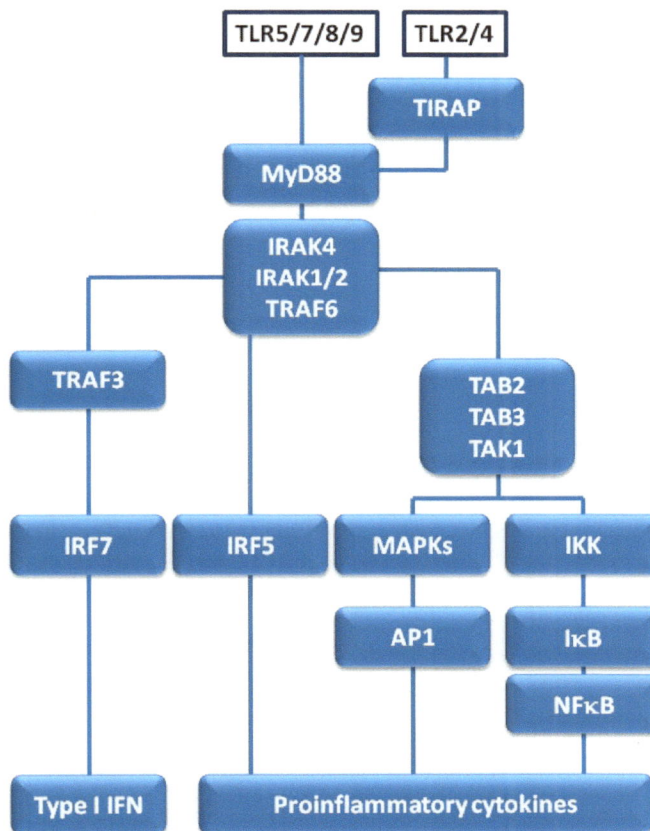

Figure 3: MyD88-dependent signaling.

7.2. TRIF-Dependent

Signaling *via* TRIF (sometimes referred to as MyD88-independent signaling) leads to activation of the IRF transcription factors or NFκB *via* the so-called 'non-canonical' pathway with consequent induction of type I interferons and inflammatory cytokines, respectively [63] (Fig. **4**). TRIF recruits TRAF6 to activate NFκB and MAPKs as described above. It can also activate this axis *via* interaction with TRADD, Pellino and RIP1. TRAF3 can mediate TRIF's activation of IKKi and TBK1 which phosphorylate and activate IRF3 and induce type 1 interferon expression.

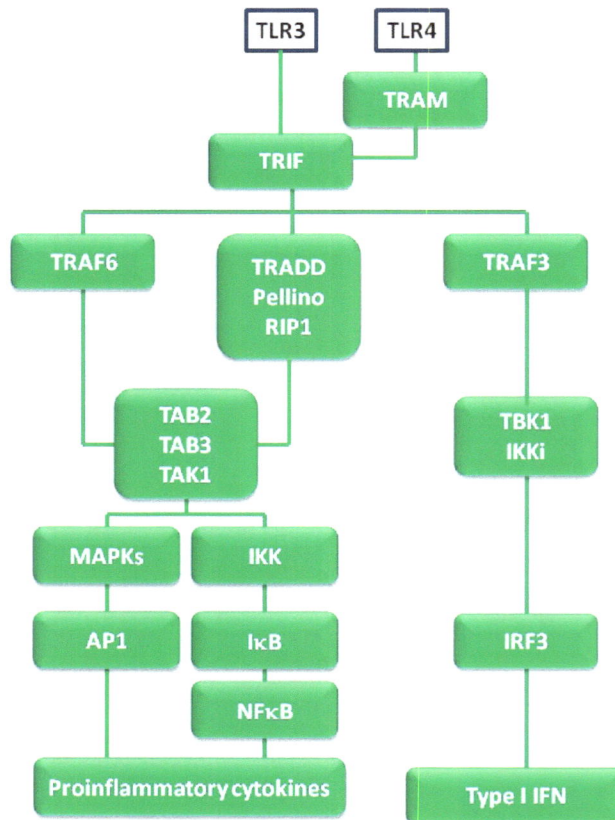

Figure 4: TRIF-dependent signaling.

8. CONCLUSION

TLRs control a complex and well co-ordinated network. Their primary role as sensors of microbial infection is indispensible for effective innate immunity. With respect to sterile inflammation, TLRs have also emerged as key factors, and together with their central role in activating the adaptive immune response, it is apparent that they occupy a pivotal position in the control of inflammatory and immune responses. How the expression and function of different TLRs can contribute to pulmonary disease, and whether therapeutics that harness or exploit the TLR network have potential for certain of these diseases is explored in the following chapters.

REFERENCES

[1]   Medzhitov R, Preston-Hurlburt P, Janeway CA, Jr. A human homologue of the *Drosophila* Toll protein signals activation of adaptive immunity. Nature 1997; 388: 394-7.

[2]   Anderson KV, Jurgens G, Nusslein-Volhard C. Establishment of dorsal-ventral polarity in the *Drosophila* embryo: genetic studies on the role of the Toll gene product. Cell 1985; 42: 779-89.

[3]   Lemaitre B, Nicolas E, Michaut L, Reichhart JM, Hoffmann JA. The dorsoventral regulatory gene cassette spatzle/Toll/cactus controls the potent antifungal response in *Drosophila* adults. Cell 1996; 86: 973-83.

[4]   O'Neill LA, Greene C. Signal transduction pathways activated by the IL-1 receptor family: ancient signaling machinery in mammals, insects, and plants. J Leukoc Biol 1998; 63: 650-7.

[5]   Gay NJ, Keith FJ. *Drosophila* Toll and IL-1 receptor. Nature 1991; 351: 355-6.

[6]   Poltorak A, He X, Smirnova I *et al.* Defective LPS signaling in C3H/HeJ and C57BL/10ScCr mice: mutations in Tlr4 gene. Science 199; 282: 2085-8.

[7]　Kim HM, Park BS, Kim JI *et al.* Crystal structure of the TLR4-MD-2 complex with bound endotoxin antagonist Eritoran. Cell 2007; 130: 906-17.

[8]　Park BS, Song DH, Kim HM, Choi BS, Lee H, Lee JO. The structural basis of lipopolysaccharide recognition by the TLR4-MD-2 complex. Nature 2009; 458: 1191-5.

[9]　Jin MS, Kim SE, Heo JY *et al.* Crystal structure of the TLR1-TLR2 heterodimer induced by binding of a tri-acylated lipopeptide. Cell 2007; 130: 1071-82.

[10]　Kang JY, Nan X, Jin MS *et al.* Recognition of lipopeptide patterns by Toll-like receptor 2-Toll-like receptor 6 heterodimer. Immunity 2009; 31: 873-84.

[11]　Zhu J, Brownlie R, Liu Q, Babiuk LA, Potter A, Mutwiri GK. Characterization of bovine Toll-like receptor 8: ligand specificity, signaling essential sites and dimerization. Mol Immunol 2009; 46: 978-90.

[12]　Shimazu R, Akashi S, Ogata H *et al.* MD-2, a molecule that confers lipopolysaccharide responsiveness on Toll-like receptor 4. J Exp Med 1999; 189: 1777-82.

[13]　Piccinini AM, Midwood KS. DAMPening inflammation by modulating TLR signaling. Mediators Inflamm 2010; 2010.

[14]　O'Neill LA. Signal transduction pathways activated by the IL-1 receptor/toll-like receptor superfamily. Curr Top Microbiol Immunol 2002; 270: 47-61.

[15]　Kim YM, Brinkmann MM, Paquet ME, Ploegh HL. UNC93B1 delivers nucleotide-sensing toll-like receptors to endolysosomes. Nature 2008; 452: 234-8.

[16]　Tabeta K, Hoebe K, Janssen EM *et al.* The Unc93b1 mutation 3d disrupts exogenous antigen presentation and signaling *via* Toll-like receptors 3, 7 and 9. Nat Immunol 2006; 7: 156-64.

[17]　Takahashi K, Shibata T, Akashi-Takamura S *et al.* A protein associated with Toll-like receptor (TLR) 4 (PRAT4A) is required for TLR-dependent immune responses. J Exp Med 2007; 204: 2963-76.

[18]　Kiyokawa T, Akashi-Takamura S, Shibata T *et al.* A single base mutation in the PRAT4A gene reveals differential interaction of PRAT4A with Toll-like receptors. Int Immunol 2008; 20: 1407-15.

[19]　Yang Y, Liu B, Dai J *et al.* Heat shock protein gp96 is a master chaperone for toll-like receptors and is important in the innate function of macrophages. Immunity 2007; 26: 215-26.

[20]　Park B, Brinkmann MM, Spooner E, Lee CC, Kim YM, Ploegh HL. Proteolytic cleavage in an endolysosomal compartment is required for activation of Toll-like receptor 9. Nat Immunol 2008; 9: 1407-14.

[21]　Ewald SE, Lee BL, Lau L *et al.* The ectodomain of Toll-like receptor 9 is cleaved to generate a functional receptor. Nature 2008; 456: 658-62.

[22]　Ewald SE, Engel A, Lee J, Wang M, Bogyo M, Barton GM. Nucleic acid recognition by Toll-like receptors is coupled to stepwise processing by cathepsins and asparagine endopeptidase. J Exp Med 2011; 208: 643-51.

[23]　Matsumoto F, Saitoh S, Fukui R *et al.* Cathepsins are required for Toll-like receptor 9 responses. Biochem Biophys Res Commun 2008; 367: 693-9.

[24]　Sepulveda FE, Maschalidi S, Colisson R *et al.* Critical role for asparagine endopeptidase in endocytic Toll-like receptor signaling in dendritic cells. Immunity 2009; 31: 737-48.

[25]　Hughes AL, Piontkivska H. Functional diversification of the toll-like receptor gene family. Immunogenetics 2008; 60: 249-56.

[26]　Wetzler LM. The role of Toll-like receptor 2 in microbial disease and immunity. Vaccine 2003; 21: S55-60.

[27]　Aliprantis AO, Yang RB, Mark MR *et al.* Cell activation and apoptosis by bacterial lipoproteins through toll-like receptor-2. Science 1999; 285: 736-9.

[28]　Brightbill HD, Libraty DH, Krutzik SR *et al.* Host defense mechanisms triggered by microbial lipoproteins through toll-like receptors. Science 1999; 285: 732-6.

[29]　Miyake K. Innate immune sensing of pathogens and danger signals by cell surface Toll-like receptors. Semin Immunol 2007; 19: 3-10.

[30]　Tapping RI. Innate immune sensing and activation of cell surface Toll-like receptors. Semin Immunol 2009; 21: 175-84.

[31]　Gallorini S, Berti F, Mancuso G *et al.* Toll-like receptor 2 dependent immunogenicity of glycoconjugate vaccines containing chemically derived zwitterionic polysaccharides. Proc Natl Acad Sci U S A 2009; 106: 17481-6.

[32]　Liang S, Hosur KB, Nawar HF, Russell MW, Connell TD, Hajishengallis G. *In vivo* and *in vitro* adjuvant activities of the B subunit of Type IIb heat-labile enterotoxin (LT-IIb-B5) from *Escherichia coli*. Vaccine 2009; 27:4302-8.

[33]　Liu X, Wetzler LM, Massari P. The PorB porin from commensal *Neisseria lactamica* induces Th1 and Th2 immune responses to ovalbumin in mice and is a potential immune adjuvant. Vaccine 2008; 26: 786-96.

[34]   Triantafilou M, Gamper FG, Haston RM *et al.* Membrane sorting of toll-like receptor (TLR)-2/6 and TLR2/1 heterodimers at the cell surface determines heterotypic associations with CD36 and intracellular targeting. J Biol Chem 2006; 281: 31002-11.

[35]   Gantner BN, Simmons RM, Canavera SJ, Akira S, Underhill DM. Collaborative induction of inflammatory responses by dectin-1 and Toll-like receptor 2. J Exp Med 2003; 197: 1107-17.

[36]   Alexopoulou L, Holt AC, Medzhitov R, Flavell RA. Recognition of double-stranded RNA and activation of NF-kappaB by Toll-like receptor 3. Nature 2001; 413: 732-8.

[37]   Reynolds A, Anderson EM, Vermeulen A *et al.* Induction of the interferon response by siRNA is cell type- and duplex length-dependent. RNA. 2006; 12: 988-93.

[38]   Sugiyama T, Hoshino K, Saito M *et al.* Immunoadjuvant effects of polyadenylic:polyuridylic acids through TLR3 and TLR7. Int Immunol 2008; 20: 1-9.

[39]   Qureshi ST, Lariviere L, Leveque G *et al.* Endotoxin-tolerant mice have mutations in Toll-like receptor 4 (Tlr4). J Exp Med 1999; 189: 615-25.

[40]   Chow JC, Young DW, Golenbock DT, Christ WJ, Gusovsky F. Toll-like receptor-4 mediates lipopolysaccharide-induced signal transduction. J Biol Chem 1999; 274: 10689-92.

[41]   Hoshino K, Takeuchi O, Kawai T *et al.* Cutting edge: Toll-like receptor 4 (TLR4)-deficient mice are hyporesponsive to lipopolysaccharide: evidence for TLR4 as the Lps gene product. J Immunol 1999; 162: 3749-52.

[42]   Vogel SN, Johnson D, Perera PY *et al.* Cutting edge: functional characterization of the effect of the C3H/HeJ defect in mice that lack an Lpsn gene: *in vivo* evidence for a dominant negative mutation. J Immunol 1999; 162: 5666-70.

[43]   Malley R, Henneke P, Morse SC, Cieslewicz MJ *et al.* Recognition of pneumolysin by Toll-like receptor 4 confers resistance to pneumococcal infection. Proc Natl Acad Sci U S A 2003; 100: 1966-71.

[44]   Rassa JC, Meyers JL, Zhang Y, Kudaravalli R, Ross SR. Murine retroviruses activate B cells *via* interaction with toll-like receptor 4. Proc Natl Acad Sci U S A 2002; 99: 2281-6.

[45]   Gomi K, Kawasaki K, Kawai Y, Shiozaki M, Nishijima M. Toll-like receptor 4-MD-2 complex mediates the signal transduction induced by flavolipin, an amino acid-containing lipid unique to *Flavobacterium meningosepticum*. J Immunol 2002; 168: 2939-43.

[46]   Sasu S, LaVerda D, Qureshi N, Golenbock DT, Beasley D. *Chlamydia pneumoniae* and chlamydial heat shock protein 60 stimulate proliferation of human vascular smooth muscle cells *via* toll-like receptor 4 and p44/p42 mitogen-activated protein kinase activation. Circ Res 2001; 89: 244-50.

[47]   Kurt-Jones EA, Popova L, Kwinn L *et al.* Pattern recognition receptors TLR4 and CD14 mediate response to respiratory syncytial virus. Nat Immunol 2000; 1: 398-401.

[48]   Kawasaki K, Akashi S, Shimazu R, Yoshida T, Miyake K, Nishijima M. Mouse toll-like receptor 4-MD-2 complex mediates lipopolysaccharide-mimetic signal transduction by Taxol. J Biol Chem. 2000; 275: 2251-4.

[49]   Zimmer SM, Liu J, Clayton JL, Stephens DS, Snyder JP. Paclitaxel binding to human and murine MD-2. J Biol Chem 2008; 283: 27916-26.

[50]   Hayashi F, Smith KD, Ozinsky A *et al.* The innate immune response to bacterial flagellin is mediated by Toll-like receptor 5. Nature 2001; 410: 1099-103.

[51]   Andersen-Nissen E, Smith KD, Bonneau R, Strong RK, Aderem A. A conserved surface on Toll-like receptor 5 recognizes bacterial flagellin. J Exp Med 2007; 204: 393-403.

[52]   Diebold SS, Kaisho T, Hemmi H, Akira S, Reis e Sousa C. Innate antiviral responses by means of TLR7-mediated recognition of single-stranded RNA. Science 2004; 303: 1529-31.

[53]   Heil F, Hemmi H, Hochrein H *et al.* Species-specific recognition of single-stranded RNA *via* toll-like receptor 7 and 8. Science 2004; 303: 1526-9.

[54]   Hemmi H, Takeuchi O, Kawai T *et al.* A Toll-like receptor recognizes bacterial DNA. Nature 2000; 408: 740-5.

[55]   Coban C, Ishii KJ, Kawai T *et al.* Toll-like receptor 9 mediates innate immune activation by the malaria pigment hemozoin. J Exp Med 200; 201: 19-25.

[56]   Hasan U, Chaffois C, Gaillard C *et al.* Human TLR10 is a functional receptor, expressed by B cells and plasmacytoid dendritic cells, which activates gene transcription through MyD88. J Immunol 2005; 174: 2942-50.

[57]   Zhang D, Zhang G, Hayden MS *et al.* A toll-like receptor that prevents infection by uropathogenic bacteria. Science 2004; 303: 1522-6.

[58]   Lauw FN, Caffrey DR, Golenbock DT. Of mice and man: TLR11 (finally) finds profilin. Trends Immunol 2005; 26: 509-11.

[59]   Yamamoto M, Sato S, Mori K *et al.* Cutting edge: a novel Toll/IL-1 receptor domain-containing adapter that preferentially activates the IFN-beta promoter in the Toll-like receptor signaling. J Immunol 2002; 169: 6668-72.

[60]   Oshiumi H, Matsumoto M, Funami K, Akazawa T, Seya T. TICAM-1, an adaptor molecule that participates in Toll-like receptor 3-mediated interferon-beta induction. Nat Immunol 2003; 4: 161-7.

[61]   Jenkins KA, Mansell A. TIR-containing adaptors in Toll-like receptor signaling. Cytokine 2010; 49: 237-44.

[62]   Yamamoto M, Takeda K. Current views of toll-like receptor signaling pathways. Gastroenterol Res Pract 2010; 2010: 240365.

[63]   Ostuni R, Zanoni I, Granucci F. Deciphering the complexity of Toll-like receptor signaling. Cell Mol Life Sci 2010; 67: 4109-34.

CHAPTER 2

TLRs in the Lung in Health and Disease

Toshihiro Ito and Steven L. Kunkel[*]

Department of Pathology, University of Michigan Medical School, Ann Arbor, Michigan 48109, USA

Abstract: Toll-like receptors (TLRs) have been shown to play a pivotal role in both innate and acquired immune responses. TLRs recognize various pathogen-associated molecular patterns (PAMPs) such as bacterial lipopolysaccharide (LPS), viral RNA, CpG-containing DNA, and flagellin, among others. Their activation and signaling lead to the induction of inflammatory cytokines and type I interferons for host defense. In addition, the responses of the innate immune system are important not only in the elimination of pathogens but also in the development of antigen-specific acquired immunity mediated by B and T cells. TLRs are also involved in non-infectious diseases such as lung injury, COPD, fibrosis, allergy, autoimmunity, and cancer. Here we describe some features of the regulation of TLRs in a variety of lung diseases.

Keywords: TLRs, exogenous and endogenous ligands, signaling, innate and acquired, immunity lung disease.

1. INTRODUCTION

The lung, with its enormous surface area, is continuously exposed to a variety of potentially harmful agents including pathogenic microorganisms, allergens, and particle pollutants [1]. The lungs are defended from these harmful agents by the host immune system which consists of two components: innate immunity and acquired immunity. The innate immune system is the first line of defense that protects hosts from invading microbial pathogens [2]. Innate immune cells express various pattern-recognition receptors (PRRs), which recognize signature molecules of pathogens [3-5]. A variety of intracellular and extra-cellular PRRs have been described such as Toll-like receptors (TLRs), Retinoic acid-inducible gene (RIG)-I-like receptors (RLRs), and Nucleotide-binding oligomerization domain (NOD)-like receptor (NLRs) [6]. Structurally conserved molecules derived from invading pathogens, known as pathogen-associated molecular patterns (PAMPs), are specifically recognized by each PRR and are considered to be an essential component for the survival of the pathogen. The interaction of PAMPs with PRRs induces the release of inflammatory cytokines and type I interferons and initiates host defense against the pathogen [4].

TLRs are the best-characterized PRRs. To date, the TLR family consists of ten members in humans (TLR1-TLR10), and twelve members in mice (TLR1-TLR9, TLR11-TLR13) [7]. Each TLR specifically recognizes various PAMPs, which can be found on gram-positive and –negative bacteria, DNA and RNA viruses, fungi, and parasitic-protozoa, among others (Table **1**). TLRs are classified into several groups based on the types of PAMPs they recognize. For example, TLR1, -2, -4, and -6 recognize lipids. Specifically, TLR4, together with extracellular components MD-2 and CD14, recognizes lipopolysaccharide (LPS) from Gram-negative bacteria [2]. TLR2, in combination with TLR1 or TLR6, can recognize triacyl- and diacyl-lipopeptide, respectively [8]. TLR5 and TLR11 recognize protein ligands, while TLR5 recognizes flagellin, a monomeric constituent of bacterial flagella [9]. Human TLR11 recognizes uropathogenic *Escherichia coli* [10], and mouse TLR11 recognizes a profilin-like protein, a class of actin-binding proteins present in the protozoan parasite *Toxoplasma gondii* [11, 12]. In addition, a third class of TLRs, TLR3, -7, -8, -9 which are endosomally localized, recognize nucleic acids derived from viruses and bacteria [8]. TLR3 recognizes double-stranded (ds)RNA, which is produced from many viruses during replication. TLR7 recognizes synthetic imidazoquionoline-like molecules, guanosine- or uridine rich single stranded (ss)RNA from various viruses, as well as small interfering RNA [13]. TLR8 mediates the recognition of imidazoquinolines and ssRNA [13, 14]. TLR9 reconizes the CpG motif of bacterial and viral DNA [15].

---

*Address correspondence to Steven L. Kunkel: Department of Pathology, University of Michigan Medical School, Ann Arbor, Michigan 48109, USA E-mail: slkunkel@umich.edu

Catherine M. Greene (Ed)

Table 1: Exogenous Ligands of TLRs

TLR	Exogenous Ligands
TLR1	Triacyl lipopeptides, lipoproteins
TLR2	Lipoproteins, lipoteichoic acid, peptidoglycan, GPI anchors lipoarabinomannan, , phenol-soluble modulin, zymosan, glycolipids
TLR3	dsRNA (virus)
TLR4	LPS, envelop proteins
TLR5	Flagellin
TLR6	Diacetylated lipopeptides
TLR7	ssRNA
TLR8	ssRNA
TLR9	CpG motifs, dsDNA
TLR10	?
TLR11	Profilin-like protein

After recognition of PAMPs by the appropriate TLR, the activation of intracellular signaling cascades is facilitated by a set of intracellular Toll/IL-1R (TIR)-domain-containing adaptors, including myeloid differentiation primary response protein 88 (MyD88), MyD88 adaptor-like (MAL), also known as TIR domain-containing adaptor protein (TIRAP), TIR domain-containing adaptor-inducing IFN-β (TRIF), and TRIF-related adaptor molecule (TRAM) [16]. These signaling cascades lead to the production of pro-inflammatory cytokines such as tumor necrosis factor α (TNF-α), interleukin (IL)-1β, IL-6, and IL-12. Furthermore, several TLRs such as TLR3, -4, -7, -8, and -9 are capable of inducing antiviral type I interferons (multiple IFN-α and single IFN-β) [8].

In recent years it has become clear that the activation of TLRs in not restricted to the recognition of microbial pathogens. It is also plausible that TLRs might function in non-infectious diseases as well as in the maintenance of normal homeostasis (Table **2**) [17, 18].

Table 2: Selected Endogenous Ligands of TLRs

TLR	Endogenous Ligands
TLR2	Eosinophil-derived neurotoxin, HMGB, Hsp60, Hsp70, versican
TLR3	dsRNA (necrotic cells)
TLR4	HSP60, HSP70, fibronectin, hyalunoran
TLR7	Imidazoquinolines
TLR8	Imidazoquinolines
TLR9	DNA-containing immunocomplexes (*e.g.* CpG ODN)

In this chapter we will describe recent advances in our understanding of how the regulation of TLRs is related to innate and acquired immunity in lungs.

2. TLRS OF THE INNATE IMMUNE SYSTEM OF THE LUNG

2.1. Innate Immunity and TLRs at a Glance

Innate immunity is the first line of host defense directed against invading pathogens, and is designed to maintain host integrity [19]. Unlike acquired immunity which is present only in vertebrates, innate immunity is found in all mammals, is activated immediately upon infection, is not antigen-specific, has no memory requirement, and requires large numbers of cells for pathogen recognition [20]. Only if the invading pathogen is able to escape or overwhelm the innate response is acquired immunity activated. In some of these latter cases the host immune response becomes excessive, leading to manifest inflammation that may be considered pathological [19].

TLRs are named after their similarity to Toll, an essential receptor of the innate immune system against fungal infection in *Drosophila* [21]. In recent years the family of mammalian TLRs expressed on dendritic cells (DCs) and macrophages have been found to be key PRRs with central roles in the induction of the innate immune response. The principal functions of macrophages and DCs are phagocytosis and the elimination of microorganisms [22]. These cells also possess secondary functions including the production of cytokines, chemokines and chemotactic lipids, which direct certain circulating cells to migrate to the site of infection and participate in the elimination of pathogens. DCs also play an important role in communicating and presenting antigens to lymphocytes, thus linking the innate and adaptive immune responses

2.2. TLR Signaling at a Glance

The TLR signaling pathways are now well known and have been extensively reviewed elsewhere [2, 7, 23]. Ligand recognition by TLRs leads to the recruitment of various TIR domain-containing adaptors such as MyD88, MAL, TRIF, and TRAM [16] (Fig. 1 and Table 3). MyD88 is the central adaptor molecule interacting with all TLRs except TLR3 [2]. In addition to MyD88, TLR1, TLR2, TLR4, and TLR6 recruit MAL/TIRAP, a linker adaptor between the TIR domain of TLRs and MyD88 [23]. TLR3 signaling recruits TRIF, the crucial adaptor for induction of the signaling pathway that eventually leads to the induction of type I IFNs [24]. TLR4 signaling also recruits TRIF through TRAM, leading to the production of various proinflammatory molecules [25].

Table 3: Adaptor Protein Utilized by TLRs

TLR	Signaling Adaptor
TLR1	MyD88, TIRAP
TLR2	MyD88, TIRAP
TLR3	TRIF
TLR4	MyD88, TIRAP, TRIF, TRAM
TLR5	MyD88
TLR6	MyD88, TIRAP
TLR7	MyD88
TLR8	MyD88
TLR9	MyD88
TLR10	MyD88, TIRAP
TLR11	MyD88

Upon ligand activation, MyD88 recruits the IRAK family of protein kinases, including IRAK1, IRAK2, IRAK4 and IRAK-M [2]. In particular IRAK4 is essential for activation of TRAF6, a member of the TRAF family. IRAK becomes phosphorylated, dissociates from MyD88 and interacts with TRAF6, followed by TAK1/TAB1/TAB2/TAB3 complex formation and activation *via* the synthesis of lysine 63-linked ubiquitination. The TAK1 complex activates the IKK complex composed of IKKα, IKKβ, and IKKγ/NEMO, which in turn catalyze IκB phosphorylation. Phosphorylated IκB proteins are degraded by the proteasome-dependent pathway, allowing NF-κB to translocate into the nuclei. TAK1 also activates the MAPK pathway, which mediates AP-1 activation. IRF5 is also recruited to the MyD88-IRAK4-TRAF6 complex, phosphorylated and translocated to the nucleus. NF-κB, AP-1, and IRF5 regulate proinflammatory cytokine production such as such as TNF-α, IL-1β, IL-6, and IL-12 [2, 23].

Activated TRIF, recruited to TLR3 and TLR4, interacts with TBK1 and IKKi, and then mediates IRF3 phosphorylation. Phosphorylated IRF3 dimerizes and translocates to the nucleus mediating type I IFN induction [26, 27]. TRIF also interacts with TRAF6 and RIP1, which mediate NF-κB activation [28-30]. TLR4, but not TLR3, utilizes TRAM for activation of the TRIF-dependent pathway [25].

TLRs 7, 8 and 9 are located within endosomes and utilize MyD88 to signal *via* TRAF6 and IRAK4 to induce inflammatory gene expression and Type I interferons. Tables **4** and **5** detail the involvement of TLRs in non-infectious and non-infectious lung diseases

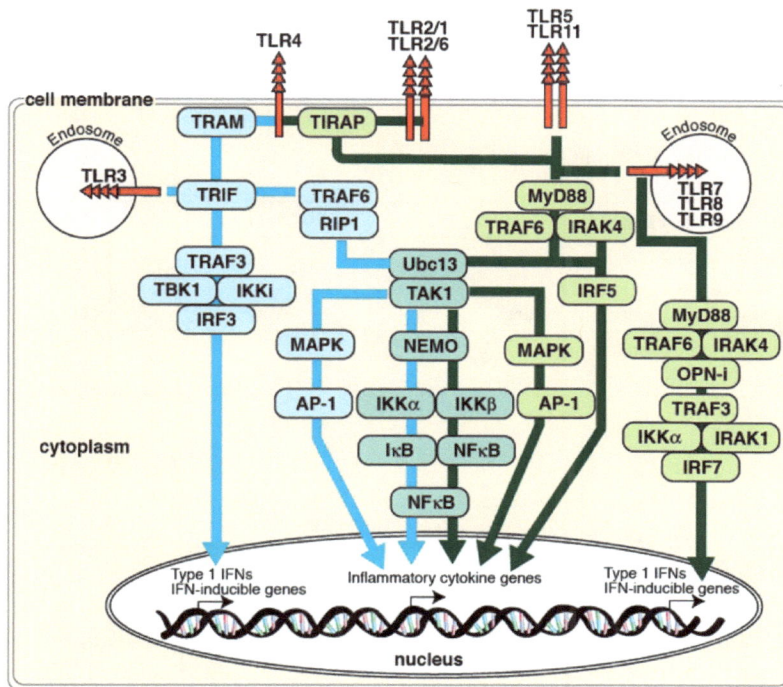

Figure 1: TLR signaling pathways.

TLR1

TLR1 is anchored in the plasma membrane and is functionally associated with TLR2 [6, 31, 32]. The TLR1/TLR2 complex recognizes triacyl lipopeptides and lipoproteins from mycobacteria. Macrophages from TLR1-deficient mice have demonstrated the importance of TLR1 in the recognition of the lipoproteins LprG, LpqH, and PhoS1, but not LprA from *Mycobacterium tuberculosis* [33]. Increased mRNA levels of TLR1 have been found in fresh unstimulated whole blood from patients with progressive pulmonary tuberculosis [34].

TLR2

Activated TLR2 functions as a heterodimer with TLR1, TLR6 or TLR10. Several lines of evidence demonstrate that TLR2 recognizes components from a variety of microbial pathogens. For example, TLR2 recognizes major cell wall constitutents of gram-positive microorganisms such as lipoproteins, lipoteichoic acid, and peptidoglycan. As mentioned above TLR1/2 recognizes triacyl lipopeptides. In contrast TLR2/6 recognizes diacylated lipopeptides [35]. In addition numerous other ligands for TLR2 have been found. These ligands include lipoproteins from pathogens such as Gram-negative bacteria, lipoarabinomannan from mycobateria, glycosylphosphatidylinositol anchors from *Trypanosoma cruzi* and *Schistosoma mansoni*, a phenol-soluble modulin from *Staphylococcus epidermis*, zymosan from fungi, and glycolipids from *Treponema maltophilum* [7, 35-40].

There are a number of studies using TLR2 knockout mice in experimental models of lung disease. For instance during pulmonary infection, the contribution of TLR2 to the immune response has been evaluated in pulmonary infection models using *Staphylococcus aureus* [41, 42], *Burkholderia pseudomallei* (Meliodosis) [43], *Legionella pneumophilia* [44, 45], *Mycobacterium tuberculosis* [46, 47], *Mycoplasma pneumoniae* [48], *Toxoplasma gondii* [49], *Cryptococcus neoformans* [50], *Aspergillus fumigatus* [51, 52], or *Paracoccidioides brasiliensis* [53] Additionally, TLR2 has been demonstrated to be required for controlling respiratory syncytial virus (RSV) replication in lung tissue [54]. In addition a variety of endogenous ligands for TLR2 have been recognized including eosinophil derived neurotoxin [55], HMGB1 (high mobility group box) [56], and other heat shock proteins [57]. A recent study has shown that the carcinoma-produced factor, versican, is a TLR2 agonist and lung carcinoma metastasis-enhancing factor [58]. Furthermore, TLR2 has been shown to be associated with the reduction of bleomycin-induced pulmonary fibrosis [59] and with sepsis-induced respiratory failure [60].

Table 4: Involvement of TLRs in Non-infectious Lung Diseases

TLR	Non-infectious Disease	References
TLR2	Metastatic lung cancer	[58]
	Lung fibrosis	[59]
	Sepsis-induced respiratory failure	[60]
TLR3	Hyperoxia-induced lung injury	[66]
	Sepsis-induced respiratory failure	[67]
TLR5	COPD	[79]
	Acute lung injury (ALI)	[80]
	Hyperoxia-induced lung injury	[81]
	Ozone-induced hyperresponsiveness	[82]
	Lung ischemia-reperfusion injury	[83]

TLR3

TLR3 differs from all the other TLRs. It is the only TLR not to signal *via* MyD88 but instead exclusively uses TRIF, mainly leading to the production of type I interferon regulated genes. TLR3 recognizes double-stranded RNA (dsRNA) from viral sources but also endogenous dsRNA from necrotic cells [61, 62]. However, the involvement of TLR3 in anti-viral responses still remains unclear and in some cases seems to have detrimental rather than protective effects: TLR3 knockout mice do not show higher susceptibility to pulmonary infection by influenza virus [63] or RSV [64]. In fact, deletion of TLR3 leads to increases in mucus production in the airways of RSV-infected mice [64], demonstrating that TLR3 might not be required for viral clearance although it is necessary to maintain the proper immune environment in the lung to avoid developing pathologic symptoms of disease. On the other hand, TLR3 has a protective role during the Th2-driven pulmonary granulomatous response induced by *Schistosoma mansoni* eggs that contain dsRNA [65]. Regarding the recognition of endogenous dsRNA from necrotic cells by TLR3, TLR3-deficient mice have shown less inflammation using both a murine model of hyperoxia-induced lung injury [66] and sepsis [67], indicating that TLR3 regulates amplification events during inflammation mediated by nonviral dsRNA stimulants and contributes to the observed pathology.

TLR4

TLR4 recognizes LPS, a major component of the outer membrane of gram-negative bacteria. For signaling, TLR4 is dependent on the presence of CD14 and MD-2 with which it forms a complex [68]. For example the contribution of TLR4 has been demonstrated using a pulmonary infectious gram-negative pneumonia model induced by *Klebsiella pneumoniae* [69], *Haemophilus influenzae* [70], and *Bordetella bronchiseptica* [71]. It has also been shown that TLR4 is required to control pulmonary infection against *Pneumocystis carinii* [72] and *Mycobacterium tuberculosis* [73]. However, differences in experimental models using *Mycobacterium tuberculosis* have yielded conflicting results, so the role of TLR4 for immune responses to *Mycobacterium tuberculosis* still remains controversial [74, 75]. TLR4 also responds to some viral proteins, and TLR4-dependent signaling is required to limit viral replication and disease mortality in a pulmonary infectious model using vaccinia [76], coronavirus (MHV-1) [77], and RSV [78]. In addition, a number of endogenous ligands for TLR4 have been described. For instance heat shock proteins (HSP60 and HSP70) and extracellular matrix (ECM) components such as fibronectin and hyalunoran have been described as TLR4 ligands [7]. HSPs serve as danger signals to the innate immune system, and ECM components are produced in response to lung injury and contribute to tissue remodeling in response to inflammation. The contribution of TLR4 has also been shown in non-infectious experimental models such as chronic obstructive pulmonary disease (COPD) [79], acute lung injury (ALI) [80], hyperoxia-induced lung injury [81], ozone-induced hyperresponsiveness [82], and lung ischemia-reperfusion injury [83].

TLR5

TLR5 recognizes a highly conserved cluster of 13 amino acid residues in flagellin, the major protein of the flagella of gram-negative bacteria [9]. TLR5 is highly expressed in human and murine lung tissue by airway epithelial cells, neutrophils, and alveolar macrophages [84]. Several observations support a role of TLR5 in the host defense to lung infectious pneumonia induced by *Legionella pnemophila* [85] and *Pseudomonas aeruginosa* [84].

TLR6

TLR6 forms heterodimers with TLR2 and as mentioned, this complex specifically recognizes diacylated lipopeptides. TLR6 has been described to be essential for the recognition of mycoplasma-derived diacyl lipopeptides [86], while the contribution of TLR6 in lung diseases still remains unknown.

TLR7

TLR7 shares its ligand with TLR8. TLR7 has been shown to recognize guanosine- or uridine-rich single stranded RNA (ssRNA) [13] from viruses such as human immunodeficiency virus [13] and influenza virus [87]. TLR7 also recognizes imidazoquinolines, which are potent activators of immune cells with anti-viral and anti-tumor properties. TLR7 agonists have demonstrated immunotherapeutic activity for infectious models using *Bacillus anthracis* spores or influenza virus [88] and for an allergic asthma model [89].

Table 5: TLR and Infectious Lung Diseases

TLR	Infectious Disease	References
TLR1	*Mycobacterium tuberculosis*	[33]
TLR2	*Staphylococcus aureus*	[41, 42]
	Burkholderia Pseudomallei	[43]
	Legionella pneumoniae	[44, 45]
	Mycobacterium tuberculosis	[46, 47]
	Mycoplasma pnemoniae	[48]
	Toxoplasma gondii	[49]
	Cryptococcus neoformans	[50]
	Aspergillus fumigutus	[51,52]
	Paracoccidioides brasiliensis	[53]
TLR3	Influenza virus	[63]
	RSV	[64]
	Shistosoma mansoni eggs (Th2-type granuloma)	[65]
TLR4	*Klebsiella pneumoniae*	[69]
	Haemophilus influenzae	[70]
	Bordetella bronchiseptica	[71]
	Pneumocystis carinii	[72]
	Mycobacterium tuberculosis	[73]
	Vaccinia	[76]
	Coronavirus	[77]
	RSV	[78]
TLR5	*Legionella pneumoniae*	[85]
	Pseudomonas aeruginosa	[84]
TLR9	*Klebsiella pnemoniae*	[94]
	Legionella pneumoniae	[95]

Staphylococcus pneumoniae	[96]
Mycobacterium tuberculosis	[97]
Aspergillus fumigutus	[98]
HSV	[99]
Mycobacteria bovis (Th1-type granuloma)	[100]
Shistosoma mansoni eggs (Th2-type granuloma)	[101]

TLR8

TLR8 and TLR7 are closely related, sharing an intracellular endosomal location. TLR8 has been shown to recognize the imidazoquinolines and ssRNA, which are ligands for TLR7 [13]. However, recent finding shows that TLR7-deficient mice are unresponsive to TLR8 agonists [89]. Similarly, natural ssRNA cannot activate murine TLR8, leading to the belief that murine TLR8 is nonfunctional [14, 90]. There seems to be flexibility in the specificity of TLR7 and TLR8 for their ligands, depending on characteristics of the ligands and the environment. The contribution of TLR8 itself to lung diseases is still unknown.

TLR9

TLR9 is essential for the recognition of the CpG motif that is present in high frequency in DNA from various microbes, including bacteria, viruses, and certain fungi [15]. The activation of TLR9 requires the uptake of microbes (or synthetic CpG oligodeoxynucleotides) within endosomes, the formation of DNA:TLR9 complexes within the endocytic vesicles, and the subsequent acidification and maturation of the endosomes [91-93]. Some observations support a role for TLR9 in the host response to lung infectious pneumonia induced by a variety of microbes such as *Klebisiella pneumoniae* [94], *Legionella pnemophila* [95], *Streptococcus pneumonia* [96], *Mycobacterium tuberculosis* [97], *Aspergillus fumigatus* [98], and Herpes simplex virus [99]. TLR9 also plays an important role in triggering a Th1 skewed immune response (See TLRs and acquired immunity). Our laboratory has demonstrated that TLR9 activation is important for the maintenance not only of mycobacteria-elicited (Th1-type) pulmonary granulomatous responses [100], but also of *Schistosoma mansoni* egg-induced (Th2-type) pulmonary granulomatous responses [101]. These findings demonstrated that TLR9 deficiency resulted in an accelerated granulomatous response, a decreased Th1 profile, and an increased Th2 cytokine profile during pulmonary granuloma formation.

TLR10

Human TLR10 has been identified as a member that is closely related to TLR1 and TLR6 [6]. The ligand of TLR10 is still unknown. A mouse homologue of TLR10 has not yet been identified.

TLR11

TLR11 recognizes a profilin-like protein, a class of actin-binding proteins present in the protozoan parasite *Toxoplasma gondii* [12]. However, the contribution of TLR11 to the pathology of lung disease remains unknown.

2.3. Adaptor Molecules in Lung Diseases

MyD88-Dependent Pathway

The adaptor molecule, MyD88, is essential for all the TLR signaling pathways that induce proinflammatory cytokines except for TLR3. Therefore, the absence of MyD88 results in a dramatic reduction of host resistance to a variety of agents. Many reports have confirmed the importance of MyD88 using pulmonary infectious models induced by pathogens such as *Staphylococcus aureus* [42], *Listeria monocytogenes* [102], *Klebsiella pneumoniae* [103], *Pseudomonas aeruginosa* [104], *Legionella pneumophilia* [105], *Chlamydia pneumoniae* [106, 107], *Chlamydia muridarum* [108], *Mycobacterium tuberculosis* [109], *Mycobacterium avium* [110], *Aspergillus fumigatus* [111], *Cryptococcus neoformans* [112], *Saccharopolyspora rectivirgula* (animal model of hypersensitivity pneumonitis) [113], RSV [114], SARS-CoA [115], MHV68 [116]. MyD88 also has been shown to be essential for non-infectious models of lung fibrosis [117] and ozone-induced airway hyperresponsiveness [82].

TRIF-Dependent Pathway

The TRIF pathway originates from TLR3 and TLR4, and induces type I interferons *via* activation of IRF3 [7]. The contribution of TRIF to lung diseases has been shown in gram-negative bacterial infections such as *Escherichia coli* [118], *Pseudomonas aeruginosa* [119], and *Klebsiella pneumoniae* [103], suggesting that the TRIF-dependent TLR4-mediating signaling cascade serves to augment pulmonary host defense against gram-negative pathogens. In addition, Imai *et al.* demonstrated that TLR4-TRIF-TRAF6 signaling is a key disease pathway that controls the severity of acute lung injury (ALI) induced by acid aspiration and influenza H5N1 [80], indicating that this pathway is essential for triggering the oxidative stress machinery set off by both chemical and viral lung pathogens. However the importance of the TLR3-TRIF-TRAF pathway for induction of type I interferons in pulmonary virus infection remains unknown because of the presence of a TLR-independent viral recognition system, the RIG-I like pathways, as described elsewhere [120].

3. TLRs OF THE ACQUIRED IMMUNE SYSTEMS OF THE LUNG

Acquired Immunity and TLRs

Several studies have provided evidence that signaling *via* TLRs is critical for the development of T helper (Th)-dependent immune responses. CD4$^+$ T cells (Th cells) are essential regulators of immune responses and inflammatory diseases and can differentiate into either Th1 or Th2 cells, depending on local environmental influences [121]. Th1 cells mainly produce IFN-γ, which is important for macrophage activation and clearance of intracellular pathogens, whereas Th2 cells produce IL-4, IL-5, and IL-13, shown to be critical for IgE production, eosinophil recruitment and clearance of extracellular parasites [122]. For example, the activation of TLRs on antigen-presenting cells such as DCs can lead to the expression of IL-12 and subsequently activate the expression of IFN-γ in Th1 cells. Interestingly, the lack of IL-12 production *via* limited TLR activation during the inflammatory/immune response appears to lead to Th2 responses, suggesting that this type of response is a default pathway that occurs in the absence of IL-12 [123]. Studies have demonstrated that MyD88 knockout mice were not able to generate a Th1 response when challenged with an infectious agent [124-126]. Also, MyD88-mediated cytokines appear to provide a suppressive signal for a Th2-type response. The caveat in these studies is that not all Th1-inducing stimuli default to Th2 responses in the absence of IL-12, suggesting that other signals may exist on antigen-presenting cells to elicit a Th1 response.

Linkage of TLRs to Notch System

Just as the study of TLRs had its origin in developmental biology and then transitioned into inflammation and immunity, so also did the field of Notch and Notch ligands originate in developmental biology and now appears to play a key role in antigen-presenting cells and T-cell communication circuits. Studies suggest that the Notch ligands Delta-like-1–4 and Jagged, expressed on DCs, can provide novel activation signals for the development of either Th1 or Th2 cells, respectively [127]. Interestingly, the expression of Delta-like-4 (DLL4) on DCs is rigorously induced *via* TLRs that use the MyD88 pathway [114]. Our studies using antibodies directed against DLL4 determined the role of this membrane-bound Notch ligand in polarizing cytokine production. Lymphocytes recovered from the lung or lymph nodes of animals treated with high-titer antibodies to DLL4 after RSV infection in the lungs demonstrated an altered response when challenged *in vivo* with antigen compared to control antibody treated animals [128]. This study showed that production of the Th2 cytokines IL-4, IL-5, and IL-13 was enhanced in antigen-challenged lymphocytes recovered from animals treated with antibody to DLL4 compared to control antibody-treated animals. Furthermore, IL-17-producing T cells have been recently described and named Th17 [129]. Th17 cells are preferential producers of IL-17A and IL-17F and play an essential role in host defense *via* protection against bacterial pathogens [129-131]. Our recent study suggests that DLL4 also specifically regulates Th17 activation in an *in vivo* experimental model of mycobacteria protein-induced pulmonary granuloma formation. These studies underscore the importance of a novel immune-activating system during the development of lung inflammation [132]. These results further identify a critical role for DLL4 in the regulation and/or development of Th1-, Th2-, and Th17-mediated responses.

4. FUTURE PROSPECTS

The identification of TLRs and the analysis of their roles in the immune system have provided us with the opportunity to reassess the pathology of inflammatory lung disease, a window into the biology of both innate and acquired immunity [133]. It is likely that TLR proteins contribute in some manner to all of these complex responses, participating in ways that can be both beneficial and detrimental to the host [134]. Key questions that remain are whether TLR proteins will prove to be important targets for the development of novel therapies and whether TLR polymorphisms will prove to be useful markers of disease in humans. To date, TLR agonists have been used mainly pharmacologically due to their immunostimulatory properties. For instance, the TLR9-mediated activation of the vertebrate immune system suggests that using CpG ODNs (short phosphorothioate-stabilized oligodeoxynucleotides), a TLR9 agonist, may prove to be an effective vaccine adjuvant for infectious disease, and for the treatment of cancer and asthma/allergy as has been shown in animal models [135]. Even though studies in human disease and animal models strongly suggest a pathogenic role of TLRs in a variety of lung diseases, direct connections and the specifics of functional pathways are still largely unknown. Future studies will hopefully define the clinical relevance of altered activation of TLRs and their pathways, while therapeutic modifications of TLR pathways offer clinical potential that has yet to be explored.

REFERENCES

[1]   Suzuki T, Chow CW, Downey GP. Role of innate immune cells and their products in lung immunopathology. Int J Biochem Cell Biol 2008; 40: 1348-61.

[2]   Kawai T, Akira S. TLR signaling. Semin Immunol 2007; 19: 24-32.

[3]   Akira S, Uematsu S, Takeuchi O. Pathogen recognition and innate immunity. Cell 2006; 124: 783-801.

[4]   Kumar H, Kawai T, Akira S. Toll-like receptors and innate immunity. Biochem Biophys Res Commun 2009; 388: 621-5.

[5]   Medzhitov R. Recognition of microorganisms and activation of the immune response. Nature 2007; 449: 819-26.

[6]   Ospelt C, Gay S. TLRs and chronic inflammation. Int J Biochem Cell Biol 2010: 42:495-505.

[7]   Takeda K, Akira S. Toll-like receptors. Curr Protoc Immunol. 2007; Chapter 14: Unit 14 2.

[8]   Miggin SM, O'Neill LA. New insights into the regulation of TLR signaling. J Leukoc Biol 2006; 80: 220-6.

[9]   Hayashi F, Smith KD, Ozinsky A *et al*. The innate immune response to bacterial flagellin is mediated by Toll-like receptor 5. Nature 2001; 410: 1099-103.

[10]   Zhang D, Zhang G, Hayden MS *et al*. A toll-like receptor that prevents infection by uropathogenic bacteria. Science 2004; 303: 1522-6.

[11]   Lauw FN, Caffrey DR, Golenbock DT. Of mice and man: TLR11 (finally) finds profilin. Trends Immunol 2005; 26: 509-11.

[12]   Yarovinsky F, Zhang D, Andersen JF *et al*. TLR11 activation of dendritic cells by a protozoan profilin-like protein. Science 2005; 308: 1626-9.

[13]   Heil F, Hemmi H, Hochrein H, Ampenberger F *et al*. Species-specific recognition of single-stranded RNA *via* toll-like receptor 7 and 8. Science 2004; 303: 1526-9.

[14]   Forsbach A, Nemorin JG, Montino C *et al*. Identification of RNA sequence motifs stimulating sequence-specific TLR8-dependent immune responses. J Immunol 2008; 180: 3729-38.

[15]   Hemmi H, Takeuchi O, Kawai T *et al*. A Toll-like receptor recognizes bacterial DNA. Nature 2000; 408: 740-5.

[16]   O'Neill LA, Fitzgerald KA, Bowie AG. The Toll-IL-1 receptor adaptor family grows to five members. Trends Immunol 2003; 24: 286-90.

[17]   Jiang D, Liang J, Li Y, Noble PW. The role of Toll-like receptors in non-infectious lung injury. Cell Res 2006; 16: 693-701.

[18]   Wissinger E, Goulding J, Hussell T. Immune homeostasis in the respiratory tract and its impact on heterologous infection. Semin Immunol 2009; 21: 147-55.

[19]   Si-Tahar M, Touqui L, Chignard M. Innate immunity and inflammation--two facets of the same anti-infectious reaction. Clin Exp Immunol 2009; 156: 194-8.

[20]   Kabelitz D, Medzhitov R. Innate immunity--cross-talk with adaptive immunity through pattern recognition receptors and cytokines. Curr Opin Immunol 2007; 19: 1-3.

[21]   Lemaitre B, Nicolas E, Michaut L, Reichhart JM, Hoffmann JA. The dorsoventral regulatory gene cassette spatzle/Toll/cactus controls the potent antifungal response in D*rosophila* adults. Cell 1996; 86: 973-83.

[22]   Takeda K, Akira S. Toll-like receptors in innate immunity. Int Immunol 2005; 17: 1-14.

[23]   Kawai T, Akira S. TLR signaling. Cell Death Differ 2006; 13: 816-25.

[24]   Yamamoto M, Sato S, Mori K *et al.* Cutting edge: a novel Toll/IL-1 receptor domain-containing adapter that preferentially activates the IFN-beta promoter in the Toll-like receptor signaling. J Immunol 2002; 169: 6668-72.

[25]   Yamamoto M, Sato S, Hemmi H *et al.* TRAM is specifically involved in the Toll-like receptor 4-mediated MyD88-independent signaling pathway. Nat Immunol 2003; 4: 1144-50.

[26]   Fitzgerald KA, McWhirter SM, Faia KL *et al.* IKKepsilon and TBK1 are essential components of the IRF3 signaling pathway. Nat Immunol 2003; 4: 491-6.

[27]   McWhirter SM, Fitzgerald KA, Rosains J, Rowe DC, Golenbock DT, Maniatis T. IFN-regulatory factor 3-dependent gene expression is defective in Tbk1-deficient mouse embryonic fibroblasts. Proc Natl Acad Sci U S A 2004; 101: 233-8.

[28]   Cusson-Hermance N, Khurana S, Lee TH, Fitzgerald KA, Kelliher MA. Rip1 mediates the Trif-dependent toll-like receptor 3- and 4-induced NF-{kappa}B activation but does not contribute to interferon regulatory factor 3 activation. J Biol Chem 2005; 280: 36560-6.

[29]   Meylan E, Burns K, Hofmann K, Blancheteau V *et al.* RIP1 is an essential mediator of Toll-like receptor 3-induced NF-kappa B activation. Nat Immunol 2004; 5: 503-7.

[30]   Sato S, Sugiyama M, Yamamoto M, Watanabe Y *et al.* Toll/IL-1 receptor domain-containing adaptor inducing IFN-beta (TRIF) associates with TNF receptor-associated factor 6 and TANK-binding kinase 1, and activates two distinct transcription factors, NF-kappa B and IFN-regulatory factor-3, in the Toll-like receptor signaling. J Immunol 2003; 171: 4304-10.

[31]   Takeuchi O, Sato S, Horiuchi T *et al.* Cutting edge: role of Toll-like receptor 1 in mediating immune response to microbial lipoproteins. J Immunol 2002; 169: 10-4.

[32]   Wyllie DH, Kiss-Toth E, Visintin A *et al.* Evidence for an accessory protein function for Toll-like receptor 1 in anti-bacterial responses. J Immunol 2000; 165: 7125-32.

[33]   Drage MG, Pecora ND, Hise AG *et al.* TLR2 and its co-receptors determine responses of macrophages and dendritic cells to lipoproteins of *Mycobacterium tuberculosis*. Cell Immunol 2009; 258: 29-37.

[34]   Chang JS, Huggett JF, Dheda K, Kim LU, Zumla A, Rook GA. *Myobacterium tuberculosis* induces selective up-regulation of TLRs in the mononuclear leukocytes of patients with active pulmonary tuberculosis. J Immunol 2006; 176: 3010-8.

[35]   Ozinsky A, Underhill DM, Fontenot JD *et al.* The repertoire for pattern recognition of pathogens by the innate immune system is defined by cooperation between toll-like receptors. Proc Natl Acad Sci U S A 2000; 97: 13766-71.

[36]   Campos MA, Almeida IC, Takeuchi O *et al.* Activation of Toll-like receptor-2 by glycosylphosphatidylinositol anchors from a protozoan parasite. J Immunol 2001; 167: 416-23.

[37]   Ouaissi A, Guilvard E, Delneste Y *et al.* The *Trypanosoma cruzi* Tc52-released protein induces human dendritic cell maturation, signals *via* Toll-like receptor 2, and confers protection against lethal infection. J Immunol 2002; 168: 6366-74.

[38]   Schwandner R, Dziarski R, Wesche H, Rothe M, Kirschning CJ. Peptidoglycan- and lipoteichoic acid-induced cell activation is mediated by toll-like receptor 2. J Biol Chem 1999; 274: 17406-9.

[39]   Underhill DM, Ozinsky A, Smith KD, Aderem A. Toll-like receptor-2 mediates mycobacteria-induced proinflammatory signaling in macrophages. Proc Natl Acad Sci U S A 1999; 96: 14459-63.

[40]   van der Kleij D, Latz E, Brouwers JF *et al.* A novel host-parasite lipid cross-talk. Schistosomal lyso-phosphatidylserine activates toll-like receptor 2 and affects immune polarization. J Biol Chem 2002; 277: 48122-9.

[41]   Knapp S, Wieland CW, van 't Veer C *et al.* Toll-like receptor 2 plays a role in the early inflammatory response to murine pneumococcal pneumonia but does not contribute to antibacterial defense. J Immunol 2004; 172: 3132-8.

[42]   Takeuchi O, Hoshino K, Akira S. Cutting edge: TLR2-deficient and MyD88-deficient mice are highly susceptible to *Staphylococcus aureus* infection. J Immunol 2000; 165: 5392-6.

[43]   Wiersinga WJ, Wieland CW, Dessing MC *et al.* Toll-like receptor 2 impairs host defense in gram-negative sepsis caused by *Burkholderia pseudomallei* (Melioidosis). PLoS Med 2007; 4: e248.

[44]   Archer KA, Roy CR. MyD88-dependent responses involving toll-like receptor 2 are important for protection and clearance of *Legionella pneumophila* in a mouse model of Legionnaires' disease. Infect Immu. 2006; 74: 3325-33.

[45]   Fuse ET, Tateda K, Kikuchi Y *et al.* Role of Toll-like receptor 2 in recognition of *Legionella pneumophila* in a murine pneumonia model. J Med Microbiol 2007; 56: 305-12.

[46]   Drennan MB, Nicolle D, Quesniaux VJ *et al.* Toll-like receptor 2-deficient mice succumb to *Mycobacterium tuberculosis* infection. Am J Pathol 2004; 164: 49-57.

[47]   Sugawara I, Yamada H, Li C, Mizuno S, Takeuchi O, Akira S. Mycobacterial infection in TLR2 and TLR6 knockout mice. Microbiol Immunol 2003; 47: 327-36.

[48]   Chu HW, Jeyaseelan S, Rino JG *et al.* TLR2 signaling is critical for *Mycoplasma pneumoniae*-induced airway mucin expression. J Immunol 2005; 174: 5713-9.

[49]   Mun HS, Aosai F, Norose K *et al.* TLR2 as an essential molecule for protective immunity against *Toxoplasma gondii* infection. Int Immunol 2003; 15: 1081-7.

[50]   Biondo C, Midiri A, Messina L al. MyD88 and TLR2, but not TLR4, are required for host defense against *Cryptococcus neoformans*. Eur J Immunol 2005; 35: 870-8.

[51]   Balloy V, Si-Tahar M, Takeuchi O *et al.* Involvement of toll-like receptor 2 in experimental invasive pulmonary aspergillosis. Infect Immun 2005; 73: 5420-5.

[52]   Buckland KF, O'Connor E, Murray LA, Hogaboam CM. Toll like receptor-2 modulates both innate and adaptive immune responses during chronic fungal asthma in mice. Inflamm Res 2008; 57: 379-87.

[53]   Loures FV, Pina A, Felonato M, Calich VL. TLR2 is a negative regulator of Th17 cells and tissue pathology in a pulmonary model of fungal infection. J Immunol 2009; 183: 1279-90.

[54]   Murawski MR, Bowen GN, Cerny AM *et al.* Respiratory syncytial virus activates innate immunity through Toll-like receptor 2. J Virol 2009; 83: 1492-500.

[55]   Yang D, Chen Q, Su SB *et al.* Eosinophil-derived neurotoxin acts as an alarmin to activate the TLR2-MyD88 signal pathway in dendritic cells and enhances Th2 immune responses. J Exp Med 2008; 205: 79-90.

[56]   Park JS, Gamboni-Robertson F, He Q *et al.* High mobility group box 1 protein interacts with multiple Toll-like receptors. Am J Physiol Cell Physiol 2006; 290: C917-24.

[57]   Asea A, Rehli M, Kabingu E *et al.* Novel signal transduction pathway utilized by extracellular HSP70: role of toll-like receptor (TLR) 2 and TLR4. J Biol Chem 2002; 277: 15028-34.

[58]   Kim S, Takahashi H, Lin WW *et al.* Carcinoma-produced factors activate myeloid cells through TLR2 to stimulate metastasis. Nature 2009; 457: 102-6.

[59]   Yang HZ, Cui B, Liu HZ *et al.* Targeting TLR2 attenuates pulmonary inflammation and fibrosis by reversion of suppressive immune microenvironment. J Immunol 2009; 182: 692-702.

[60]   Petersen B, Bloch KD, Ichinose F *et al.* Activation of Toll-like receptor 2 impairs hypoxic pulmonary vasoconstriction in mice. Am J Physiol Lung Cell Mol Physiol 2008; 294: L300-8.

[61]   Alexopoulou L, Holt AC, Medzhitov R, Flavell RA. Recognition of double-stranded RNA and activation of NF-kappaB by Toll-like receptor 3. Nature 2001; 413: 732-8.

[62]   Brentano F, Schorr O, Gay RE, Gay S, Kyburz D. RNA released from necrotic synovial fluid cells activates rheumatoid arthritis synovial fibroblasts *via* Toll-like receptor 3. Arthritis Rheum 2005; 52: 2656-65.

[63]   Le Goffic R, Balloy V, Lagranderie M *et al.* Detrimental contribution of the Toll-like receptor (TLR)3 to influenza A virus-induced acute pneumonia. PLoS Pathog 2006; 2: e53.

[64]   Rudd BD, Smit JJ, Flavell RA *et al.* Deletion of TLR3 alters the pulmonary immune environment and mucus production during respiratory syncytial virus infection. J Immunol 2006; 176: 1937-42.

[65]   Joshi AD, Schaller MA, Lukacs NW, Kunkel SL, Hogaboam CM. TLR3 modulates immunopathology during a *Schistosoma mansoni* egg-driven Th2 response in the lung. Eur J Immunol 2008; 38: 3436-49.

[66]   Murray LA, Knight DA, McAlonan L *et al.* Deleterious role of TLR3 during hyperoxia-induced acute lung injury. Am J Respir Crit Care Med 2008; 178: 1227-37.

[67]   Cavassani KA, Ishii M, Wen H *et al.* TLR3 is an endogenous sensor of tissue necrosis during acute inflammatory events. J Exp Med 2008; 205: 2609-21.

[68]   Shimazu R, Akashi S, Ogata H *et al.* MD-2, a molecule that confers lipopolysaccharide responsiveness on Toll-like receptor 4. J Exp Med 1999; 189: 1777-82.

[69]   Branger J, Knapp S, Weijer S *et al.* Role of Toll-like receptor 4 in gram-positive and gram-negative pneumonia in mice. Infect Immun 2004; 72: 788-94.

[70]   Wang X, Moser C, Louboutin JP *et al.* Toll-like receptor 4 mediates innate immune responses to *Haemophilus influenzae* infection in mouse lung. J Immunol 2002; 168: 810-5.

[71]   Mann PB, Wolfe D, Latz E, Golenbock D, Preston A, Harvill ET. Comparative toll-like receptor 4-mediated innate host defense to *Bordetella* infection. Infect Immun 2005; 73: 8144-52.

[72]   Ding K, Shibui A, Wang Y, Takamoto M, Matsuguchi T, Sugane K. Impaired recognition by Toll-like receptor 4 is responsible for exacerbated murine *Pneumocystis* pneumonia. Microbes Infect 2005; 7: 195-203.

[73] Abel B, Thieblemont N, Quesniaux VJ *et al.* Toll-like receptor 4 expression is required to control chronic *Mycobacterium tuberculosis* infection in mice. J Immunol 2002; 169: 3155-62.

[74] Holscher C, Reiling N, Schaible UE *et al.* Containment of aerogenic *Mycobacterium tuberculosis* infection in mice does not require MyD88 adaptor function for TLR2, -4 and -9. Eur J Immuno. 2008; 38: 680-94.

[75] Shim TS, Turner OC, Orme IM. Toll-like receptor 4 plays no role in susceptibility of mice to *Mycobacterium tuberculosis* infection. Tuberculosis (Edinb) 2003; 83: 367-71.

[76] Hutchens MA, Luker KE, Sonstein J, Nunez G, Curtis JL, Luker GD. Protective effect of Toll-like receptor 4 in pulmonary vaccinia infection. PLoS Pathog 2008; 4: e1000153.

[77] Khanolkar A, Hartwig SM, Haag BA, Meyerholz DK, Harty JT, Varga SM. Toll-like receptor 4 deficiency increases disease and mortality after mouse hepatitis virus type 1 infection of susceptible C3H mice. J Virol 2009; 83: 8946-56.

[78] Kurt-Jones EA, Popova L, Kwinn L *et al.* Pattern recognition receptors TLR4 and CD14 mediate response to respiratory syncytial virus. Nat Immunol 2000; 1: 398-401.

[79] Zhang X, Shan P, Jiang G, Cohn L, Lee PJ. Toll-like receptor 4 deficiency causes pulmonary emphysema. J Clin Invest 2006; 116: 3050-9.

[80] Imai Y, Kuba K, Neely GG *et al.* Identification of oxidative stress and Toll-like receptor 4 signaling as a key pathway of acute lung injury. Cell 2008; 133: 235-49.

[81] Ogawa Y, Tasaka S, Yamada W *et al.* Role of Toll-like receptor 4 in hyperoxia-induced lung inflammation in mice. Inflamm Res 2007; 56: 334-8.

[82] Williams AS, Leung SY, Nath P *et al.* Role of TLR2, TLR4, and MyD88 in murine ozone-induced airway hyperresponsiveness and neutrophilia. J Appl Physiol 2007; 103: 1189-95.

[83] Shimamoto A, Pohlman TH, Shomura S, Tarukawa T, Takao M, Shimpo H. Toll-like receptor 4 mediates lung ischemia-reperfusion injury. Ann Thorac Surg 2006; 82: 2017-23.

[84] Morris AE, Liggitt HD, Hawn TR, Skerrett SJ. Role of Toll-like receptor 5 in the innate immune response to acute *P. aeruginosa* pneumonia. Am J Physiol Lung Cell Mol Physiol 2009; 297: L1112-9.

[85] Hawn TR, Berrington WR, Smith IA *et al.* Altered inflammatory responses in TLR5-deficient mice infected with *Legionella pneumophila*. J Immunol 2007; 179: 6981-7.

[86] Takeuchi O, Kawai T, Muhlradt PF *et al.* Discrimination of bacterial lipoproteins by Toll-like receptor 6. Int Immunol 2001; 13: 933-40.

[87] Diebold SS, Kaisho T, Hemmi H, Akira S, Reis e Sousa C. Innate antiviral responses by means of TLR7-mediated recognition of single-stranded RNA. Science 2004; 303: 1529-31.

[88] Wu CC, Hayashi T, Takabayashi K *et al.* Immunotherapeutic activity of a conjugate of a Toll-like receptor 7 ligand. Proc Natl Acad Sci U S A 2007; 104: 3990-5.

[89] Camateros P, Tamaoka M, Hassan M *et al.* Chronic asthma-induced airway remodeling is prevented by toll-like receptor-7/8 ligand S28463. Am J Respir Crit Care Med 2007; 175: 1241-9.

[90] Gorden KK, Qiu XX, Binsfeld CC, Vasilakos JP, Alkan SS. Cutting edge: activation of murine TLR8 by a combination of imidazoquinoline immune response modifiers and polyT oligodeoxynucleotides. J Immunol 2006; 177: 6584-7.

[91] Latz E, Schoenemeyer A, Visintin A *et al.* TLR9 signals after translocating from the ER to CpG DNA in the lysosome. Nat Immunol 2004; 5: 190-8.

[92] Wagner H. The immunobiology of the TLR9 subfamily. Trends Immunol 2004; 25: 381-6.

[93] Yasuda K, Ogawa Y, Yamane I, Nishikawa M, Takakura Y. Macrophage activation by a DNA/cationic liposome complex requires endosomal acidification and TLR9-dependent and -independent pathways. J Leukoc Biol 2005; 77: 71-9.

[94] Bhan U, Lukacs NW, Osterholzer JJ *et al.* TLR9 is required for protective innate immunity in Gram-negative bacterial pneumonia: role of dendritic cells. J Immunol 2007; 179: 3937-46.

[95] Bhan U, Trujillo G, Lyn-Kew K *et al.* Toll-like receptor 9 regulates the lung macrophage phenotype and host immunity in murine pneumonia caused by *Legionella pneumophila*. Infect Immun 2008; 76: 2895-904.

[96] Albiger B, Dahlberg S, Sandgren A *et al.* Toll-like receptor 9 acts at an early stage in host defence against pneumococcal infection. Cell Microbiol 2007; 9: 633-44.

[97] Bafica A, Scanga CA, Feng CG, Leifer C, Cheever A, Sher A. TLR9 regulates Th1 responses and cooperates with TLR2 in mediating optimal resistance to *Mycobacterium tuberculosis*. J Exp Med 2005; 202: 1715-24.

[98] Ramaprakash H, Ito T, Standiford TJ, Kunkel SL, Hogaboam CM. Toll-like receptor 9 modulates immune responses to *Aspergillus fumigatus* conidia in immunodeficient and allergic mice. Infect Immun 2009; 77: 108-19.

[99] Lund J, Sato A, Akira S, Medzhitov R, Iwasaki A. Toll-like receptor 9-mediated recognition of Herpes simplex virus-2 by plasmacytoid dendritic cells. J Exp Med 2003; 198: 513-20.

[100] Ito T, Schaller M, Hogaboam CM, Standiford TJ, Chensue SW, Kunkel SL. TLR9 activation is a key event for the maintenance of a mycobacterial antigen-elicited pulmonary granulomatous response. Eur J Immunol 2007; 37: 2847-55.

[101] Ito T, Schaller M, Raymond T *et al.* Toll-like receptor 9 activation is a key mechanism for the maintenance of chronic lung inflammation. Am J Respir Crit Care Med 2009; 180: 1227-38.

[102] Seki E, Tsutsui H, Tsuji NM *et al.* Critical roles of myeloid differentiation factor 88-dependent proinflammatory cytokine release in early phase clearance of *Listeria monocytogenes* in mice. J Immunol 2002; 169: 3863-8.

[103] Cai S, Batra S, Shen L, Wakamatsu N, Jeyaseelan S. Both TRIF- and MyD88-dependent signaling contribute to host defense against pulmonary *Klebsiella* infection. J Immunol 2009; 183: 6629-38.

[104] Power MR, Marshall JS, Yamamoto M, Akira S, Lin TJ. The myeloid differentiation factor 88 is dispensable for the development of a delayed host response to *Pseudomonas aeruginosa* lung infection in mice. Clin Exp Immunol 2006; 146: 323-9.

[105] Archer KA, Alexopoulou L, Flavell RA, Roy CR. Multiple MyD88-dependent responses contribute to pulmonary clearance of *Legionella pneumophila*. Cell Microbiol 2009; 11: 21-36.

[106] Naiki Y, Michelsen KS, Schroder NW *et al.* MyD88 is pivotal for the early inflammatory response and subsequent bacterial clearance and survival in a mouse model of *Chlamydia pneumoniae* pneumonia. J Biol Chem 2005; 280: 29242-9.

[107] Rodriguez N, Mages J, Dietrich H *et al.* MyD88-dependent changes in the pulmonary transcriptome after infection with *Chlamydia pneumoniae*. Physiol Genomics 2007; 30: 134-45.

[108] Zhang X, Gao L, Lei L *et al.* A MyD88-dependent early IL-17 production protects mice against airway infection with the obligate intracellular pathogen *Chlamydia muridarum*. J Immunol 2009; 183: 1291-300.

[109] Fremond CM, Yeremeev V, Nicolle DM, Jacobs M, Quesniaux VF, Ryffel B. Fatal *Mycobacterium tuberculosis* infection despite adaptive immune response in the absence of MyD88. J Clin Invest 2004; 114: 1790-9.

[110] Feng CG, Scanga CA, Collazo-Custodio CM *et al.* Mice lacking myeloid differentiation factor 88 display profound defects in host resistance and immune responses to *Mycobacterium avium* infection not exhibited by Toll-like receptor 2 (TLR2)- and TLR4-deficient animals. J Immunol 2003; 171: 4758-64.

[111] Bretz C, Gersuk G, Knoblaugh S *et al.* MyD88 signaling contributes to early pulmonary responses to *Aspergillus fumigatus*. Infect Immun 2008; 76: 952-8.

[112] Yauch LE, Mansour MK, Shoham S, Rottman JB, Levitz SM. Involvement of CD14, toll-like receptors 2 and 4, and MyD88 in the host response to the fungal pathogen *Cryptococcus neoformans in vivo*. Infect Immun 2004; 72: 5373-82.

[113] Nance SC, Yi AK, Re FC, Fitzpatrick EA. MyD88 is necessary for neutrophil recruitment in hypersensitivity pneumonitis. J Leukoc Biol 2008; 83: 1207-17.

[114] Rudd BD, Schaller MA, Smit JJ *et al.* MyD88-mediated instructive signals in dendritic cells regulate pulmonary immune responses during respiratory virus infection. J Immunol 2007; 178: 5820-7.

[115] Sheahan T, Morrison TE, Funkhouser W *et al.* MyD88 is required for protection from lethal infection with a mouse-adapted SARS-CoV. PLoS Pathog 2008; 4: e1000240.

[116] Gargano LM, Moser JM, Speck SH. Role for MyD88 signaling in murine gammaherpesvirus 68 latency. J Virol 2008; 82: 3853-63.

[117] Gasse P, Mary C, Guenon I *et al.* IL-1R1/MyD88 signaling and the inflammasome are essential in pulmonary inflammation and fibrosis in mice. J Clin Invest 2007; 117: 3786-99.

[118] Jeyaseelan S, Young SK, Fessler MB *et al.* Toll/IL-1 receptor domain-containing adaptor inducing IFN-beta (TRIF)-mediated signaling contributes to innate immune responses in the lung during *Escherichia coli* pneumonia. J Immunol 2007; 178: 3153-60.

[119] Power MR, Li B, Yamamoto M, Akira S, Lin TJ. A role of Toll-IL-1 receptor domain-containing adaptor-inducing IFN-beta in the host response to *Pseudomonas aeruginosa* lung infection in mice. J Immunol 2007; 178: 3170-6.

[120] Kawai T, Akira S. Toll-like receptor and RIG-I-like receptor signaling. Ann N Y Acad Sci 2008; 1143: 1-20.

[121] Goldstein DR. Toll-like receptors and other links between innate and acquired alloimmunity. Curr Opin Immunol 2004; 16: 538-44.

[122] Zhu J, Paul WE. Heterogeneity and plasticity of T helper cells. Cell Res 20: 4-12.

[123] Raymond T, Schaller M, Hogaboam CM, Lukacs NW, Rochford R, Kunkel SL. Toll-like receptors, Notch ligands, and cytokines drive the chronicity of lung inflammation. Proc Am Thorac Soc 2007; 4: 635-41.

[124] Debus A, Glasner J, Rollinghoff M, Gessner A. High levels of susceptibility and T helper 2 response in MyD88-deficient mice infected with *Leishmania major* are interleukin-4 dependent. Infect Immun 2003; 71: 7215-8.

[125] Sun J, Walsh M, Villarino AV *et al.* TLR ligands can activate dendritic cells to provide a MyD88-dependent negative signal for Th2 cell development. J Immunol 2005; 174: 742-51.

[126] Ulevitch RJ. Therapeutics targeting the innate immune system. Nat Rev Immunol 2004; 4: 512-20.

[127] Amsen D, Antov A, Flavell RA. The different faces of Notch in T-helper-cell differentiation. Nat Rev Immunol 2009; 9: 116-24.

[128] Schaller MA, Neupane R, Rudd BD *et al.* Notch ligand Delta-like 4 regulates disease pathogenesis during respiratory viral infections by modulating Th2 cytokines. J Exp Med 2007; 204: 2925-34.

[129] Stockinger B, Veldhoen M. Differentiation and function of Th17 T cells. Curr Opin Immunol 2007; 19: 281-6.

[130] Harrington LE, Hatton RD, Mangan PR *et al.* Interleukin 17-producing CD4+ effector T cells develop *via* a lineage distinct from the T helper type 1 and 2 lineages. Nat Immunol 2005; 6: 1123-32.

[131] Weaver CT, Harrington LE, Mangan PR, Gavrieli M, Murphy KM. Th17: an effector CD4 T cell lineage with regulatory T cell ties. Immunity 2006; 24: 677-88.

[132] Ito T, Schaller M, Hogaboam CM *et al.* TLR9 regulates the mycobacteria-elicited pulmonary granulomatous immune response in mice through DC-derived Notch ligand delta-like 4. J Clin Invest 2009; 119: 33-46.

[133] Chaudhuri N, Whyte MK, Sabroe I. Reducing the toll of inflammatory lung disease. Chest 2007; 131: 1550-6.

[134] Basu S, Fenton MJ. Toll-like receptors: function and roles in lung disease. Am J Physiol Lung Cell Mol Physiol 2004; 286: L887-92.

[135] Jurk M, Vollmer J. Therapeutic applications of synthetic CpG oligodeoxynucleotides as TLR9 agonists for immune modulation. BioDrugs 2007; 21: 387-401.

CHAPTER 3

Role of Toll-Like Receptors in Asthma

S. Sagar[1,2], N.A. Georgiou[1,2], G. Folkerts[1], J. Garssen[1,2] and A.D. Kraneveld[1*]

[1]*Division of Pharmacology, Utrecht Institute for Pharmaceutical Sciences, Faculty of Science, Utrecht University, Utrecht, The Netherlands and* [2]*Danone Research - Centre for Specialised Nutrition, Wageningen, The Netherlands*

Abstract: Asthma is a chronic inflammatory airway disease characterized by episodes of reversible airway narrowing, bronchial hyperresponsiveness and chronic pulmonary inflammation. The prevalence of asthma has been increasing since the 1980s with more than 150 million people affected worldwide. Developed and westernized countries have higher asthma prevalence. To date, asthma is the most common chronic disease in children. More than 50% of asthma cases are the atopic/allergic form triggered by environmental allergens. In the last decade, much attention has been focused on the role of toll-like receptors (TLRs) in the pathogenesis of allergic asthma where it has been suggested that TLRs form the link between the innate and the adaptive immune responses. Toll-like receptors exhibit an important role in the activation of cells of the innate immune system, such as monocytes, macrophages, dendritic cells, mast cells and neutrophils. This chapter will discuss the current knowledge on the different TLRs and their possible roles in allergic asthma.

Keywords: Asthma, allergic lung, CpG-ODN therapy, probiotics.

1. INTRODUCTION

Pathophysiology and Population Frequencies of Asthma

Asthma is a chronic inflammatory airway disease characterized by episodes of reversible airway narrowing, bronchial hyperresponsiveness and chronic pulmonary inflammation. Asthma can be classified either according to frequency of symptoms (clinical) or according to triggers causing the airway symptoms. Clinical classification of asthma severity is as follows:

1. Intermittent, where patients suffer less than once a week from symptoms and having a forced expiratory volume in 1 sec (FEV1) of more than 80% predicted.

2. Mild, where patients suffer from symptoms more than once per week, but less than once per day, and have a FEV1 of more than 80% predicted.

3. Moderate persistent, where patients suffer daily from symptoms and have a FEV1 of 60-80% predicted.

4. Severe persistent, where patients suffer daily from symptoms also at nighttime and have a FEV1 less than 60% predicted.

Asthma may also be classified as atopic, where symptoms are induced by allergens or non-atopic where symptoms are induced by non-specific triggers. Workplace exposures are the world's most common cause of so-called occupational asthma. 15-23% of new-onset asthma cases in adults are work-related.

During remission, patients suffer from symptoms such as nighttime coughing and shortness of breath when exercising. Exacerbation of the disease consists of an acute asthma attack during which patients are short of breath, suffer from chest tightness, have a rapid heart rate (tachycardia) and wheezing can occur. The

*Address Correspondence to A.D. Kraneveld: Division of Pharmacology, Utrecht Institute for Pharmaceutical Sciences, Faculty of Science, Utrecht University, PO box 80082, 3508 TB Utrecht, The Netherlands. Tel:+31302534509; E-mail: A.D.Kraneveld@uu.nl

Catherine M. Greene (Ed)

prevalence of asthma has been increasing since the 1980s, particularly in children and young adults. To date, asthma is the most common chronic disease in children. More than 150 million people worldwide are diagnosed with asthma with developed and westernized countries having a higher asthma prevalence. More than 50% of the cases of asthma are of the atopic/allergic form. In the pathology of asthma, the airway inflammation is characterized by the influx of several inflammatory cells such as mast cells, eosinophils, B-lymphocytes and T-lymphocytes. The mechanism of allergic asthma will be discussed in detail in this chapter.

2. HYGIENE HYPOTHESIS

Since 1960, the prevalence of asthma and allergy has markedly increased in the western world [4]. Asthma is associated with a western life style and this has been shown clearly, for example, by the rapid increase in the prevalence of asthma in children who have migrated from developing countries to developed countries [5]. Four reasons could be involved in the increased prevalence of asthma associated with western lifestyle [6]:

1. Exposure to house dust mite, a major allergen, has increased due to modern housing and increasing time spent indoors.

2. Exposure to a wide range of microorganisms has changed because of improved hygiene and wide spread antibiotic use.

3. The prevalence of obesity has increased in children.

4. Changes in the western diet, for example the decline of fresh and/or raw vegetables in the diet.

3. CURRENT STATUS OF THERAPY OF ALLERGIC ASTHMA

Classically, asthma has been regarded as a bronchoconstrictive disease and is predominantly treated with bronchodilators, such as β2 agonists [7]. Currently, the chronic inflammatory process is targetted with inhaled corticosteroids. For the management of asthma, patients take regularly inhaled corticosteroids with or without long acting β2 agonists. However, 50% of the patients are poorly controlled and there is still a need for new therapies. Because corticosteroids have long term side effects, patients are apprehensive of their long term use and often show poor compliance [8]. Furthermore, the long-term safety of long acting β2 agonists, which have been linked to increased risk of mortality and desensitization of the β2 receptor, is of concern [9, 10].

Blocking the synthesis or receptor for a single mediator (such as lipid mediators) involved in asthma seems unlikely to be very effective. Anti-leukotrienes that block cysteinyl leukotriene receptor 1 (CysLt1), are currently used in therapy, but these drugs are less effective than inhaled corticosteroids [7]. In addition, leukotriene B4 (LTB4) receptor antagonists have shown no effect in mild asthma [11]. Compounds targeting another arachidonic metabolite and its receptor, prostaglandin D2, are now in clinical development for asthma. Since cytokines play a crucial role in orchestrating chronic inflammation, they have become important targets for asthma treatments. However, over 50 cytokines have been implicated in asthma (including interleukin (IL)-4, IL-5, IL-13, tumor necrosis factor α (TNFα), and C-C chemokine receptor type 3(CCR3)) and several cytokine and chemokine blocking antibodies are now in clinical development but clinical studies in asthmatic patients have been disappointing [7]. Antibodies blocking IgE are only used in the treatment of patients with severe asthma, due to the high cost of treatment and the unclear mechanism of clinical efficacy.

The most promising anti-inflammatory therapy is by the use of phosphodiesterase (PDE)4 inhibitors targeting T cells, eosinophils, smooth muscle cells and epithelial cells. Roflumilast, an oral PDE4 inhibitor, demonstrated inhibitory effects on allergen-induced responses in asthma similar to low doses of inhaled corticosteroids [12]. However, side effects such as nausea, headaches and diarrhea are the major limitations for using of the drug. Kinases play a crucial role in regulating the expression of inflammatory genes in asthma and are therefore also a promising target. Several kinase inhibitors are currently in clinical development [13].

A different approach is specific immune therapy, whereby asthmatic patients are exposed in a controlled way to allergens or allergen-peptides, (either subcutaneously or sublingually) to induce tolerance and desensitization. Some efficacy by this approach has been demonstrated, however, longer studies and comparison with inhaled corticosteroids are needed to determine efficacy [7].

A limited number of clinical studies have been reported that specifically target the innate immune system. In this chapter, the innate immune system in asthma, specifically as regulated by TLRs will be reviewed and possible targeting of TLRs for the prevention and treatment of asthma will be addressed.

4. TLR INVOLVEMENT IN ASTHMA

Toll-like receptors have an important role in the activation of cells of the innate immune system, such as monocytes, macrophages, dendritic cells (DCs), mast cells and neutrophils. TLRs play pivotal roles in the detection of and response to pathogens and they are implicated in both infective and non-infective inflammatory responses in the lung [14, 15]. In addition to their protective role against microbial infections, it is also becoming clear that these receptors exhibit homeostatic roles. In the lung, for example, breakdown products of the extracellular matrix component hyaluranon have been shown to to signal *via* TLRs [16]. Signaling *via* TLRs also seems to be required for maintaining epithelial integrity in health and for epithelial survival and proliferation after injury [16]. The latter is in turn necessary for restoration of normal tissue architecture [16-18].

In the pathology of asthma, the inflammation in the airways is characterized by the presence of several inflammatory cells such as mast cells, eosinophils, B-lymphocytes and T-lymphocytes. The mechanism of allergic asthma involves an exaggerated immune response to inhaled allergens, inducing the production of antigen-specific T-helper 2 (Th2) lymphocytes [19, 20]. Upon inhalation of a specific allergen, antigen-presenting cells (APCs) in the airway such as DCs, migrate to the draining lymph nodes where they present the antigen to precursor Th cells. Immature pulmonary DCs express TLRs on their surface and these become activated during infection or inflammation leading to upregulation of co-stimulatory molecules. The precursor Th cells then differentiate and mature into a population of CD4[+] Th2 cells. Generation of these antigen-specific Th2 cells leads to the production and activation of eosinophils, release of cytokines, such as IL-4 and IL-13, and the activation of the humoral immune system resulting in the development of antigen-specific B cells that in turn become plasma cells producing antigen-specific immunoglobulin E (IgE) (Fig. **1a**) [1, 7, 14, 19, 21-23]. Possibly, TLR-primed DCs also present antigen to antigen-specific T cells leading to proliferation of these cells and the release of Th2 cytokines, such as IL-4, IL-5 and IL-13. The release of these cytokines causes eosinophil proliferation and infiltration and enhanced mucus production resulting in chronic airway inflammation, (Fig. **1b**) [1, 14, 21-23].

Murine studies have demonstrated that in addition to DCs, mast cells also play an important role in the induction of allergic airway inflammation [1, 24]. Mast cells play a crucial role in both acute and allergic inflammation and additionally they express the high-affinity receptor receptors for IgE (FcεRI) on their surface. Extravascularly, IgE binds to mast cells and re-exposure to the same antigen will bind IgE-armed mast cells resulting in mast cell activation. In general, mast cell activation can be divided into three different phases. In the first phase degranulation takes place. During this process preformed mediators, such as histamine, serotonin, prostaglandins, leukotrienes, IL-4, IL-5, IL-9 and IL-13 stored in granules are rapidly released in a matter of seconds. The release of these vasoactive substances increases the vascular permeability allowing the flow of inflammatory mediators, eosinophils and more antigen-specific Th2 cells, into the antigen-encountered site resulting in bronchoconstriction [24-26]. In the second phase of mast cell activation, arachidonic acid metabolites are formed. The *de novo* production of chemokines and cytokines takes place in the third phase. In conjunction with the arachidonic acid metabolites, these chemokines and cytokines recruit inflammatory cells leading to induction of chronic inflammation (Fig. **2**) [24-26]. Interleukin-5 is the main cytokine involved in the differentiation of eosinophils from bone marrow precursor cells and prolongs eosinophil survival.

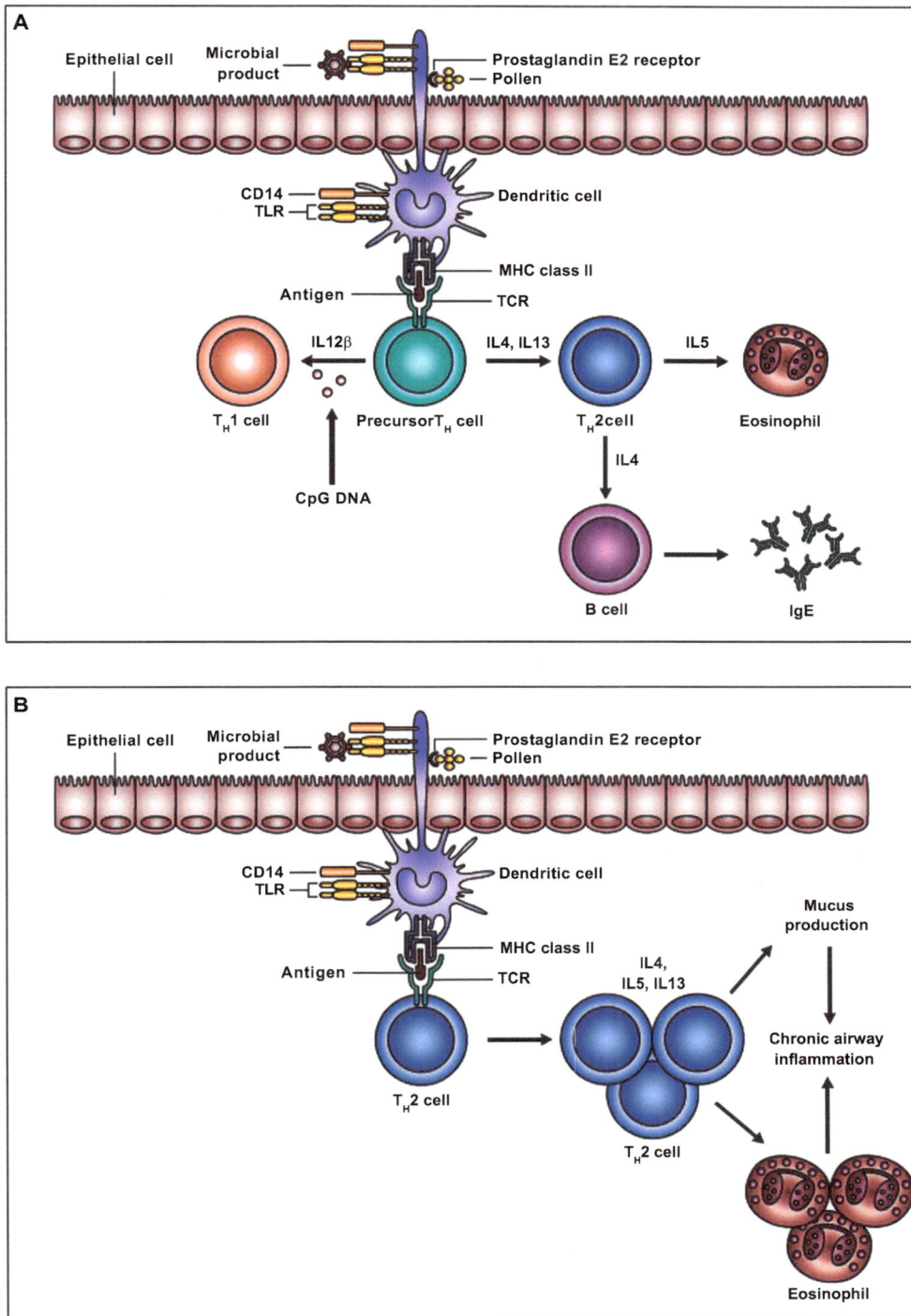

Figure 1: Role of dendritic cells in airway inflammation. (**A**) Upon inhalation of an allergen, the DCs migrate to the draining lymph nodes where they present the antigen to precursor Th cells. Precursor Th cells then maturate and differentiate into Th2 cells leading to the production and activation of eosinophils, the release of IL-4, IL-13 and the development of antigen-specific B cells. The B cells become plasma cells which produce antigen-specific IgE. Possibly, TLR9 ligands (CpG DNA) restore the immune balance by shifting the balance from a Th2 response to a Th1 response. (**B**) Immature DCs express TLRs on their surface. These TLRs become activated during infection or inflammation. TLR-primed DCs also present the antigen to antigen-specific Th2 cells leading to proliferation of these cells, release of IL-4, IL-5 and IL-13, eosinophil proliferation. All these events lead to enhanced mucus production and eventually airway inflammation. The figure is adapted from [1, 2].

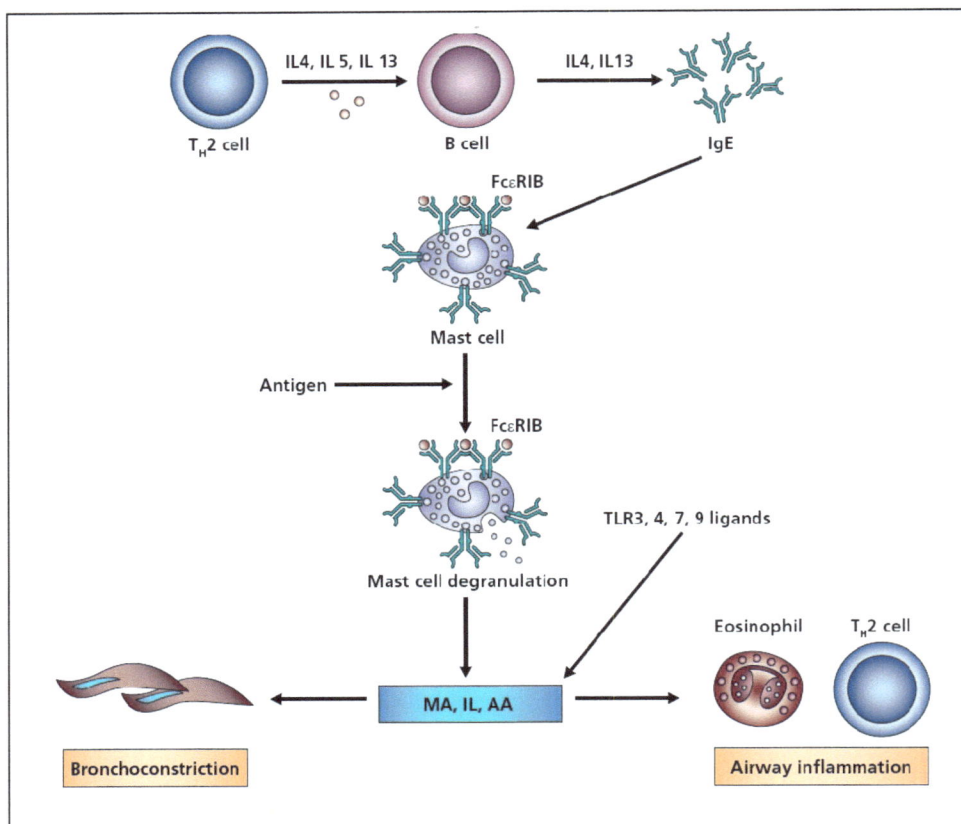

Figure 2: Role of mast cells in airway inflammation. Th2 cells release IL-4, IL-5 and IL-13 leading to the development of antigen-specific B cells which differentiate into IgE-producing plasma cells. MCs express receptors for IgE on their surface. Binding of IgE to MCs leads to activation of MCs followed by degranulation. During degranulation of MCs monoamines (MA; histamine, serotonin, prostaglandins), interleukins (IL; IL-4, IL-5, IL-13) and arachidonic acid metabolites (AA) are released resulting in increased flow of inflammatory mediators and cells into the antigen-encountered site leading to bronchoconstriction. The released of chemokines, cytokines recruit eosinophils and Th2 cells leading to chronic inflammation. TLR3, TLR4, TLR7 and TLR9 ligands seem to induce MCs activation and the release of cytokines and chemokines without the induction of degranulation and arachidonic acid metabolism. The figure is adapted from [1, 2].

The activation of residential mast cells (acute response) and infiltrated eosinophils and Th2 cells (late response) leads to airway narrowing because of mucosal edema, smooth muscle constriction and mucus hyper-secretion [26]. Chronic inflammation persists due to the involvement of antigen-specific Th2 cells and eosinophils, leading to characteristic structural changes in the asthmatic airway such as collagen deposition at the basolateral side of the epithelium (basement membrane thickening), angiogenesis and increased airway smooth muscle as a result of hypertrophy and hyperplasia, resulting in airway hyperresponsiveness [26].

In addition, it has been demonstrated that mast cell activation and the secretion of pro-inflammatory cytokines and chemokines by these cells is directly induced by TLR3, TLR4, TLR7 and TLR9 ligands. These ligands seem to induce these events without the induction of degranulation and arachidonic acid metabolism (Fig. **2**) [24-32].

The functions of the distinct TLRs in allergic airway inflammation are mediated by the activation of cells of the innate immune system, such as DCs, mast cells and neutrophils. So far, DCs and mast cells have been described to be the major players in allergic asthma. However, our understanding of the exact functions of TLRs in allergic airway inflammation is complicated by the fact that TLRs often act together by forming heterodimers or homodimers expanding the range of TLR ligands which have to be studied in order to elucidate the functional role of TLRs in disease pathogenesis. These observations about the role of TLRs in homeostasis highlight the importance of elucidating the functional role of TLRs in health and disease before the development of TLR-based therapies can be considered.

5. EXPRESSION, FUNCTION AND ACTIVATION OF TLRs IN THE ASTHMATIC/ALLERGIC LUNG

The various TLRs exhibit different cell- and stimulus specific patterns of expression in various tissues. The **TLR1** gene is ubiquitously expressed and at a higher level than the other TLRs [33, 34]. The exact role of TLR1 in asthma still needs to be elucidated. Recently, a German case-control study was carried out in which all human TLR genes were systematically investigated for polymorphisms [35]. Functional genetic variants in the TLR genes were evaluated for their association with different asthma phenotypes in children with asthma, bronchial hyperresponsiveness (BHR) or both [35]. It was shown in this study that single nucleotide polymorphisms (SNPs) in the TLR1 gene have protective effects on atopic asthma. Moreover, it was also demonstrated that TLR1 SNPs increase proinflammatory and Th1 cytokine interferon-γ (IFN-γ) expression levels and reduce Th2 associated IL-4 production [35]. Thus, TLR1 SNPs seem to have protective effects on atopic asthma by skewing the Th1/Th2 balance toward Th1.

In contrast to TLR1, **TLR2** has a restricted pattern of expression and it is present in human monocytes, polymorphonuclear (PMN) and DCs [33, 36]. Moreover, TLR2 acts as a heterodimer with TLR1, TLR6 and possibly TLR10 [37, 38]. These TLR2 heterodimers recognize different structures of lipopeptides and lipoproeins [39-41]. TLR2 has been demonstrated to play an important role in host defense mechanisms during lung inflammation [42]. In addition, the expression of TLR2 in human airway smooth muscle cells (ASMCs) of patients undergoing lung transplantation or surgical resection for carcinoma was shown to be regulated by TNF-α and the TLR3 ligand double-stranded RNA (dsRNA). Both of these stimuli showed synergistic effects with the cytokine IFN-γ on TLR2 mRNA expression. Moreover, stimulation of ASMCs with the TLR2 ligand peptidoglycan (PGN) induced the release of IL-8 from ASMCs whilst the corticosteroid dexamethasone inhibited cytokine- and TLR2 ligand-induced TLR2 mRNA expression in those ASMCs [43]. Furthermore, expression of TLR2 mRNA and protein was shown to be synergistically enhanced by dexamethasone in combination with the cytokines TNF-α and IFN-γ in the human bronchial epithelial cell line (BEAS-2B) [42]. On the other hand, murine models of allergic asthma have shown that TLR2 agonists have the potential to both inhibit and promote the development of allergic immune responses [44]. For example, intratracheal treatment of asthmatic mice with a TLR2/TLR6 agonist in combination with the Th1-cytokine IFN-γ resulted in reduction of airway hyperresponsiveness, eosinophilia and the Th2 cytokines IL-5 and IL-13 in bronchoalveolar lavage (BAL) fluid [44, 45]. In another murine model of asthma, a synthetic TLR2/1 ligand was shown to reverse established ovalbumin (OVA)-induced airways inflammation in mice [44, 46]. In addition, intranasal challenge of OVA sensitized mice with OVA allergen and a TLR2/4 agonist resulted in suppression of airway inflammation represented by decreased airway eosinophilia and Th2 cytokines [41, 44]. Contradictory results were reported in another study where allergic asthma was aggravated in mice immunized with OVA allergen in combination with a TLR2/1 agonist by inducing a Th2 immune response [44, 47]. Moreover, a TLR2/6 agonist was shown to reduce eosinophilic infiltration in a murine model of chronic allergic airway inflammation in which mice were intranasally sensitized to Timothy grass pollen antigens [48].

TLR6 has a restricted pattern of expression and was shown to be highly expressed on human B cells and at lower levels on monocytes and NK cells [33, 49]. In addition, TLR6 was also demonstrated to be expressed on human cord blood-derived mast cells mast (CBMCs) [50]. TLR6 signals as a heterodimer with TLR2 and binds specifically to di-acetylated lipopeptides [37, 49]. In the German case-control study in children with asthma, SNPs in the TLR6 gene were shown to have protective effects on atopic asthma. TLR6 SNPs increased pro-inflammatory and Th1 cytokine IFN-γ expression and reduced Th2 associated IL-4 production [35]. Moreover, Tantisira and co-workers described 53 SNPs in the DNA samples of three distinct ethnic groups, African Americans, European Americans and Hispanic Americans. Preliminary analysis in this study demonstrated one non-synonymous TLR6 SNP (Ser249Pro), in the region encoding the extracellular domain of the TLR6 protein, to be significantly associated with protection from asthma in African Americans in a case-control disease-association study in asthmatic and healthy African Americans

[51]. Similar results were described by Hoffjan and co-workers. The 249Ser allele was shown to be weakly, but significantly associated with childhood asthma in a study which involved unrelated adult asthma patients, unrelated children with asthma and healthy control subjects [52]. Murine models of allergic asthma have shown that when administered intra-tracheally to asthmatic mice, the combination of TLR2/6 agonist and IFN-γ reduced airway hyperresponsiveness, eosinophilia and the Th2 cytokines IL-5 and IL-13 in the BAL fluid [45, 48].

In summary, the evidence surrounding the involvement of TLR2 is broad with some studies reporting improvement and others worsening of the disease symptoms in animal models where specific ligands were tested. This seems to depend partly on which TLR2 heterodimer, TLR1/2 or TLR2/TLR6, is addressed. SNPs in TLR6 were shown to have protective effects on allergic asthma.

TLR3 has a selective pattern of expression and was shown to be exclusively expressed by human immature DCs. Moreover, TLR3 mRNA expression was significantly decreased in mature DCs [33, 36]. The exact role of TLR3 in the pathogenesis of allergic asthma still needs to be elucidated. However, its role in the exacerbations of pulmonary diseases has been studied in murine airway inflammation models as well as *in vitro* studies. A known ligand of TLR3 is polyinosine-polycytidylic acid poly (I:C), a synthetic analog of dsRNA, a molecular pattern associated with viral infection. Stowell and co-workers have demonstrated that intranasal administration of poly (I:C), into wild-type mice resulted in up regulation of expression of TLR2, TLR3, TLR7 and TLR9 as well as up regulation of chemokines, cytokines and signaling molecules in the lung [53]. Additionally, poly(I:C)-treated mice showed a significant increase in the total cell number, especially neutrophils, in the BAL fluid. Moreover, poly (I:C) stimulation induced bronchial epithelial cell hypertrophy in wild-type mice leading to impairment of the pulmonary function in those mice. However, in TLR3 knock out (KO) mice poly (I:C)-induced inflammatory cell influx was attenuated and the mice were protected from bronchial epithelial cell hypertrophy and changes in the lung function. These data suggest that viral activation of TLR3 can play a critical role in exacerbation of respiratory diseases such as asthma [53]. On the other hand, the expression of TLR3 in ASMCs of patients undergoing lung transplantation or surgical resection for carcinoma was shown to be regulated by TNF-α and poly (I:C). Stimulation of ASMCs with the TLR3 ligand induced the release of the chemokine IL-8 in ASMCs of these patients [43]. The dsRNA was shown to be an effective epithelial activator in both BEAS-2B airway epithelial cell line and human primary bronchial epithelial cells (PBEC). In addition, activation of TLR3 by dsRNA increased the expression of TLR3 and triggered strongly the expression of IL-8, macrophage inflammatory protein 3-α (MIP-3α) and granulocyte macrophage colony-stimulating factor (GM-CSF). MIP-3α and GM-CSF may play a role in immature DCs migration and maturation. These data are consistent with data from murine models of airway inflammation and suggest a pro-inflammatory role of TLR3 agonists [54]. In addition, the influences of human thymic stromal lymphopoietin (TSLP) and TLR3 ligand stimulation on DCs activation was also investigated. TLSP is expressed in the lungs of asthmatic patients and activates a specific subset of DCs (CD11c+) to give rise to proallergic T cell responses [55-57]. TLR3 ligands in combination with TSLP were shown to activate human DCs and thereby promote the differentiation of Th17 cells suggesting a role of TLR3 ligands in the pathogenesis of severe asthma [55, 58]. Together these data suggest a pro-inflammatory role of TLR3 in allergic asthma and other respiratory diseases.

TLR4 is the most well studied TLR. TLR4 is expressed in a variety of human cell types including macrophages, DCs and endothelial cells and is activated by lipopolysaccharide (LPS), an outer cell wall component of gram-negative bacteria [43]. Recently, the expression profile of TLRs and the TLR ligand-activated production profile of asthma-related inflammatory cytokines, such as TNF-α, IL-10 and IL-1β, was investigated in PBMCs of asthmatic patients. TLR4 expression on monocytes, lymphocytes and DCs in asthmatic patients was shown to be significantly lower compared to the control subjects. Moreover, the *ex vivo* production of TNF-α, IL-10 and IL-1β by PBMCs stimulated with LPS was also shown to be significantly lower in asthmatic patients. It was suggested that the observed reduction in TLR4 activation leads to reduced release of the Th1-related cytokine IL-1β and anti-inflammatory cytokine IL-10 and thereby contributes to the immunological mechanisms of asthma [59].

On the other hand, Sukkar and co-workers demonstrated the expression of TLR4 in human ASMCs of patients undergoing lung transplantation or surgical resection for carcinoma which was shown to be synergistically regulated by the cytokines TNF-α, IFN-γ and dsRNA [43]. Moreover, stimulation of the ASMCs with LPS induced the release of IL-8 in ASMCs of these patients. House dust mite (HDM) has been suggested to induce asthma *via* TLR4 triggering of airway neutrophils and monocytes. It has been shown that TLR4 expression in irradiated chimeric mice is necessary for DCs activation and the priming of T helper responses to HDM in the asthmatic lung [60]. Administration of the TLR4 antagonist, an under-acylated form of *Rhodobacter sphaeroides* LPS, by inhalation at the time of HDM injections reduced the features of asthma. Mice treated with this TLR4 antagonist showed reduced eosinophilia and lymphocytosis, reduced levels of Th2 cytokines IL-5, IL-13 and IFN-γ in the BAL fluid, decreased goblet cell hyperplasia and also lower airway hyper-responsiveness [60]. The molecular mechanism of allergic asthma induced by LPS has been extensively studied in murine models of allergic asthma. It was demonstrated that the dose of LPS would determine which type of immune response, Th1 or Th2, will be induced. In addition, the combination of low dose of LPS with OVA was shown to enhance antigen-induced inflammation in lung tissue of asthmatic mice [61]. Significant inflammatory infiltration of both eosinophils and neutrophils in the lung tissue of asthmatic mice was observed. This was accompanied by high levels of Th2 cytokines in the BAL fluid [61]. Mice exposed to OVA containing low dose of LPS demonstrated increased mucus secretion. However, a high dose of LPS induced a Th1 response with recruitment of neutrophils into lung tissue and increased IFN- γ levels in BAL fluid. In another study, the expression of TLR4 mRNA in alveolar macrophages showed no correlation with the dose of LPS and an up-regulation of TLR4 was observed in the lungs of all asthmatic mice regardless of the LPS dose received [61]. In murine models of allergic asthma, the dose of LPS seems to partly determine the involvement of TLR4. Data from *in vitro* studies showed a broad role of TLR4 in allergic asthma with some studies reporting improvement and others worsening of disease symptoms.

TLR5 has a restricted pattern of expression and is expressed on human monocytes, immature DCs, epithelial cells, NK cells and T cells [33, 36, 49]. Binding of flagellin, a structural component of flagellated bacteria and the only known TLR5 ligand so far, to TLR5 homodimers stimulates the activation of NF-κB [37, 62]. In addition, in models of human intestinal epithelia flagellin was demonstrated to activate basolaterally expressed TLR5 which induced epithelial secretion of IL-8 *via* activation of NF-κB signaling pathway [63]. In addition, binding of flagellin to TLR5 heterodimers results in the production of type-1 interferons and nitric oxide (NO). The latter was shown to be induced by signaling *via* heteromeric TLR4/TLR5 complexes in HeNC2 cells, a murine macrophage cell line that expresses wild-type TLR4 [37, 62]. Furthermore, flagellin was shown to stimulate the maturation of human monocyte-derived DCs from healthy volunteers but not murine DCs [64]. Nevertheless, very little is known about the function of TLR5 in allergic asthma. Recently, decreased functional response of TLR5 was demonstrated in asthmatic patients. Compared with healthy subjects, the *ex vivo* flagellin-stimulated production of TNF-α, IL-10 and IL-1β by PBMCs was shown to be significantly lower in asthmatic patients. In addition, the expression of TLR5 was also found to be significantly decreased in monocytes, lymphocytes and DCs of asthmatic patients. It was suggested that the observed reduction in TLR5 activation leads to reduced release of Th1-related cytokine IL-1β and anti-inflammatory cytokine IL-10 and thereby contributes to the immunological mechanisms of asthma [59]. The exact function of TLR5 in allergic asthma still needs to be investigated.

TLR7 is expressed on human B cells and plasmacytoid precursor DCs [33, 49]. In the general context of allergic disorders and specifically in that of asthma, little attention has been given to the TLR7. However, a family based association analysis has identified TLR7 as a novel risk gene in asthma. In this study, significant associations were observed for the rs179008 SNP of TLR7, a non-synonymous change altering a glutamic acid to leucine residue in the signal peptide sequence of TLR7 at amino acid position 11 (Glu11Leu), in four allergic phenotypes including asthma [65]. Moreover, the function of TLR7 was found to be reduced in adolescents with asthma compared to healthy individuals [66]. Furthermore, the synthetic TLR7 ligand R-837 was shown to activate human eosinophils from allergic patients and healthy subjects. The TLR responses of eosinophils were higher in allergic patients and activation of TLR7 by R-837 resulted in the activation of eosinophils at several levels, including prolonged survival, enhanced migration and induction of IL-8 release. These data suggest that during viral respiratory infections TLR7-mediated activation of eosinpohils may contribute to allergic exacerbations [67]. A murine model of allergic asthma has demonstrated that at birth intranasal sensitization of mice with endotoxin[low] OVA in the presence of single stranded RNA (ssRNA), a ligand of TLR7, and challenge with endotoxin[low] OVA increased airway and tissue eosinophils, mucus-producing cells and the production of antigen-specific IL-13. Activation of TLR7 in early life seems to promote the development of Th2 cells resulting in allergic airway inflammation upon allergen challenge in later life [68]. On the other hand, the synthetic compound S28463 (resiquimod, R-848) which is a TLR7/TLR8 ligand was shown to prevent chronic asthma-induced airway remodeling in rats. The development of goblet cell hyperplasia and the increase in airway smooth muscle mass was inhibited by the compound. In addition, the protein expression of both the Th1 cytokine IFN-γ as well as the Th2 cytokines IL-4, IL-5 and IL-13 was reduced in the lungs of rats [69]. Overall data from human studies have shown that TLR7 might play a role in the exacerbation of allergic asthma. However, data from murine models of allergic asthma are contradictory emphasizing the caveats of using animal models to determine human diseases but possibly suggesting a dual role of TLR7 in allergic asthma.

Similar to TLR7, **TLR8** has a restricted pattern of expression and is highly expressed on human monocytes and at lower levels on NK and T cells [33, 49]. The exact role of TLR8 in allergic asthma still needs to be elucidated. However, a family based association analysis has identified TLR8 as a novel risk gene in asthma. Significant associations were observed for the rs5741883 SNP of TLR8, located at the promoter region of the TLR8 gene affecting potential transcription binding sites, in four allergic phenotypes including asthma [65].

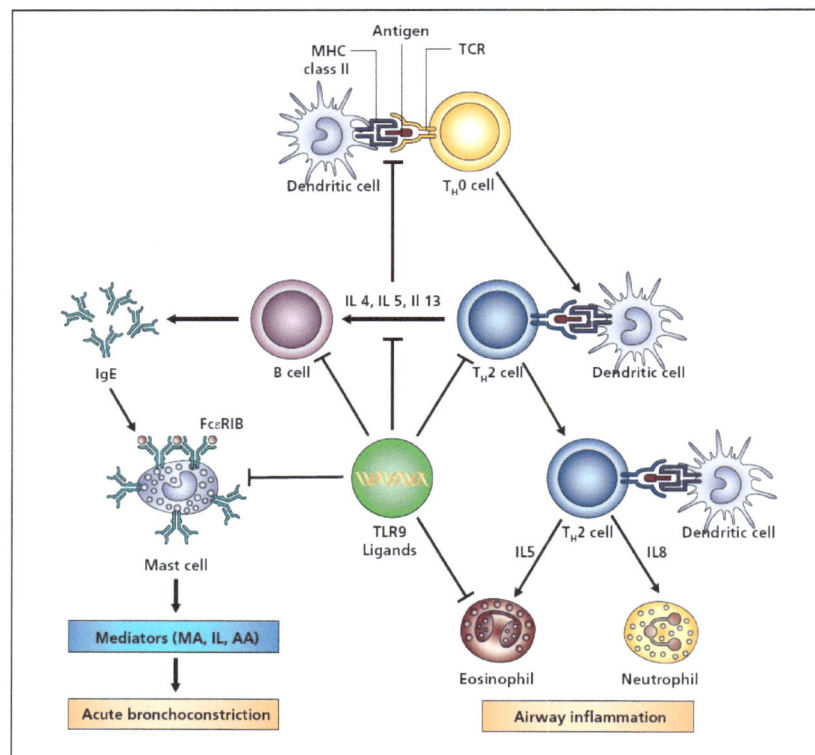

Figure 3: Modulation of allergic inflammation and immunopathology by TLR ligands. Acute bronchoconstriction is modulated by inhibition of Th2 cytokine release, activation of B cells, IgE production and release of monoamines (MA; histamine, serotonin, prostaglandins), interleukins (IL; IL-4, IL-5, IL-13) and arachidonic acid metabolites (AA) by mast cells. TLR9 ligands modulate airway inflammation by inhibition of Th0 cells differentiation into Th2, release of IL-8 and Il-5 and recruitment of neutrophils and eosinophils. The figure is adapted from [3].

The **TLR9** receptor, besides TLR2 and TLR4, is one of the most extensively studied TLRs in asthma. TLR9 is expressed on human plasmacytoid precursor DCs, B cells, macrophages, polymorphonuclear leukocytes (PMLs) and microglial cells amongst others [33, 70, 71]. The receptor recognizes unmethylated bacterial cytosine-guanine repeat (CpG) dideoxynucleotides; these motifs are mostly methylated and less common in vertebrates [72, 73]. TLR9 agonists are highly effective immune modulators with applications as vaccine adjuvants, as stand-alone therapy or in combination with other therapies for the treatment of cancer, infectious diseases, allergy and asthma. In the specific context of asthma, CpG ODN demonstrated benefit in various rodent and primate models of asthma and they have shown positive results in a number of early human clinical trials (Fig. **3**) [3, 74].

CpG DNA motifs can activate NK cells *via* stimulation of DCs leading to the induction of a Th1 innate response. The latter is characterized by the production of IFN-γ, as well as IL-10 and IL-12 and can counterbalance the allergic Th2 dominated phenotype [75-77]. For example, CpG was demonstrated to activate human eosinophils from allergic patients and healthy subjects. The TLR responses of eosinophils were higher in allergic patients and activation of TLR9 by CpG resulted in the activation of eosinophils at several levels, including prolonged survival, enhanced migration and induction of IL-8 release. These data suggest that during viral respiratory infections TLR9-mediated activation of eosinpohils may contribute to allergic exacerbations [67]. In agreement with the hygiene hypothesis, which states that lack of exposure to microbial agents at early childhood contribute to increased susceptibility to the development of allergic diseases [78], maternal TLR signaling was shown to be required for prenatal asthma protection in mice. The progeny from mothers intranasally exposed to the cowshed-derived bacterium *Acinetobacter lowffii* F78 (*A. lwoffii* F78) were protected against the development of asthma. Although maternal exposure to *A. lwoffii* F78 resulted in transiently increased lung and serum TNF-α and IL-6 and up regulation of lung TLR2, 3, 6, 7 and 9 mRNA expression, suppression of TLRs was observed in placental tisssue. Moreover, the offspring from *A. lwoffii* F78-treated TLR2/3/4/7/9$^{-/-}$ mothers were no longer protected against asthma [79].

In summary, the TLR9 ligand, CpG ODN, demonstrated benefit in various rodent and primate models of allergic asthma and they have shown positive results in a number of early human clinical trials. TLR9 is discussed in more detail later in relation to preclinial and clinical evidence of its beneficial use as TLR-targeted therapy for the treatment of allergic symptoms.

TLR10 is the most recently discovered human TLR and it is highly expressed on B cells and at lower levels on plasmacytoid precursor DCs [33, 49]. The ligand of TLR10 has not been identified yet, it is an orphan receptor, and it has no rodent homologue. TLR10 may signal in heterodimers with TLR1 and TLR2 [37, 38]. To date, very little is known about TLR10 and its role in allergic asthma. However SNPs in the TLR10 gene have been reported to have protective effects on atopic asthma. TLR10 SNPs increased pro-inflammatory and Th1 cytokine IFN-γ expression and reduced Th2 associated IL-4 production [35]. Moreover, Lazarus and co-workers have described TLR10 as highly polymorphic and in 47 subjects (24 African American and 23 European American) 78 SNPs of TLR10 were found. From these SNPs, two SNPs (1031G>A, 2322A>G) showed significant association with asthma in a case-control study in European American subjects, including 517 asthma cases and 519 control subjects [80].

To sum up, the various TLRs exhibit different cell- and stimulus specific pattern of expression. According to their cellular expression pattern, TLRs can be categorized as either ubiquitous (TLR1), restricted (TLR2, 4, 5, 6, 7, 8, 9 and 10) or selective (TLR3). Besides their protective role against microbial infections, TLRs also exhibit homeostatic roles. Functional genetic variations in TLR1, TLR6 and TLR10 genes have protective effects on atopic asthma in human. However, TLR2 and TLR4 have the potential to both inhibit and promote the development of allergic immune responses and in the case of TLR4, the dose of LPS appears to determine whether a Th1- or Th2-mediated allergic response is induced. On the other hand, the activation of TLR4 and TLR5 is reduced in asthmatic patients suggesting a pro-inflammatory role of these two receptors in the immunological mechanisms of asthma. In addition, TLR3 agonists seem to play a pro-inflammatory role in respiratory diseases and TLR3 contributes to exacerbations of these diseases including asthma. TLR7 and TLR8 have been identified as novel risk genes in asthma. However, the function of TLR7 was shown to be reduced in adolescents with asthma and consistently a TLR7 ligand was described to inhibit airway remodeling features in a rodent allergic asthma model. To date, the TLR9 receptor is one of the most extensively studied TLRs in asthma. CpG ODN, ligands of TLR9, demonstrated benefit in various rodent and primate models of asthma and they have shown positive results in a number of early human clinical trials. It is thought that TLR9 modulates allergic responses by skewing the balance from a Th2 towards a Th1 response. The expression, function and role of the different TLRs is summarized in Table **1**.

Table 1: Role of TLRs and NLRs in Allergic Asthma

Receptor	Cell Type	Human Studies	Animal Studies	Role in Allergic Asthma	References
TLR1	Ubiquitous	↑ Th1 ↓ Th2		Protective role of SNPs	[33-35]
TLR2	Monocytes, PMN , DCs	↑ IL-8 in ASMCs by PGN	↑↓ airway inflammation by TLR1/TLR2 ↓ Th2 by TLR2/TLR4 ↓ AHR and Th2 by TLR2/TLR6	Protective effect of TLR2/TLR4 and TLR2/TLR6 Dual role of TLR1/TLR2	[33, 36-50]
TLR3	Immature DCs	↑ IL-8 in ASMCs by poly (I:C)	↑ airway inflammation by poly (I:C)	Exacerbation of the disease	[33, 36, 43, 53-58]
TLR4	Macrophages, DCs, endothelial cells	↓ Th1 in PBMCs ↑ IL-8 in ASMCs by LPS	↑ Th2 by low dose LPS with OVA ↑ Th1 by high dose LPS with OVA	Induction of airway inflammation	[23, 33, 36, 43, 59, 61]
TLR5	Monocytes, immature DCs, epithelial cells, NK cells, T cells	↓ Th1 in PBMCs		Promotion of the disease	[33, 36, 37, 49, 59, 62-64]
TLR6	High expression in B cells, lower expression in monocytes and NK cells	↑ Th1 ↓ Th2	↓ AHR and Th2 by TLR2/TLR6	Protective role	[35, 37, 45, 48, 49, 51, 52]
TLR7	B cells, plasmacytoid precursor DCs	Risk gene ↑ IL-8 in eosinophils by R-837	↑ Th2 by ssRNA in later life ↓ Th1 and Th2 expression by R-848	Exacerbation of the disease	[33, 49, 65-69]
TLR8	High expression in monocytes, low expression in NK cells, T cells	Risk gene	↓ Th1 and Th2 expression by R-848	Not known yet	[33, 49, 65, 69]
TLR9	plasmacytoid precursor dendritic cells, B cells, macrophages, PMN, micoglial cells	Positive disease modulation in early clinical trials	↑ Th1 and ↓ Th2 by CpG DNA Prenatal protection	Modulation of the disease	[3, 33, 67, 70-79, 81, 82]
TLR10	High expression in B cells, low expression in plasmacytoid precursor DC	↑ Th1 and ↓ Th2 by SNPs Association of SNPs with asthma		Not known yet	[33, 35, 37, 38, 49, 80]
NOD-1	Expression in various tissues	Lower frequency of allergies in farming children by SNPs		Protective role of SNPs	[83-85]
NOD-2	monocytes, granulocytes, DCs, epithelial cells	Association of SNPs with asthma		Development of allergic asthma	[86-94]

6. EXPRESSION, FUNCTION AND ACTIVATION OF OTHER PATTERN RECOGNITION RECEPTORS IN THE ASTHMATIC/ALLERGIC LUNG

In addition to the TLRs, the nod-like receptors (NLRs) are another family of pattern recognition receptors. Genetic studies have linked the function of these receptors with susceptibility towards the development of allergic diseases, including asthma [84, 86]. Nod-like receptor 1 (NOD1) and 2 (NOD2) also known as nucleotide-binding oligomerization domain protein 4 (CARD4) and 15 (CARD15) respectively, are both cytosolic pattern recognition receptors [83, 87].

NOD1/CARD4 is expressed in various types of tissues and it interacts with muropeptides which are a component of gram-negative bacteria [83, 85]. Strong associations between polymorphisms in CARD4/ NOD1 and the presence of asthma and elevated IgE levels were shown in three independent panels of healthy and asthmatic subjects [84]. Similar results were shown in another study where polymorphisms in CARD4 were shown to significantly modify the protective effects of exposure to a farming environment [83]. This study included 668 Australian and German farming children and children not raised on a farm and have reported a very common polymorphism in CARD4/NOD1 (CARD4/-21596) to significantly contribute to the lower frequency of allergies in children heavily exposed to microbial products [83].

NOD2/CARD15, on the other hand, functions as a cytosolic receptor for LPS and peptidoglycan [87, 88]. This receptor is expressed in monocytes, granulocytes, DCs and epithelial cells [89, 90]. Three different relevant polymorphisms in CARD15 were shown to be associated with atopic diseases including asthma [91]. In this study 1872 school children from East and West Germany were genotyped for three functional CARD15 polymorphisms (C2104T, G2722C and 3020iC) previously related to the development of Crohn's disease [91-94] and it was shown that these polymorphisms may increase the severity of asthma. These results suggest that atopic diseases including asthma share their genetic background with Crohn's disease which might be caused by an impaired recognition of microbial exposures [91, 92] Similar results were reported in other study which included a population-based cohort of 1875 German adults where eight polymorphisms in CARD15 showed association with the development of asthma [91]. To date, no studies have been published showing the exact mechanism on cellular or molecular level of the polymorphisms of CARD4 or CARD15 in relation to allergic asthma.

Overall the functions of the CARD4/NOD1 and CARD15/NOD2 members of the NLR family, have also been linked with susceptibility towards the development of allergic asthma. Genetic studies have reported protective roles of polymorphisms in CARD4 and these gene variations were shown to lower the frequency of allergies in farming children. However, polymorphisms in CARD15 were associated with the development of allergic asthma. The expression, function and role of CARD4 and CARD15 is summarized in Table **1**.

7. TOLL-LIKE RECEPTOR LIGANDS AS TARGETS IN ALLERGIC ASTHMA

The expression of various pattern recognition receptors has been described in asthmatics and it has been suggested that modulating TLR-mediated inflammatory signals can influence the management of the disease [95]. In the study conducted by Chun *et al.* [95] expression of TLR4 on PBMCs collected from mild to moderate asthmatics, as well as *ex vivo* stimulation of TNF-α by LPS were significantly higher than in severe asthmatics. TLR-mediated inflammatory signals contribute to the development and severity of asthma and are not reduced by glucocorticoid treatment [95].

The involvement of TLRs in allergic asthma stem primarily from preclinical models of asthma. A significant amount of data generated over the last few years supports the concept that that TLR-based immunotherapy is effective in the prevention and treatment of animal models of allergic disorders. In a model of chronic allergic airway inflammation induced by intranasal administration of Timothy grass pollen allergen extract eosinophilic inflammation was reduced by administration of the TLR2/6 ligand, macrophage-activating lipopeptide of 2 kDa (MALP-2) [48].

TLR3 KO mice were found to be protected from synthetic dsRNA analog poly(I:C) changes in lung function at baseline, which correlated with milder inflammation in the lung, and significantly reduced epithelial cell hypertrophy [53]. TLR3 activation may be one mechanism through which viral infections contribute towards exacerbation of respiratory disease [53]. The role of viral infections and especially of viral TLR ligands in allergy exacerbation has been reported [53]. Viral TLR ligands involve dsRNA and ssRNA which are recognized by TLR3 (poly(I:C)) or TLR7 (R-848), respectively. In a model of experimental asthma, TLR3 and TLR7 activation by viral TLR ligands was shown to have both preventive as well as suppressive effects, mediated by the additive effects of IL-12 and IL-10 [96]. During the sensitization phase, either ligand prevented the production of OVA-specific IgE and IgG1 antibodies and subsequently abolished all features of experimental asthma including airway hyperresponsiveness and allergic airway inflammation [96]. Furthermore, administration of poly(I:C) or R-848 into animals with already established primary allergic responses revealed a markedly reduced secondary response following allergen aerosol re-challenges [96].

Regarding the involvement of TLR4 in allergic asthma, low levels of inhaled LPS signaling through TLR4 was necessary to induce Th2 responses to inhaled antigens in a mouse model of allergic sensitization [97]. The mechanism by which LPS signaling results in Th2 sensitization involved the activation of antigen-containing DCs. On the contrary, inhalation of high levels of LPS with antigen resulted in Th1 responses. The level of LPS exposure can be the determining factor in which type of inflammatory response is generated and this could provide a potential mechanistic explanation of epidemiological data on endotoxin exposure and asthma prevalence [97].

8. THE USE OF CPG-ODN, THE TLR9 LIGAND IN ALLERGIC ASTHMA: PRECLINICAL AND CLINICAL EVIDENCE

The most extensively studied synthetic TLR ligand in preclinical models of allergic asthma as well as in the clinical setting are ODNs, which contain unmethylated motifs centered on CG dinucleotides. These CpG ODNs (resembling bacterial DNA) engage TLR9 on B cells and DCs and potently induce Th1 cytokines, suppress Th2 cytokines and can prevent manifestations of asthma in animal models. These agents have the potential to reverse Th2 responses to allergens and thus restore the balance of the immune system [98]. Klinman *et al.* reported that CpG–ODNs induce the production of IL-6, IFN-γ and IL-12 by NK cells, B cells and CD4+ T lymphocytes both *in vivo* and *in vitro* [99]. CpG–ODN also induces IL-12 secretion by activated macrophages and other antigen presenting cells. IL-12 in turn stimulates the secretion of IFN-γ by NK cells and T-lymphocytes, resulting in a Th1 inflammatory response which would be favorable in allergic asthma. The stimulation of regulatory T cell production has also been reported after DC stimulation with CpG-ODN *via* enhanced IL12 and IL10 production [100]. Indoleamine 2,3-dioxygenase (IDO), the rate-limiting enzyme of tryptophan, is induced by TLR9 ligands and mediates, in part, anti-inflammatory responses reported by its administration.

Preclinical models of asthma have demonstrated that CpG–ODN are potent inhibitors of atopic responses, suppressing Th2 cytokine [101] and reducing airway eosinophilia [102], systemic levels of IgE, and bronchial hyperreactivity [98], in short the critical attributes of the asthmatic phenotype in models of chronic allergen exposure. CpG–ODN are also effective in preventing the development of airway remodeling by reducing goblet cell hyperplasia, subepithelial fibrosis, airway hyperreactivity, peribronchial smooth muscle layer thickening, peribronchial fibrosis, mucus production, peribronchial myofibroblast accumulation and levels of the pro-fibrotic cytokine transforming growth factor (TGF)-β1 [7, 8].

In established asthma, CpG–ODN can reverse manifestations of disease, both when used alone or in combination with allergen immunotherapy. Early clinical trials have had mixed results, including a significant benefit when CpG–ODN were conjugated to ragweed allergen in an allergic rhinitis immunotherapy study by shifting a Th2 dominant to a Th1 dominant response [103], but only limited efficacy seen when administered prior to allergen challenge in asthmatics [104]. In clinical studies, the administration of CpG-ODN did not result in adverse effects. Further study of CpG–ODNs for the treatment of asthma and other atopic disorders is warranted by existing data [105].

9. PROBIOTICS IN ASTHMA

The United Nations Food and Agricultural Organization and the World Health Organization define probiotics as "live microorganisms, which, when administered in adequate amounts, confer a health benefit to the host" [106]. Recently an international expert group from the International Life Sciences Institute (ILSI) evaluated the published evidence of the functionality of probiotics in allergy, chronic intestinal inflammatory and functional disorders, infections and metabolic processes [107]. They have stated that there is substantial evidence from clinical studies to suggest a role of probiotics in the prevention and management of allergy [108]. The rationale for a potential effect stems from the fact that probiotics, as gram-positive bacteria, contain TLR ligands and thus can potentiate a TLR-driven response as well as shifting the balance from a Th2 to a Th1 response. Probiotics have been shown to have the ability to differentially induce regulatory T cell response in humans [109, 110] and induce the expression of FoxP3 in intestinal lamina propria cells in a murine asthma model [111].

Evidence for the potential use of probiotics in the treatment of allergy arises predominantly from clinical studies with children suffering from atopic disease. It has been shown that the composition of the gut microbiota differs between healthy and allergic infants and in countries of high and low prevalence of allergy [112-116]. Over 25 randomized, double-blind controlled clinical trials have been conducted to study the effects of various probiotics on treatment and prevention of allergic disease. A systematic review of randomized controlled trials with probiotics for the treatment of allergic rhinitis and asthma has been published by Vliagoftis *et al.* [117] showing an overall beneficial effect in allergic rhinitis patients by symptom severity reduction and reduction of medication use.

There is pre-clinical evidence that the use of probiotics in asthma may have therapeutic benefit. A well established model of allergic airway disease is the OVA-sensitized mouse model whereby mice are sensitized by intraperitoneal injection of OVA followed by intranasal OVA challenge after a few weeks. Airway hyperresponsiveness to increasing concentrations of methacholine can be measured in these animals. In a study conducted by Forsythe *et al.*, two probiotic strains *Lactobacillus reuteri* and *Lactobacillus salivarius* have been compared for their ability to attenuate antigen-induced eosinophil influx to the airway as well as local cytokine responses and hyperresponsiveness to methacholine in an OVA-sensitized mouse model of allergic airway disease [118]. Live and heat killed *L. reuteri* but not *L. salivarius* significantly attenuated the influx of eosinophils to the airway lumen and parenchyma and reduced the levels of TNF-α, monocyte chemoattractant protein-1, IL-5, and IL-13 in bronchoalveolar lavage fluid of antigen-challenged animals, but there was no change in eotaxin or IL-10. *L. reuteri* but not *L. salivarius* also decreased allergen-induced airway hyperresponsiveness and this was associated with increased activity of IDO [118]. These responses were dependent on TLR9, as ingestion by TLR9 knockout mice did not result in attenuation of eosinophil influx, BAL cytokine levels or airway hyperesponsiveness to metacholine [118]. In another comparative study using the OVA-sensitized model of allergic airway disease, a panel of six probiotics was compared in their anti-allergic effects. Measurements of anti-allergic effects and pulmonary inflammation were carried out by analyzing bronchoalveolar lavage fluid for the presence of eosinophils, neutrophils, macrophages and lymphocytes and for IL-4, IL-5, IL-10 and IFN-γ. In addition, OVA-specific IgE, IgG1 and IgG2a were measured in serum and allergic skin reaction test [119]. Oral administration of *B. breve* M-16V and *L. plantarum* NumRes8 resulted in a reduced eosinophil and lymphocyte Influx into the airways. In addition, the *B. breve* M-16V significantly reduced the increased airway response to methacholine at the highest concentration of methacholine, as did the levels of IL-4 and IL-5 in the serum of animals, levels of OVA-specific IgE and ear swelling [119].

10. RECENT ADVANCES IN THE AREA TARGETING TLRS IN ASTHMA

Sublingual immunotherapy (SLIT), TLR9 vaccines using cytosine CpG–allergen conjugates, and anti-IL-5 are three novel approaches for the treatment of allergic asthma [120]. Their safety and effectiveness still has to be fully assessed. SLIT provides a novel oral route of administering an allergen to induce tolerance to inhaled allergens. Studies of SLIT in allergic rhinitis demonstrated that it reduces symptoms and medication use and is associated with a low incidence of systemic allergic reactions. Another candidate adjuvant for sublingual allergy vaccines is the synthetic TLR2 agonist triacylated lipopeptide Pam3CSK4. Sublingual administration of Pam3CSK4 together with the antigen in BALB/c mice sensitized to OVA, decreases airway hyperresponsiveness as well as OVA-specific Th2 responses in cervical lymph nodes dramatically [121, 122]. Recently the use of probiotics were tested as candidate adjuvants for sublingual allergy vaccines [123]. In OVA-sensitized mice, sublingual administration of *L.helventicus*, shown to be a potent inducer of IL-12p70 and IL-10 in DCs *in vitro*, supported IFN-γ and IL-10 production in CD4+ T cells, reduced airway hyperresponsiveness, bronchial inflammation and proliferation of specific T cells in cervical lymph nodes [123]. The pure Th1 inducer *L.casei* did not achieve allergic symptom reduction [123] and did not potentiate tolerance *via* the sublingual route.

Initial phase II studies with TLR9 vaccines conjugated to a ragweed allergen demonstrated that they reduce symptoms of allergic rhinitis during the ragweed season [124]. Th1-skewing was noted in the same study population [125].

The beneficial role of probiotics in allergy has recently been reviewed by an international expert group from ILSI and recommendations were given regarding the uniform interpretation of clinical studies outcomes [107, 108]. There is a need for identifying the clusters of target populations based on similar symptom scoring techniques, tackling the variability in microbiota between different subjects and in addition, the co-administration of anti-allergic medication should be scored as well as lifestyle. Uniformity of study populations would result in more reliable interpretation of results and would facilitate inter-study comparisons [108]. In addition, studies investigating the possible role of TLR in the complex working mechanisms of probiotic strains that are effective in the prevention or treatment of asthma, are also needed. Drugable TLR-targets using small molecular weight compounds such as TLR ligands or TLR antagonists are worth exploring as future candidates for the prevention or treatment of asthma.

REFERENCES

[1]   Schroder NW, Maurer M. The role of innate immunity in asthma: leads and lessons from mouse models. Allergy 2007; 62: 579-90.

[2]   Vercelli D. Discovering susceptibility genes for asthma and allergy. Nat Rev Immunol 2008; 8: 169-82.

[3]   Hayashi T, Raz E. TLR9-based immunotherapy for allergic disease. Am J Med 2006; 119: 897 e1-6.

[4]   Devenny A, Wassall H, Ninan T, Omran M, Khan SD, RussellG. Respiratory symptoms and atopy in children in Aberdeen: questionnaire studies of a defined school population repeated over 35 years. BMJ 2004; 329: 489-90.

[5]   Waite DA, Eyles EF, Tonkin SL, O'Donnell TV. Asthma prevalence in Tokelauan children in two environments. Clin Allergy 1980; 10: 71-5.

[6]   Devereux G. The increase in the prevalence of asthma and allergy: food for thought. Nat Rev Immunol 2006; 6: 869-74.

[7]   Barnes PJ. New therapies for asthma: is there any progress? Trends Pharmacol Sci. 2010; 31: 335-43.

[8]   Gamble J, Stephenson M, McClean E, Heaney LG. The prevalence of nonadherence in difficult asthma. Am J Respir Crit Care Med 2009; 180: 817-22.

[9]   Weatherall M, Wijesinghe M, Perrin K, Harwood M, Beasley R. Meta-analysis of the risk of mortality with salmeterol and the effect of concomitant inhaled corticosteroid therapy. Thorax 2010; 65: 39-43.

[10]   Charlton SJ. Agonist efficacy and receptor desensitization: from partial truths to a fuller picture. Br J Pharmacol 2009; 158: 165-8.

[11]   Evans DJ, Barnes PB, Spaethe SM, van Alstyne EL, Mitchell MI, O'Connor BJ. Effect of a leukotriene B4 receptor antagonist, LY293111, on allergen induced responses in asthma. Thorax 1996; 51: 1178-84.

[12]   Bousquet J, Aubier M, Sastre J. *et al.* Comparison of roflumilast, an oral anti-inflammatory, with beclomethasone dipropionate in the treatment of persistent asthma. Allergy 2006; 61: 72-8.

[13]   Cuenda A, Rousseau S. p38 MAP-kinases pathway regulation, function and role in human diseases. Biochim Biophys Acta 2007; 1773: 1358-75.

[14]   Chaudhuri N, Dower SK, White MK, Sabroe I. Toll-like receptors and chronic lung disease. Clin Sci (Lond) 2005; 109: 125-33.

[15]   Sabroe I, Dower SK, Whyte MK. The role of Toll-like receptors in the regulation of neutrophil migration, activation, and apoptosis. Clin Infect Dis 2005; 41: S421-6.

[16]   Jiang, D, Liang J, Fan J *et al*. Regulation of lung injury and repair by Toll-like receptors and hyaluronan. Nat Med 2005; 11: 1173-9.

[17]   Sabroe I, Parker LC, Dower SK, Whyte MK. The role of TLR activation in inflammation. J Pathol 2008; 214: 126-35.

[18]   O'Neill LA. TLRs play good cop, bad cop in the lung. Nat Med 2005; 11: 1161-2.

[19]   Wills-Karp M. Interleukin-13 in asthma pathogenesis. Immunol Rev 2004; 202: 175-90.

[20]   Barnes PJ. Immunology of asthma and chronic obstructive pulmonary disease. Nat Rev Immunol 2008; 8: 183-92.

[21]   Lambrecht BN, De Veerman M, Coyle AJ , Gutierrez-Ramos JC, Thielemans K, Pauwels RA. Myeloid dendritic cells induce Th2 responses to inhaled antigen, leading to eosinophilic airway inflammation. J Clin Invest 2000; 106: 551-9.

[22]   Lambrecht BN. Dendritic cells and the regulation of the allergic immune response. Allergy 2005; 60: 271-82.

[23]   Hammad H, Lambrecht BN, Pochard B *et al*. Monocyte-derived dendritic cells induce a house dust mite-specific Th2 allergic inflammation in the lung of humanized SCID mice: involvement of CCR7. J Immunol 2002; 169: 1524-34.

[24]   Kambayashi T, Larosa DF, Silverman MA, Koretzky GA. Cooperation of adapter molecules in proximal signaling cascades during allergic inflammation. Immunol Rev 2009; 232: 99-114.

[25]   Hines C. The diverse effects of mast cell mediators. Clin Rev Allergy Immunol 2002; 22: 149-60.

[26]   Barnes P.J. The cytokine network in asthma and chronic obstructive pulmonary disease. J Clin Invest 2008; 118: 3546-56.

[27]   Kulka M, Alexopoulou L, Flavell RA, Metcalfe DD. Activation of mast cells by double-stranded RNA: evidence for activation through Toll-like receptor 3. J Allergy Clin Immunol 2004; 114: 174-82.

[28]   Matsushima H, Yamada N, Matsue H, Shimada S. TLR3-, TLR7-, and TLR9-mediated production of proinflammatory cytokines and chemokines from murine connective tissue type skin-derived mast cells but not from bone marrow-derived mast cells. J Immunol 2004; 173: 531-41.

[29]   Mrabet-Dahbi S, Metz M, Dudeck A, Zuberbier T, Maurer M. Murine mast cells secrete a unique profile of cytokines and prostaglandins in response to distinct TLR2 ligands. Exp Dermatol, 2009. 18(5): p. 437-44.

[30]   Zaidi AK, Thangam ER, Ali H. Distinct roles of Ca2+ mobilization and G protein usage on regulation of Toll-like receptor function in human and murine mast cells. Immunology 2006; 119: 412-20.

[31]   Qiao H, Andrade MV, Lisboa FA, Morgan K, Beaven MA. FcepsilonR1 and toll-like receptors mediate synergistic signals to markedly augment production of inflammatory cytokines in murine mast cells. Blood 2006; 107: 610-8.

[32]   McCurdy JD, Lin TJ, Marshall JS. Toll-like receptor 4-mediated activation of murine mast cells. J Leukoc Biol 2001; 70: 977-84.

[33]   Janssens S, Beyaert R. Role of Toll-like receptors in pathogen recognition. Clin Microbiol Rev 2003; 16: 637-46.

[34]   Rock FL, Hardiman G, Timans JC, Kastelein RA, Bazan JF. A family of human receptors structurally related to *Drosophila* Toll. Proc Natl Acad Sci U S A, 1998; 95: 588-93.

[35]   Kormann MS, Depner M, Hartl D *et al*. Toll-like receptor heterodimer variants protect from childhood asthma. J Allergy Clin Immunol 2008; 122: 86-92.

[36]   Muzio M, Bosisio D, Polentarutti N *et al*. Differential expression and regulation of toll-like receptors (TLR) in human leukocytes: selective expression of TLR3 in dendritic cells. J Immunol 2000; 164: 5998-6004.

[37]   Ospelt C, Gay S. TLRs and chronic inflammation. Int J Biochem Cell Biol 2010; 42: 495-505.

[38]   Hasan U, Chaffois C, Gaillard C *et al*. Human TLR10 is a functional receptor, expressed by B cells and plasmacytoid dendritic cells, which activates gene transcription through MyD88. J Immunol 2005; 174: 2942-50.

[39]   Wilde I, Lotz S, Englemann D *et al*. Direct stimulatory effects of the TLR2/6 ligand bacterial lipopeptide MALP-2 on neutrophil granulocytes. Med Microbiol Immunol 2007; 196: 61-71.

[40]   Into T, Dohkan J, Inomata M, Nakashima M, Shibata K, Matsushita K. Synthesis and characterization of a dipalmitoylated lipopeptide derived from paralogous lipoproteins of *Mycoplasma pneumoniae*. Infect Immun 2007; 75: 2253-9.

[41]   Revets H, Pynaert G, grooten J, De Baetselier P. Lipoprotein I, a TLR2/4 ligand modulates Th2-driven allergic immune responses. J Immunol 2005; 174: 1097-103.

[42]   Homma T, Kato A, Hashimoto N *et al*. Corticosteroid and cytokines synergistically enhance toll-like receptor 2 expression in respiratory epithelial cells. Am J Respir Cell Mol Biol 2004; 31: 463-9.

[43]   Sukkar MB, Xie S, Khorasani NM *et al*. Toll-like receptor 2, 3, and 4 expression and function in human airway smooth muscle. J Allergy Clin Immunol 2006; 118: 641-8.

[44]   Fuchs B, Braun A. Modulation of asthma and allergy by addressing toll-like receptor 2. J Occup Med Toxicol 2008; 3: S5.

[45]   Weigt H, Nassenstein, Tschernig T, Mühlradt PF, Krug N, Braun A. Efficacy of macrophage-activating lipopeptide-2 combined with interferon-gamma in a murine asthma model. Am J Respir Crit Care Med 2005; 172: 566-72.

[46]   Patel M, Xu D, Kewin P *et al.* TLR2 agonist ameliorates established allergic airway inflammation by promoting Th1 response and not *via* regulatory T cells. J Immunol 2005; 174: 7558-63.

[47]   Redecke V, Hacker H, Datta SK *et al.* Cutting edge: activation of Toll-like receptor 2 induces a Th2 immune response and promotes experimental asthma. J Immunol 2004; 172: 2739-43.

[48]   Fuchs B, Knothe S, Rochlitzer S *et al.* A Toll-Like Receptor 2/6 Agonist Reduces Allergic Airway Inflammation in Chronic Respiratory Sensitisation to Timothy Grass Pollen Antigens. Int Arch Allergy Immunol 2009; 152: 131-139.

[49]   Hornung V, Rothenfusser S, Britsch S *et al.* Quantitative expression of toll-like receptor 1-10 mRNA in cellular subsets of human peripheral blood mononuclear cells and sensitivity to CpG oligodeoxynucleotides. J Immunol 2002; 168: 4531-7.

[50]   McCurdy JD, Olynych TJ, Maher LH, Marchall JS. Cutting edge: distinct Toll-like receptor 2 activators selectively induce different classes of mediator production from human mast cells. J Immunol 2003; 170: 1625-9.

[51]   Tantisira K, Klimecki WT, Lazarus R *et al.* Toll-like receptor 6 gene (TLR6): single-nucleotide polymorphism frequencies and preliminary association with the diagnosis of asthma. Genes Immun 2004; 5: 343-6.

[52]   Hoffjan S, Stemmler S, parwez Q *et al.* Evaluation of the toll-like receptor 6 Ser249Pro polymorphism in patients with asthma, atopic dermatitis and chronic obstructive pulmonary disease. BMC Med Genet 2005; 6: 34.

[53]   Stowell NC, Seideman J, Raymond HA *et al.* Long-term activation of TLR3 by poly(I:C) induces inflammation and impairs lung function in mice. Respir Res 2009; 10: 43.

[54]   Sha Q, Truong-Tran AQ, Plitt J, Beck LA, Schleimer RP. Activation of airway epithelial cells by toll-like receptor agonists. Am J Respir Cell Mol Biol 2004; 31: 358-64.

[55]   Tanaka J, Watanabe N, Kido M *et al.* Human TSLP and TLR3 ligands promote differentiation of Th17 cells with a central memory phenotype under Th2-polarizing conditions. Clin Exp Allergy 2009; 39: 89-100.

[56]   Liu YJ, Soumelis V, Watanabe N *et al.* TSLP: an epithelial cell cytokine that regulates T cell differentiation by conditioning dendritic cell maturation. Annu Rev Immunol 2007; 25: 193-219.

[57]   Ying S, O'Connor B, Ratoff J *et al.* Thymic stromal lymphopoietin expression is increased in asthmatic airways and correlates with expression of Th2-attracting chemokines and disease severity. J Immunol 2005; 174: 8183-90.

[58]   Shannon J, Ernst P, Yamauchi Y *et al.* Differences in airway cytokine profile in severe asthma compared to moderate asthma. Chest 2008; 133: 420-6.

[59]   Lun SW, Wong CK, Ko FW, Hui DS, Lam CW. Expression and functional analysis of toll-like receptors of peripheral blood cells in asthmatic patients: implication for immunopathological mechanism in asthma. J Clin Immunol 2009; 29: 330-42.

[60]   Hammad H, Chieppa M, Perros F, Willart MA, Germain RN, Lambrecht BN. House dust mite allergen induces asthma *via* Toll-like receptor 4 triggering of airway structural cells. Nat Med 2009; 15: 410-6.

[61]   Dong L, Li H, Wang S, Li Y. Different doses of lipopolysaccharides regulate the lung inflammation of asthmatic mice *via* TLR4 pathway in alveolar macrophages. J Asthma 2009; 46: 229-33.

[62]   Mizel SB, Honko AN, Moors MA, Smith PS, West AP. Induction of macrophage nitric oxide production by Gram-negative flagellin involves signaling *via* heteromeric Toll-like receptor 5/Toll-like receptor 4 complexes. J Immunol 2003; 170: 6217-23.

[63]   Gewirtz AT, Navas TA, Lyons S, Godowski PJ, Madara JL. Cutting edge: bacterial flagellin activates basolaterally expressed TLR5 to induce epithelial proinflammatory gene expression. J Immunol 2001; 167: 1882-5.

[64]   Means TK, Hayashi F, Smith KD, Aderem A, Luster AD. The Toll-like receptor 5 stimulus bacterial flagellin induces maturation and chemokine production in human dendritic cells. J Immunol 2003; 170: 5165-75.

[65]   Moller-Larsen S, Nyegaard M, Haagerup A, Vestbo J, Kruse TA, Børglum AD. Association analysis identifies TLR7 and TLR8 as novel risk genes in asthma and related disorders. Thorax 2008; 63: 1064-9.

[66]   Roponen M, Yerkovich ST, Hollams E, Sly PD, Holt PG, Upham JW. Toll-like receptor 7 function is reduced in adolescents with asthma. Eur Respir J 2010; 35: 64-71.

[67]   Mansson A, Cardell LO. Role of atopic status in Toll-like receptor (TLR)7- and TLR9-mediated activation of human eosinophils. J Leukoc Biol 2009; 85: 719-27.

[68]   Phipps S, Hansbro N, Lam CE, Foo SY, Matthaei KI, Foster PS. Allergic sensitization is enhanced in early life through toll-like receptor 7 activation. Clin Exp Allergy 2009; 39: 1920-8.

[69]   Camateros P, Tamaoka M, Hassan M *et al.* Chronic asthma-induced airway remodeling is prevented by toll-like receptor-7/8 ligand S28463. Am J Respir Crit Care Med 2007; 175: 1241-9.

[70]   An H, Xu H, Yu Y *et al.* Up-regulation of TLR9 gene expression by LPS in mouse macrophages *via* activation of NF-kappaB, ERK and p38 MAPK signal pathways. Immunol Lett 2002; 81: 165-9.

[71]   Kadowaki N, Ho S, Antonenko S *et al.* Subsets of human dendritic cell precursors express different toll-like receptors and respond to different microbial antigens. J Exp Med 2001; 194: 863-9.

[72]   Zuany-Amorim C, Hastewell J, Walker C. Toll-like receptors as potential therapeutic targets for multiple diseases. Nat Rev Drug Discov 2002; 1: 797-807.

[73]   Davis HL. Use of CpG DNA for enhancing specific immune responses. Curr Top Microbiol Immunol,2000; 247: 171-83.

[74]   Vollmer J, Krieg AM. Immunotherapeutic applications of CpG oligodeoxynucleotide TLR9 agonists. Adv Drug Deliv Rev 2009; 61: 195-204.

[75]   Feleszko W, Jaworska J, Hamelmann E. Toll-like receptors--novel targets in allergic airway disease (probiotics, friends and relatives). Eur J Pharmacol 2006; 533: 308-18.

[76]   Kline JN. Eat dirt: CpG DNA and immunomodulation of asthma. Proc Am Thorac Soc 2007; 4: 283-8.

[77]   Uematsu S, Akira S. Toll-like receptors and innate immunity. J Mol Med 2006; 84: 712-25.

[78]   Strachan DP. Family size, infection and atopy: the first decade of the "hygiene hypothesis". Thorax 2000; 55: S2-10.

[79]   Conrad ML, Ferstl R, Teich R *et al.* Maternal TLR signaling is required for prenatal asthma protection by the nonpathogenic microbe *Acinetobacter lwoffii* F78. J Exp Med 2009; 206: 2869-77.

[80]   Lazarus R, Raby BA, Lange C *et al.* TOLL-like receptor 10 genetic variation is associated with asthma in two independent samples. Am J Respir Crit Care Med 2004; 170: 594-600.

[81]   Hayashi T, Beck L, Rosetto C *et al.* Inhibition of experimental asthma by indoleamine 2,3-dioxygenase. J Clin Invest 2004; 114: 270-9.

[82]   Kline JN, Krieg AM. Toll-like receptor 9 activation with CpG oligodeoxynucleotides for asthma therapy. Drug News Perspect 2008; 21: 434-9.

[83]   Eder W, Klimecki W, Yu L *et al.* Association between exposure to farming, allergies and genetic variation in CARD4/NOD1. Allergy 2006; 61: 1117-24.

[84]   Hysi P, Kabesch M, Moffatt MF *et al.* NOD1 variation, immunoglobulin E and asthma. Hum Mol Genet 2005; 14: 935-41.

[85]   Chamaillard M, Hashimoto M, Horie Y *et al.* An essential role for NOD1 in host recognition of bacterial peptidoglycan containing diaminopimelic acid. Nat Immunol 2003; 4: 702-7.

[86]   Reijmerink NE, Bottema RW, Kerkhof M *et al.* TLR-related pathway analysis: novel gene-gene interactions in the development of asthma and atopy. Allergy 2010; 65: 199-207.

[87]   Weidinger S, Klopp N, Rummler L *et al.* Association of CARD15 polymorphisms with atopy-related traits in a population-based cohort of Caucasian adults. Clin Exp Allergy 2005; 35: 866-72.

[88]   Athman R, Philpott D. Innate immunity *via* Toll-like receptors and Nod proteins. Curr Opin Microbiol 2004; 7: 25-32.

[89]   Gutierrez O, Pipaon C, Inohara N *et al.* Induction of Nod2 in myelomonocytic and intestinal epithelial cells *via* nuclear factor-kappa B activation. J Biol Chem 2002; 277: 41701-5.

[90]   Kobayashi K, Inohara N, Hernnandez LD *et al.* RICK/Rip2/CARDIAK mediates signaling for receptors of the innate and adaptive immune systems. Nature 2002; 416: 194-9.

[91]   Kabesch M, Peters W, Carr D, Leupold W, Weiland SK, von Mutius E. Association between polymorphisms in caspase recruitment domain containing protein 15 and allergy in two German populations. J Allergy Clin Immunol 2003 111: 813-7.

[92]   Hampe J, Cuthbert A, Croucher PJ *et al.* Association between insertion mutation in NOD2 gene and Crohn's disease in German and British populations. Lancet 2001; 357: 1925-8.

[93]   Hugot JP, Chamaillard M, Zouali H *et al.* Association of NOD2 leucine-rich repeat variants with susceptibility to Crohn's disease. Nature 2001; 411: 599-603.

[94]   Ogura Y, Bonen DK, Inohara N *et al.* A frameshift mutation in NOD2 associated with susceptibility to Crohn's disease. Nature 2001; 411: 603-6.

[95]   Chun E, Lee SH, Lee SY *et al.* Toll-like Receptor Expression on Peripheral Blood Mononuclear Cells in Asthmatics; Implications for Asthma Management. J Clin Immunol 2010; 30: 459-64.

[96]   Sel S, Wegmann S, Sel S *et al.* Immunomodulatory effects of viral TLR ligands on experimental asthma depend on the additive effects of IL-12 and IL-10. J Immunol 2007; 178: 7805-13.

[97]   Eisenbarth SC, Piggott DA, Huleatt JW, Visintin I, Herrick CA, Bottomly K. Lipopolysaccharide-enhanced, toll-like receptor 4-dependent T helper cell type 2 responses to inhaled antigen. J Exp Med 2002; 196: 1645-51.

[98]   Hussain I, Kline JN. CpG oligodeoxynucleotides in asthma. Curr Opin Investig Drugs 2001; 2: 914-8.

[99]   Klinman DM, Yi AK, Beaucage S, Conover J, Krieg AM. CpG motifs present in bacteria DNA rapidly induce lymphocytes to secrete interleukin 6, interleukin 12, and interferon gamma. Proc Natl Acad Sci U S A 1996; 93: 2879-83.

[100]   Jarnicki AG, Conroy H, Brereton C *et al.* Attenuating regulatory T cell induction by TLR agonists through inhibition of p38 MAPK signaling in dendritic cells enhances their efficacy as vaccine adjuvants and cancer immunotherapeutics. J Immunol 2008; 180: 3797-806.

[101]   Chu RS, Targoni OS, Kreig AM, Lehmann PV, Harding CV. CpG oligodeoxynucleotides act as adjuvants that switch on T helper 1 (Th1) immunity. J Exp Med 1997; 186: 1623-31.

[102]   Sur S, Wild JS, Choudhury BK, Sur N, Alam R, Klinman DM. Long term prevention of allergic lung inflammation in a mouse model of asthma by CpG oligodeoxynucleotides. J Immunol 1999; 162: 6284-93.

[103]   Simons FE, Shikishima Y, Van Nest G, Eiden JJ, HayGlass KT. Selective immune redirection in humans with ragweed allergy by injecting Amb a 1 linked to immunostimulatory DNA. J Allergy Clin Immunol 2004; 113: 1144-51.

[104]   Gauvreau GM, Hessel EM, Boulet LP, Coffman RL, O'Byrne PM. Immunostimulatory sequences regulate interferon-inducible genes but not allergic airway responses. Am J Respir Crit Care Med 2006; 174: 15-20.

[105]   Fonseca DE, Kline JN. Use of CpG oligonucleotides in treatment of asthma and allergic disease. Adv Drug Deliv Rev 2009; 61: 256-62.

[106]   Food and Agricultural Organisation of the United Nations and World health Organisation Expert Consultation Report. Health and Nutritional Properties of Probiotics in Food including Powder Milk with Live Lactic Acid Bacteria. 2001; http://www.who.int/foodsafety/publications/fs_management/en/probiotics.pdf

[107]   Rijkers GT, Bengmark S, Enck P *et al.* Guidance for substantiating the evidence for beneficial effects of probiotics: current status and recommendations for future research. J Nutr 2010; 140: 671S-6S.

[108]   Kalliomaki M, Antoine JM, Herz U, Rijkers GT, Wells JM, Mercenier A. Guidance for substantiating the evidence for beneficial effects of probiotics: prevention and management of allergic diseases by probiotics. J Nutr 2010; 140: 713S-21S.

[109]   de Roock S, van Elk M, van Dijk ME *et al.* Lactic acid bacteria differ in their ability to induce functional regulatory T cells in humans. Clin Exp Allergy 2010; 40: 103-10.

[110]   Fink LN. Induction of regulatory T cells by probiotics: potential for treatment of allergy? Clin Exp Allergy 2010; 40: 5-8.

[111]   Hong HJ, Kim E, Cho D, Kim DS. Differential Suppression of Heat-Killed Lactobacilli Isolated from kimchi, a Korean Traditional Food, on Airway Hyper-responsiveness in Mice. J Clin Immunol 2010; 30: 449-58.

[112]   Bjorksten B, Naaber P, Sepp E, Mikelsaar M. The intestinal microflora in allergic Estonian and Swedish 2-year-old children. Clin Exp Allergy 1999; 29: 342-6.

[113]   Watanabe S, Narisawa Y, Arase S *et al.* Differences in fecal microflora between patients with atopic dermatitis and healthy control subjects. J Allergy Clin Immunol 2003; 111: 587-91.

[114]   Kalliomaki M, Kirjavainen P, Eerola E, Kero P, Salminen S, Isolauri E. Distinct patterns of neonatal gut microflora in infants in whom atopy was and was not developing. J Allergy Clin Immunol 2001; 107: 129-34.

[115]   Bjorksten B, Sepp E, Julge K, Voor T, Mikelsaar M. Allergy development and the intestinal microflora during the first year of life. J Allergy Clin Immunol 2001; 108: 516-20.

[116]   Penders J, Thijs C, van den Brandt PA *et al.* Gut microbiota composition and development of atopic manifestations in infancy: the KOALA Birth Cohort Study. Gut 2007; 56: 661-7.

[117]   Vliagoftis H, Kouranos VD, Betsi GI, Falagas ME. Probiotics for the treatment of allergic rhinitis and asthma: systematic review of randomized controlled trials. Ann Allergy Asthma Immunol 2008; 101: 570-9.

[118]   Forsythe P, Inman MD, Bienenstock J. Oral treatment with live Lactobacillus reuteri inhibits the allergic airway response in mice. Am J Respir Crit Care Med 2007; 175: 561-9.

[119]   Hougee S, Vriesema AJ, Wijering SC *et al.* Oral treatment with probiotics reduces allergic symptoms in ovalbumin-sensitized mice: a bacterial strain comparative study. Int Arch Allergy Immunol 2010; 151: 107-17.

[120]   Broide DH. Immunomodulation of allergic disease. Annu Rev Med 2009; 60: 279-91.

[121]   Lombardi V, Van Overtvelt L, Horiot S *et al.* Toll-like receptor 2 agonist Pam3CSK4 enhances the induction of antigen-specific tolerance *via* the sublingual route. Clin Exp Allergy 2008; 38: 1819-29.

[122]   Goldman M. Sublingual immunotherapy: the quest for innovative adjuvants. Clin Exp Allergy 2008; 38: 1705-6.

[123]   Van Overtvelt L, Moussu H, Horiot S *et al.* Lactic acid bacteria as adjuvants for sublingual allergy vaccines. Vaccine 2010; 28: 2986-92.

[124] Creticos PS, Schroeder JT, Hamilton RG *et al.* Immunotherapy with a ragweed-toll-like receptor 9 agonist vaccine for allergic rhinitis. N Engl J Med 2006; 355: 1445-55.

[125] Tulic MK, Fiset PO, Christodoulopoulos P *et al.* Amb a 1-immunostimulatory oligodeoxynucleotide conjugate immunotherapy decreases the nasal inflammatory response. J Allergy Clin Immunol 2004 113: 235-41.

CHAPTER 4

TLRs and the Airway Epithelium in the Cystic Fibrosis Lung

Gerrit John[1*] and Markus O. Henke[2]

[1]Comprehensive Pneumology Center, Institute of Lung Biology and Disease, Helmholtz Zentrum München, Ingolstädter Landstraße 1, 85764 Neuherberg, Germany and [2]Philipps-University Marburg, Department of Pulmonary Medicine, Baldingerstraße 1, 35043 Marburg, Germany

Abstract: Cystic fibrosis (CF) is an autosomal recessive disorder caused by mutations in the gene, encoding the cystic fibrosis transmembrane conductance regulator (CFTR) protein. These mutations disrupt CFTR function within epithelial cells. Although the defect affects ion transport in many organs, the major cause of morbidity and mortality in individuals with CF is the progressive lung disease characterized by inflammation and unremitting bacterial infection with *Pseudomonas*, *Staphylococcus*, *Haemophilus*, *Aspergillus* and *Burkholderia* species. Although CF airways exhibit high numbers of immune cells and elevated levels of proinflammatory cytokines, the lung's innate immune defenses fail to clear bacterial infections. These observations suggest a modified immune response in the CF lung (due to the CFTR mutation and associated secondary alterations of the airway epithelium). Airway epithelial cells not only function as a physical barrier against inhaled pathogens, but also play an important role in innate immune responses of the host. Microorganisms are recognized through a variety of pattern recognition receptors (PRR), mainly Toll-like receptors (TLRs) that are abundantly expressed in airway epithelial cells. TLR activation in a milieu potentially rich in microbial (and endogenous) TLR agonists probably adds to the chronic inflammatory phenotype in CF airway epithelia. Therefore, the expression, function and activation of TLRs in CF airway epithelia have become the focus of intensive research. In this chapter, we give an overview of the current understanding of TLR signaling in CF and its potential role in the pathogenesis of CF lung disease.

Keywords: TLRs, cystic fibrosis, CFTR, therapies.

1. CYSTIC FIBROSIS, MUTATIONS AND POPULATION FREQUENCIES IN RELATION TO CF

The lethal hereditary disorder cystic fibrosis (CF) is caused by mutations in the CF transmembrane conductance regulator (CFTR) gene [1]. It is the most common genetic disease among Caucasians in most European and North American nations, where 1 in approximately 20 individuals is a heterozygous carrier of a mutant CFTR allele [2, 3]. Other races are affected in considerably smaller numbers. The carrier frequency of CFTR mutations directly correlates to the incidence of CF in different races, accounting for 1 in 2,000-3,000 live births among Caucasian newborns. In other races, live births range from 1 in 8,000 in Hispanics to 1 in 32,000 in Asians [4]. Since CF was first described as a separate disease entity in 1938, continuous refinements in both conventional and symptomatic care as well as in medications have dramatically improved the duration and quality of CF patients' lives (detailed information can be found in the annual registry reports of the American Cystic Fibrosis Foundation, www.cff.org, and the European Cystic Fibrosis Society, www.ecfs.eu). This trend toward an aging CF population is expected to continue [5, 6].

1.1. The CFTR Protein

The CF gene is located on the long arm of chromosome 7 and encodes the CFTR protein, a member of the ATP-binding cassette (ABC) transporter family [1]. It is 1480 amino acids long, has a molecular weight of 170 kDa and functions as cAMP-regulated chloride ion channel in the apical membrane of epithelia lining secretory organs such as the lung, liver, pancreas, gastrointestinal and reproductive tract, and skin. The CFTR protein consists of two transmembrane domains forming the ion channel, two nucleotide-binding domains (NBD) required for ATP binding and hydrolysis, and one regulatory (R) domain [7]. The movement of chloride ions and liquids across the epithelial cell membrane is regulated by the activity

---

*Address correspondence to Gerrit John: Comprehensive Pneumology Center, Institute of Lung Biology and Disease, Helmholtz Zentrum München, Ingolstädter Landstraße 1, 85764 Neuherberg, Germany; Tel: +49-89-31873795; E-mail: gerrit.john@helmholtz-muenchen.de

Catherine M. Greene (Ed)

and gating of the CFTR channel (Fig. **1**). These processes are tightly controlled by the balance of kinase and phosphatase activities within the cell and by cellular ATP levels. An extracellular stimulus such as a ligand binding to a receptor results in an adenylate cyclase-mediated increase in cAMP levels, which leads to cAMP binding and activation of cAMP-dependent protein kinases (PKA). This in turn causes the phosphorylation of multiple serine residues within the R domain of CFTR. In a second step, gating of the activated channel is regulated by ATP binding and hydrolysis at the NBDs. Finally, protein phosphatases dephosphorylate the R domain and return the channel to its quiescent state.

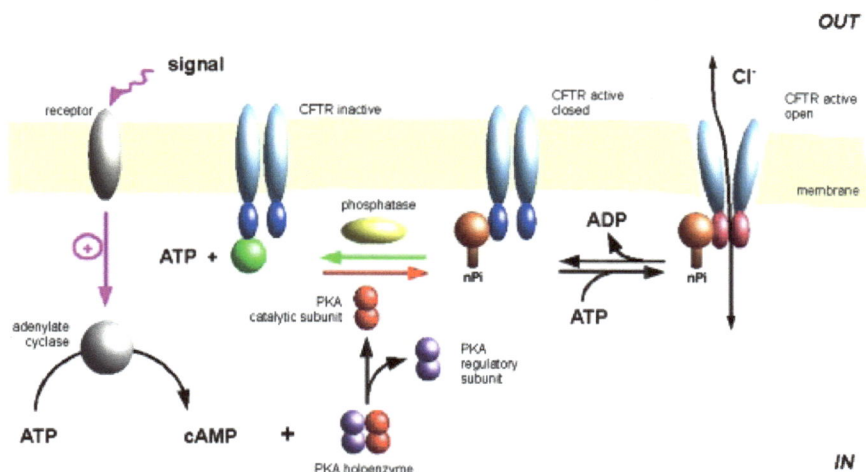

Figure 1: Schematic representation of the pathway to activate and gate the CFTR anion channel [8]; printed with permission.

1.2. CFTR Gene Mutations

In CF, mutations in the CFTR gene disrupt its protein function within epithelial cells mainly by preventing the protein from attaining its native conformation. To date, more than 1,800 disease-causing CFTR mutations have been described that vary in the severity of disease they produce, suggesting a correlation between genotype and phenotype [9]. These mutations include nonsense, frameshift, RNA splice-type or missense mutations. According to their molecular and phenotypic consequences, a classification of CFTR mutations was developed, ranging from no or defective protein product to impaired ion transport and reduced mRNA expression (Table **1**) [10-12]. Class I, II, and III mutations are associated with significant defects in CFTR production or function and usually cause severe pulmonary disease and pancreatic insufficiency. Class IV and V mutations often result in a milder, atypical, or even no disease phenotype. A novel class of mutations (putatively designated Class VI) resulting in functional but unstable CFTR present at the apical membrane was also described, with nonsense or frameshift mutations such as Q1412X, 4326delTC, and 4279insA causing a 70- to 100-bp truncation of the C-terminus of the CFTR, which leads to the marked instability of an otherwise fully processed and functional variant [13]. This is associated with a severe CF phenotype.

The most common mutation, F508del or ΔF508, is a genetically unusual codon deletion and accounts for almost 70% of CF chromosomes worldwide. The deletion of three base pairs results in the loss of a phenylalanine residue at amino acid position 508 of the CFTR protein, affecting its nucleotide-binding domain [14]. This causes misfolding and accumulation of defective and incompletely processed CFTR proteins in the endoplasmic reticulum (ER) [15-17]. Almost 100% of ΔF508 CFTR polypeptides undergo rapid proteasomal degradation before exiting from the ER, in contrast to the wild-type protein that is transported from the ER to the Golgi [18]. Under particular circumstances, *e.g.* reduced temperature or glycerol or sodium 4-phenylbutyrate treatment of cells, ΔF508 CFTR proteins are processed, transported and integrated into the epithelial membrane, where they can still exert, to some degree, their designated function [19-21]. However, these channels show significant stability defects and altered kinetics [22-25]. Although ΔF508 is by far the most common CFTR mutation, it varies in population frequency, even in

Europe where its incidence is highest. Outside Europe some continents (such as South East Asia) have a very low prevalence of ΔF508 and a low population incidence of CF. In Ashkenazi Jews, W1282X accounts for nearly 50% of mutated CFTR alleles and this is the only significant population in which ΔF508 is not the dominant CF-causing mutation [4].

Among the remaining CF alleles there is great mutational heterogeneity throughout the world. Most mutations occur with a frequency of less than 1% and the vast majority is typically limited to a small number of individuals. Recently, novel CFTR gene variants have been recognized more commonly in many non-Caucasian populations [26-29].

1.3. CF Pathophysiology

The loss of CFTR channel activity and its regulatory function on epithelial sodium channels causes abnormalities in electrolyte and fluid transport in exocrine epithelia in CF, affecting both absorptive and secretory processes [36, 37]. Although calcium-stimulated chloride channels are working properly, their activity is not sufficient to compensate for the disruption of CFTR function. The impact of this defect on transport function is tissue specific. For example, electrolyte reabsorption is decreased in the sweat duct and gives rise to elevated sweat chloride concentration. On the other hand, CF airway epithelia show an increased chloride absorption that is accompanied by an abnormal sodium and fluid influx [38, 39]. This imbalance between absorptive and secretory functions causes the thickening of secretions in CF airway epithelia and is thought to play a major role in the development of CF lung disease.

Table 1: Classes of CFTR Mutations

Class	Defect and Molecular and Phenotypic Effects	Example and References
I	Defective protein synthesis; no protein at the apical membrane; typical (severe) CF phenotype	G542X, W1282X [30]
II	Abnormal processing and trafficking; no protein at the apical membrane; typical (severe) CF phenotype	ΔF508, R1066C [11, 31]
III	Defective regulation; normal amount of nonfunctional CFTR at the apical membrane; typical (severe) CF phenotype	G551D, G1349D [32]
IV	Decreased conductance; normal amount of CFTR with some residual function at the apical membrane; milder pancreatic phenotype (pancreatic sufficiency)	R117H, R334W, R347P [33]
V	Reduced synthesis due to altered mRNA levels; reduced amount of functional CFTR at the apical membrane; mild CF phenotype, occasionally normal sweat electrolytes and single organ pathology (CBAVD[1])	3849+10kbC→T, A455E [34, 35]
VI	Decreased protein stability; mature and functional but unstable CFTR at the apical membrane; typical (severe) CF phenotype	Q1412X, 4326delTC, 4279insA [13]

[1]CBAVD, congenital bilateral absence of the vas deferens.

The CFTR defect affects ion transport in multiple organs in CF, including the lung, liver, pancreas, and gastrointestinal and reproductive tract. The clinical consequences are diverse and include pancreatic insufficiency (associated with malabsorption and malnutrition), intestinal obstruction, biliary cirrhosis, and congenital bilateral absence of the vas deferens (CBAVD), often in combination. However, the major cause of morbidity and mortality is the progressive lung disease characterized by chronic infection of the airways with *Pseudomonas*, *Staphylococcus*, *Haemophilus*, *Aspergillus* and *Burkholderia* species [3, 6]. The dehydration and thickening of airway secretions contributes to the inability of the lung to clear infections. This leads to persistent neutrophilic inflammation causing lung injury, bronchiectasis, a decrease in lung function and respiratory failure. Other complications affecting the airways in CF can include haemoptysis, pneumothorax, pulmonary hypertension and *cor pulmonale*.

However, there is a wide range of disease severity in CF. The heterogeneity of the disease phenotype can be explained, to some degree, by the distinct molecular consequences of the different classes of CFTR mutations (see Table **1**). Some disease-causing CF alleles seem to retain sufficient CFTR channel activity to give rise to less severe symptoms [40, 41]. Other mutant versions may also lead to normal sweat chloride concentrations and normal lung and pancreatic function in patients, but males suffer CBAVD [42]. Even among patients that are homozygous for the most common CF alleles there is variation in the disease phenotype. Therefore, environmental, therapeutic, and other genetic influences, especially modifier genes may affect CFTR production or function and contribute to the outcome of the disease in CF patients.

1.4. CF Diagnosis

For the majority of patients with CF, the diagnosis is based on the presence of one or more characteristic clinical features, a family history of CF, or a positive newborn screening test result and will then be confirmed by laboratory evidence of CFTR dysfunction [43]. Almost every patient with a clinical syndrome of CF has elevated sweat chloride concentrations, including those with a milder disease phenotype, *e.g.* without pancreatic complications. Abnormal CFTR function is determined by two elevated sweat chloride concentrations of ≥ 60 mEq/L obtained on separate days.

Since the discovery of the CF gene by positional cloning in 1989 [1, 14, 44], it has been possible to diagnose CF by identifying two CFTR mutations. This can also be applied to prenatal diagnosis. However, the large number of disease-causing mutations described so far has presented challenges for genetic screening programs. Genetic testing for the most common alleles will not identify all patients with CF or all heterozygous carriers. The mutations found in a population will also vary greatly in frequency and distribution among different races and ethnic groups. Therefore, other screening methods have been developed.

For patients with only one or even no common CFTR mutation and an atypical phenotype that comprises partial CF phenotype, normal or borderline sweat chloride concentrations, alternative testing can focus on abnormal nasal potential difference [45]. The nasal potential difference (NPD) test provides evidence of abnormal CFTR function, because patients with CF have abnormal levels due to elevated sodium reabsorption and reduced chloride secretion in response to cAMP [46]. However the test is technically very difficult to perform and abnormal NPD measurement must be recorded on two separate days [47], therefore, it is still only progressing from a research tool to clinical application. For over 25 years, patients have also been identified by newborn screening using a two-tier method. Analyzing serum for immunoreactive trypsinogen is used as the primary screening test, because levels are elevated in most patients with CF due to pancreatic insufficiency [48]. But since this test gives a high rate of false-positive results, further screening for CF mutations is required. Therefore, clinical features of the individual patient as well as sweat test and mutation analysis results must always be taken into consideration for a definitive diagnosis of CF.

1.5. Heterozygote Advantage

The high prevalence of the ΔF508 mutation has led to the question why such a lethal mutation has persisted and spread in the human population, probably for a long time [49, 50]. In other common autosomal recessive disorders such as sickle-cell anemia, heterozygous carriers have an increased resistance to fatal infection compared to both homozygous mutation carriers and non-carriers, a concept known as heterozygote advantage [51]. For ΔF508, the most plausible advantage is the protection against severe diarrheal diseases such as cholera, which has been supported by various studies in mice [52, 53]. However, it is not clear why this should be unique for one specific mutation out of over 1,600 reported. Furthermore, in contrast to the concept of heterozygote advantage persons heterozygous for a CF allele appear to be at increased risk for bronchiectasis, pancreatitis, sinusitis, or allergic bronchopulmonary aspergillosis [54-57]. Therefore, this hypothesis has recently been reviewed in further studies that showed no evidence for heterozygote advantage [58].

2. THE ROLE OF TLRs IN CYSTIC FIBROSIS

The main function of the lung is rapid gas exchange. Due to the respiratory process, the lung is in constant and direct contact with microorganisms and pathogens in inspired air. However, bacterial infection and especially colonization of the lung are relatively rare events. This is accomplished by a diverse innate defense system that involves all pulmonary tissues and protects the lung from infection by numerous inhaled microorganisms as well as haematogenous pathogens [59].

2.1. TLRs and Innate Immunity

The respiratory epithelium plays an important role in a dynamic host defense system. At the interface with the environment, it maintains an effective antimicrobial milieu to prevent infection. The ciliated epithelium acts as a physical barrier and removes inhaled material, such as particles and bacteria, by ciliary clearance and cough, also termed the mucociliary escalator. Furthermore, airway mucus itself has antimicrobial properties due to the presence of antimicrobial peptides such as defensins and proteins of the complement system [60, 61]. In the presence of potential pathogens, epithelial cells are capable of inducing an inflammatory response by increased production of antimicrobial factors and by recruitment of phagocytic cells such as alveolar macrophages and neutrophils [62, 63]. The inflammatory process is further activated by inflammatory mediators that are released by the recruited cells as well as from the epithelium itself. Antigen presentation by phagocytic cells also leads to the induction of cell-mediated adaptive immune responses in the lung [64]. This contains the infection and results in an effective prevention of microbial colonization to preserve proper functioning of gas exchange.

The innate immune response of the airway epithelium to bacteria in the airway surface fluid involves the activation of cell surface pattern recognition receptors (PRRs) on cells of myeloid and lymphoid origin, as well as on epithelial cells. The conserved family of Toll-like receptors (TLRs) constitutes the most significant component of pulmonary PRRs. A broad spectrum of TLRs has been shown to be expressed by airway epithelial cells [65-67], demonstrating an active involvement of these non-immune cells in TLR-mediated host defense mechanisms. TLRs are activated by both infective and inflammatory stimuli and subsequent signal transduction pathways have been identified, which result in the increased transcription of host defense response genes such as immune and proinflammatory genes.

2.2. TLR Function and Signaling

Initially identified in the fruitfly *Drosophila melanogaster* as a factor required for dorsal-ventral embryonic polarity [68], *Drosophila* or dToll acts as a key receptor in the antifungal response in the adult fly [69] and shares structural homology with an important receptor in mammalian innate immunity, the Type I IL-1 receptor (IL-1RI) [70]. The first human homologue of dToll, TLR4, was identified in 1997 [71]. To date, ten human TLRs have been identified and shown to play a significant role in innate immune responses [72].

TLRs are type I transmembrane glycoproteins, *i.e.* single pass molecules with an extracellular N-terminus. They recognize and discriminate a diverse array of pathogen-associated molecular patterns (PAMPs) derived from bacteria, viruses, mycoplasma, yeasts and protozoa (Table **2**). Heterodimerization of TLRs further increases the diversity and target specificity. Their extracellular domains consisting of leucine-rich repeat (LRR) motifs represents the characteristic feature of all TLRs and is responsible for specific ligand recognition [73]. The intracellular domain is composed of up to 200 amino acid residues that share homology with IL-1RI, therefore termed the TIR (Toll/IL-1R) domain [74]. This conserved cytosolic TIR domain is essential for TLR signaling by recruiting adaptor proteins, which leads to subsequent activation of downstream signal transduction pathways involved in the inflammatory response.

TLRs 3, 7, 8 and 9 recognize pathogenic nucleic acids. Viral double-stranded (ds)RNA, a potential by-product in virally infected cells, is sensed by TLR3 [75, 76]. TLR7 and TLR8 are structurally quite similar and sense guanosine- and uridine-rich single-stranded (ss)RNA found in many viruses [77, 78]. Unmethylated CpG dinucleotide motifs that are more frequent in DNA from bacteria than vertebrates are recognized by TLR9 [79]. Heterodimerization of TLR2 with TLR1 or TLR6 confers responsiveness to *Mycoplasma pneumonia* [80] and *Streptococcus pneumonia* [81] amongst others and to a variety of components derived from the cell wall of Gram-positive bacteria, including lipoteichoic acid, peptidoglycan, and di- and triacylated lipopeptides [82-85]. Zymosan, a component of the cell membrane of fungi, is also recognized by TLR2 [86, 87]. TLR4 and TLR5 are involved in the recognition of Gram-negative bacteria. TLR4 is the principal receptor for lipopolysaccharide (LPS) [88], but requires the presence of two accessory proteins to respond to LPS, namely the co-receptors myeloid differentiation protein-2 (MD-2), a soluble glycoprotein on the outer surface of the cell membrane [89], and CD14, a glycophospatidyl inositol-anchored receptor [90]. CD14 binds and concentrates LPS bound to LPS-binding protein to allow binding to the TLR4/MD-2 complex [91]. In addition, TLR4 can recognize other microbial agonists including *Chlamydia pneumonia* and its heat-shock protein 60 (Hsp60) [92], pneumolysin [93], flavolipin [94] and the fusion proteins of respiratory syncytial virus (RSV) and murine retro-viruses [95, 96]. Components of fungal pathogens such as mannans from *Saccharomyces cerevisiae* and

Candida albicans and glucuronoxylomannan from *Cryptococcus neoformans* are also sensed by TLR4 [97, 98]. TLR5-dependent signaling is activated by flagellin, a protein component of bacterial flagellae expressed by Gram-negative bacteria [99]. The only receptor of the human TLR family without a known ligand is TLR10 [100] (Table **2**).

Table 2: Human TLRs and Their Major Microbial Agonists

TLR	Microbial Agonist
TLR1/2	Triacylated lipopeptide
TLR2/6	Diacylated lipopeptide
TLR3	dsRNA
TLR4	LPS
TLR5	Flagellin
TLR7/TLR8	ssRNA
TLR9	CpG DNA
TLR10	Unknown

In addition to their abilities to detect pathogens, TLR4 and others, mainly TLR2, are also activated by several mammalian host molecules, mainly antimicrobial molecules and products of cell damage and death. These endogenous agonists include antimicrobial defensins [101], reactive oxygen species (ROS) [102], surfactant protein A [103], heat shock proteins (Hsp) [104, 105], the neutrophil-derived elastolytic protease neutrophil elastase [106] and breakdown products of extracellular tissue matrix, such as fragments of fibronectin [107] and hyaluronan [108].

Binding of receptor agonists leads to dimerization of TLRs, which form homodimers (such as TLR4) or heterodimers (such as TLR2 with TLR1 or TLR6). In a next step, the TIR domain of each TLR interacts with the TIR domain of a TLR signaling adaptor protein. The adaptor molecule MyD88 (myeloid differentiation factor 88) is used by all TLRs, apart from TLR3. Once the adaptor is in place, it recruits and activates a number of kinases, namely IRAK-4 and IRAK-1 of the IRAK (IL-1 receptor-associated kinase) family and TRAF6 (tumor necrosis factor receptor-associated factor 6). Further downstream kinases are subsequently activated including the IκB (inhibitor of kappa B) kinase (IKK) complex, which culminates in phosphorylation and degradation of IκB reversing its inhibitory function on the transcription factor NF-κB (nuclear factor kappa B). This allows NF-κB to translocate to the nucleus and mediate an increase in transcription of host defense response genes such as immune and proinflammatory genes [109]. Other transcription factors such as AP1 as well as the MAPKs c-Jun N-terminal kinase (JNK), p38 and extracellular signal-regulated kinase (ERK)1/2 can also be activated by TLR signaling *via* TRAF6 [110].

The selective use of different intracellular adaptor molecules further increases the diversity and specificity of TLR function [111]. TLR2 and TLR4 signaling specifically requires the recruitment of a second adaptor, MyD88 adapter like (MAL/TIRAP), that functions as a bridging adaptor for MyD88 recruitment [112, 113]. TLR3 signals through TIR domain containing adaptor inducing IFN-β (TRIF), leading to the synthesis of type I interferons such as IFN-β *via* activation of IFN-regulatory factor 3 (IRF3), as well as to NF-κB release [114]. This pathway, known as the MyD88-independent pathway, can also be activated by TLR4 using the adaptor proteins TRIF und TRAM (TRIF-related adaptor molecule) [115, 116].

Eventually, TLR signaling leads to the production and secretion of a variety of proinflammatory chemokines, cytokines and antimicrobial peptides, as well as to enhanced cell surface adhesion molecule expression. The attraction of more immune cells to the site of infection, mainly macrophages and neutrophils, induces further inflammatory processes, including cell-mediated adaptive defenses. Therefore, TLRs have an important regulatory function for both innate and adaptive immune responses, and signaling must be tightly controlled [117].

2.3. TLR Expression and Activation in the Lung

Airway epithelial cells express many of the TLRs, including TLRs 1-6 and 9, as well as TLR adaptor molecules and TLR4 co-receptors MD-2 and CD14 [65-67]. Several bacteria (*S. aureus*, *P. aeruginosa*, *Legionella pneumophila* and *Bordetella bronchispetica*) and their bacterial products LPS, (triacylated) lipopeptides, flagellin, unmethylated CpG DNA, as well as viral agonists including dsRNA and influenza A virus stimulate airway epithelial cells through these receptors to induce cytokines such as IL-8, IL-6, TNF-α, RANTES, and IFN-β, and the major adhesion molecule ICAM-1 [118-123]. IL-8 and ICAM-1 are especially relevant markers of inflammatory gene activation because these mediators function to direct neutrophil recruitment at sites of infection and participate in regulation of intense airway neutrophilia characteristically seen in patients with CF. Other chemokines induced in airway epithelial cells include macrophage inflammatory protein-3α (MIP-3α) and granulocyte-macrophage colony-stimulating factor (GM-CSF) that can be increased in response to dsRNA, LPS, zymosan and flagellin [124]. Furthermore, defensin molecules that are known for their antimicrobial activity against a broad range of bacterial, fungal, and viral pathogens are also produced by airway epithelial cells and induced *via* TLR activation. TLR2-dependent production of human β defensin 2 (HBD-2) occurs in response to peptidoglycan [125], bacterial lipopeptide [126] and lipoteichoic acid [127]. Similarly, TLR4 agonists can also induce HBD-2 expression in airway epithelial cells [128].

Evidence for endogenous ligands that might signal extreme danger conditions *via* TLRs has also been obtained (see above). In airway epithelial cells, activation of TLR4 and TLR2 occurs in response to neutrophil elastase and hyaluronan amongst others [106, 129]. This might represent an innate mechanism to recognize these danger-associated molecular patterns (DAMPs) as signals of chronic inflammation and injury of the lung [130].

2.4. TLR Agonists in the CF Lung

Innate immunity is an integral factor in the mediation and regulation of inflammatory pathways and responses to infectious agents as they occur in the pathophysiology of CF. The lung disease in CF is characterized by infection, bacterial colonization, inflammation, and mucus overproduction [6]. The accumulation of bacteria in the mucus triggers a dramatic inflammatory response to the infection and TLRs expressed by immune and epithelial cells in the CF lung contribute in large part to this response. However, in CF the lung's innate immune defenses fail to eradicate bacterial infections from the airways and TLR activation in a milieu potentially rich in microbial and endogenous TLR agonists probably adds to the chronic inflammatory phenotype in CF airway epithelia.

TLR agonists are abundantly present in CF airways. Higher than normal levels of both bacterial and yeast-derived factors have been demonstrated in the CF lung [131], including microbial- or fungal-derived TLR2 agonists (lipopeptides or lipoteichoic acids (LTA) derived from *Pseudomonas* and/or *Staphylococcus* species) as well as *Pseudomonas* DNA, flagellin and LPS [66, 132] that stimulate TLRs 9, 5 and 4, respectively. Other infective agents that act in conjunction with bacteria and have the potential to modulate TLR activity also play a critical part in the pathogenesis of pulmonary damage in CF. During the course of the disease, CF patients' airways typically exhibit high levels of immune cells and inflammatory mediators. For example, high numbers of neutrophils and elevated levels of neutrophil elastase and proinflammatory cytokines such as IL-8 could be observed in CF bronchoalveolar lavage (BAL) fluid and sputum [133-136]. Furthermore, the association of respiratory viruses with exacerbations in CF implicates an involvement of viral infection and TLR activation in CF lung disease [137].

2.5. Neutrophil Elastase

Proteases in the lung play a key role in health and disease. They regulate processes such as regeneration and repair and exert their function on tissue remodeling, mucin expression, neutrophil chemotaxis and bacterial killing [138]. When kept in fine balance by antiprotease activity (*e.g.* alpha-1 antitrypsin, A1AT; secretory leucoprotease inhibitor, SLPI; elafin; cystatins and tissue inhibitor of MMP, TIMP), proteases generally contribute to the resolution of both infection and inflammation. However, a disturbed balance due to dysregulated protease expression or activity (*i.e.* increased release of proteases or insufficient inhibition by antiproteases) has a significant impact on the inflammatory process and results in lung damage as seen in chronic inflammatory lung diseases [139]. CF is characterized by higher than normal levels of pulmonary proteases resulting in a protease-antiprotease imbalance in the lungs [140]. The neutrophil-derived elastolytic protease neutrophil elastase (NE) that belongs to the class of serine proteases is especially elevated in CF bronchoalveolar fluid and sputum [133, 134]. This is caused by the abundance and accumulation of neutrophils in the CF lung generating a milieu rich in NE due to neutrophil degranulation and necrosis. NE is one of the most prominent and important proteases controlling many aspects of infection and inflammation in the lung. It not only has important intrinsic proteolytic properties that lead to direct killing of microbes [141], but it also acts as a proinflammatory mediator. NE transcriptionally regulates the inducible expression of other classes of proteases and is capable of directly activating them. For example, transcription of cathepsin B and matrix metalloprotease MMP-2 is increased in alveolar macrophages in response to NE *via* activation of NF-κB [142], and TLR4 has been shown to be involved in this induction.

NE also contributes to innate immunity and inflammation in the lung by regulating mucin production (as an important factor in the composition of airway mucus) and by recruiting neutrophils *via* IL-8 induction [143, 144]. Since IL-8 is a potent activator and chemoattractant of neutrophils, it represents a key factor in the lungs during neutrophil-dominated inflammatory diseases such as CF [145, 146]. Signaling *via* TLR2 and/or TLR4 has been implicated in NE-induced IL-8 expression [66, 147]. Further studies also provided evidence for a role for TLRs in EGFR-mediated signaling [148] and for a direct association between EGFR and TLR4 in response to stimulation with NE [144]. Therefore, increasing interest in the context of CF is focusing on the potential of NE to modulate TLR activity and on the mechanisms to counterbalance excessive NE-mediated inflammatory processes.

2.6. Viral Infection in CF

Ongoing research suggests that viral infections have a greater impact on CF patients compared to non-CF controls [149, 150]. Viral infections are believed to significantly contribute to CF lung disease by predisposing to subsequent infection by bacteria. In CF patients, up to 40% of pulmonary exacerbations are attributed to viral infections [151-153] (with respiratory syncytial virus (RSV) and influenza being the most common pathogens) causing a pronounced increase in morbidity at short and long term. This is characterized by increased respiratory symptoms, more frequent and prolonged hospitalizations, a decrease in lung function and increased likelihood and high rate of early *Pseudomonas aeruginosa* acquisition [154-156]. In infants with CF, increased incidences of lower respiratory tract viral infections are associated with a poorer disease outcome [154, 157].

During viral respiratory infections, increased virus replication, impaired specific anti-bacterial defense and increased adherence of bacteria to the airways have been described [158, 159]. Viral infection and the co-existence of bacterial pathogens have also been directly implicated in pulmonary damage and cause a reduction in barrier functions in the airway epithelium resulting in increased transepithelial permeability [160]. The inflammatory process is further activated by the induction of IL-8 expression and infiltration of neutrophils in response to viral infection by RSV and influenza A, respectively [161, 162]. In addition, both influenza A and B and adenovirus have cytotoxic effects on airway epithelial cells [163].

As independent pulmonary pathogens, viruses express agonists for a variety of TLRs (*i.e.* TLRs 3, 7 and 8). The viruses implicated in causing respiratory symptoms in CF include respiratory syncytial virus (RSV), adenovirus, parainfluenza virus (types 1, 2 and 3), influenza A and B and rhinovirus [153, 164, 165]. They act mainly through TLR3 (influenza A, influenza B, rhinovirus) [76, 119] and TLR4 (RSV) [95] whereas signaling pathways for parainfluenza virus *via* TLRs are undetermined. Airway epithelial cells demonstrated upregulation of TLR4 and TLR3 in response to RSV and influenza A, respectively [119, 120], suggesting a strong potential of viral agonists to modulate TLR activity. In addition, human alveolar macrophages showed an impairment of cytokine responses to bacterial LPS and LTA after exposure to infectious rhinovirus [166]. Therefore, further knowledge about the role of viruses and their interaction with bacteria in CF lung disease will probably be obtained by elucidating viral signaling pathways and the involvement of TLRs and might result in new therapeutic strategies to improve prognosis of CF patients.

2.7. TLR Expression and Activation in the CF Lung

Severe inflammation occurs in response to bacteria, their products, and host factors that accumulate in the unique environment created by defective mucociliary clearance in the CF lung. Under these circumstances, it is further possible that CF cells are less capable of downregulating proinflammatory responses. As signs of early infection and excessive pulmonary inflammation, high numbers of neutrophils and elevated levels of neutrophil elastase and proinflammatory cytokines such as IL-8, amongst others, have been observed in the lungs of infants and young children with CF [133-136]. In addition, antiinflammatory cytokines such as IL-10 are present at lower levels in CF airways [167]. Especially IL-10 has been shown to exert its anti-inflammatory effects *via* downregulation of IκB alpha/beta kinases (IKK) [168] and is involved in deactivation of alveolar macrophages [62]. This imbalance of pro- and antiinflammatory cytokines could disturb the autoregulatory loop in the inflammatory process and lead to defective regulation of further innate immune responses such as TLR signaling in CF airway epithelia. Constant proinflammatory activation might cause early pulmonary tissue damage and destruction that increases susceptibility to infection and colonization even though the lung is structurally normal at birth [169]. In other organs affected by the CFTR defect, such as the intestine, pancreas and vas deferens, structural damage already occurs during gestation, causing functional insufficiency shortly after birth. However, the disease pathogenesis of these organs does not involve bacterial infection and is thought to solely result from defective electrolyte transport [2, 36].

The CF lung may create an environment that impairs the activity of primary host defenses in the airway. This can lead to increased susceptibility to airway infections and early colonization by pathogens. The loss of CFTR function, combined with the increase in sodium transport, leads to abnormal transepithelial electrolyte and fluid transport [36, 170]. As a result, the composition and volume of the airway surface fluid are altered. NaCl concentrations in airway secretions have been shown to be increased in CF patients compared with normal subjects as well as in cultured epithelial cells *in vitro* [171-173]. Because bactericidal activity in the airway surface fluid requires low NaCl concentrations, a variety of antimicrobial peptides such as defensins might be compromised in CF and the airway epithelium fails to kill bacteria [174]. Furthermore, periciliary liquid layer depletion reduces the volume of the airway surface fluid, which contributes to abnormal rheology of airway secretions and defective mucociliary clearance [175]. The result is retention of thick secretions and chronic bacterial infection that probably leads to constant activation of inflammatory responses including TLR signaling.

On the other hand, TLRs appear to be less important in early responses of the airway epithelium to luminal bacteria [123, 126, 176], with only limited and weak responses to released bacterial products [66, 67, 118]. For example, TLRs 7 and 8 are either not well expressed by lung epithelium [177] or not functional [67], even though they are expressed by immune cells within the lung where they have a known role in the antiviral response [178, 179]. Airway epithelial cells also express lower levels of TLR2 than professional immune cells of monocytic origin [126], and responsiveness of TLR2 and TLR4 to bacterial ligands seems to be limited by low expression of co-receptors [128, 177]. Furthermore, an intracellular localization and activation of TLR4 requiring internalization of LPS has been described for various pulmonary epithelial cells [180]. In CF airway epithelial cells, a reduced surface expression of TLR4 was accompanied by an increased intracellular localization of the receptor or receptor components leading to decreased MyD88-dependent inflammatory responses to LPS from gram-negative bacteria [181].

These findings suggest that the bronchial epithelium is capable of regulating its sensitivity to recognize microbes by managing expression levels of TLRs and their co-receptors. Different adaptations to modify responsiveness might even occur as a result of diverse cellular environments. However, it remains controversial whether such adaptations that affect TLR function and activation and cause delayed or even absent TLR-dependent immune responses would be beneficial in the context of early CF airway infection. It has also been reported that CFTR mutations are accompanied by mutations or polymorphisms in genes involved in inflammatory processes, including a TLR4 polymorphism, D299G, that is associated with hyporesponsiveness to the bacterial ligand LPS [182]. Although this is believed to represent another negative regulatory mechanism that attenuates the inflammatory response *via* TLR signaling to maintain the immunological balance, a protective role of the TLR4 polymorphism for the lung of CF patients has yet to be demonstrated. In the unique environment of a CF lung it is more likely that TLR hyporesponsiveness during periods of early bacterial challenge may rather increase susceptibility to airway infections and predispose the airway epithelium to bacterial colonization.

3. IMMUNOTHERAPEUTIC POSSIBILITIES AND FUTURE APPLICATIONS

TLRs are a fundamental part of the host's immune system to provoke an innate response and enhance adaptive immunity against invading pathogens. However, an imbalance between TLR activation and inhibition causes inappropriate inflammatory responses that may have severe consequences for the host. In CF, chronic inflammation of the airways is in large part due to constant TLR activation in a milieu rich in microbial and endogenous TLR agonists. Targeting this detrimental inflammatory response in the CF lung is the key to improving duration and quality of CF patients' lives. The solid knowledge of TLRs, their microbial and endogenous agonists, signaling pathways and molecules enables ongoing development and refinement of therapeutics that interfere with TLR function in the CF lung. Available therapeutics to target TLRs or their signaling pathways include inhibitory peptides, microbial and naturally-occurring endogenous inhibitors or antiproteases. Usually, most of these molecules are traditionally administered using their purified versions, whereas the expression of endogenous inhibitors can also be induced pharmacologically.

3.1. Endogenous Inhibitors

Since negative regulatory mechanisms are essential to attenuate TLR signaling to maintain an immunological balance, a variety of endogenous TLR inhibitors exist and several such factors have been identified. These molecules differ in their mode of action and include transmembrane proteins and nuclear receptors, ubiquitin-modifying and adaptor proteins, kinases and phosphatases, such as A20 [183-187], toll interacting protein (Tollip) [188, 189], single immunoglobulin IL-1-related receptor (SIGIRR) [190-192], MyD88s [193, 194], IRAK-M [195, 196], suppressors of cytokine synthesis (SOCS) [197], sterile α and HEAT-Armadillo motifs protein (SARM) [198], Src homolog protein tyrosing phosphatase 1 (Shp-1) [199], protein tyrosine phosphatase, non-receptor type 1 (PTP1B) [200], mucin 1 (MUC1) [201, 202] and peroxisome proliferator activated receptor gamma (PPARgamma) [203].

3.2. Microbial TLR Antagonists, Inhibitory Peptides, and Anti-TLR Properties of Pulmonary Antiproteases

A wide variety of TLR inhibitors have been discovered and characterized in recent years. For example microbial TLR antagonists include the viral proteins A46R, A52R and N1L from *Vaccinia* virus and RSV G/soluble G protein [204-206] and the TIR domain-containing-proteins Typhimurium large plasmid A (TlpA) from *Salmonella*, *Brucella* TIR-containing protein 1 (Btp1)/TIR domain containing-protein (Tcp)B from *Brucella* spp. and TcpC from *Escherichia coli* [207-209]. Low-molecular-weight peptides with the ability to specifically inhibit agonist binding or signal transduction can also be used as therapeutic agents for CF. These compounds exert their antiinflammatory activity by gaining access to intracellular compartments and directly interfering with signaling pathways. As of now, inhibitory peptides targeting TLRs include mimetics based on BB-loop sequences of adaptor molecules MyD88, Mal, TRIF and TRAM [210-212]. Furthermore, the pulmonary antiproteases secretory leukoprotease inhibitor (SLPI), elafin, and alpha-1 antitrypsin (A1AT) also possess antimicrobial properties and have potential anti-TLR activity [213-215].

3.3. Delivery of Therapeutics to the CF Lung

The lung's unique features of large surface area, good vascularization, immense capacity for solute exchange and ultra-thinness of the alveolar epithelium usually enable rapid drug absorption. However, physical and biochemical barriers, and lack of optimal dosage forms and delivery devices are general limiting factors for delivery of therapeutics *via* pulmonary administration especially in the context of chronic inflammatory processes. In the CF lung, bacterial biofilm formation, excessive mucus production and parenchymal damage can further negatively affect drug distribution and bioavailability.

To therapeutically target the lung, a drug can be delivered as an aerosol. The particle characteristics of the aerosol are the most important parameters defining the site of deposition and retention within the respiratory tract [216]. But despite direct administration of an aerosol to the site of action it is challenging to ensure the drug's efficacy with regards to antiinflammatory effects and pharmacokinetics due to difficulties with sampling of epithelial lining fluid.

The CFTR-dependent decrease in the airway surface liquid of the CF lung leads to thick hyperviscous mucus constituting significant barriers to efficient therapeutic drug delivery. The composition and complex biological environment of CF mucus are the main factors influencing pulmonary drug absorption. Mucins as the major macromolecular component of CF mucus determine its viscoelasticity by forming a dense matrix intertwined with other macromolecules such as actin and DNA thereby decreasing its permeability.

Due to the viscoelasticity, diffusion rates of colloidal particles are significantly reduced in CF sputum where dispersed nanoparticles (100-500 nm in diameter) are transported primarily through lower viscosity pores within a highly elastic matrix [217]. Neutral particles with a diameter of less than 200 nm undergo more rapid transport in CF sputum than charged or larger particles. Interestingly, treatment with recombinant human DNase (Pulmozyme) reduces macroviscoelastic properties of CF sputum by up to 50% *via* hydrolysis of host and bacterial DNA, thereby possibly abrogating TLR9-mediated signaling in response to unmethylated CpG DNA.

Novel promising technologies could assist inhaled therapeutics in penetrating the airway. For example polyethylene glycol (PEG)ylated poly-L-lysine nanoparticles have been shown to efficiently transfect lung epithelium following intrapulmonary administration [218]. Furthermore, novel liposomal nanoparticle formulations have been described. These particles are 300 nm in diameter and are contained in a neutral liposomal shell, which allows the drug to penetrate into bacterial biofilms [219]. Nevertheless, besides innovations in the development of lipid nanoparticle aerosols, the safety must be ascertained, both in short-term and long-term use.

Novel devices for delivery of therapeutics to the CF lung include the portable PARI Altera® nebulizer system (PARI Pharma GmbH, Gräfelfing, Germany) that uses the PARI eFlow® vibrating mesh technology to enable highly efficient aerosolization [220]. The eFlow® technology produces aerosols with a very high density of active drug, a precisely defined droplet size, and a high proportion of respirable droplets delivered in the shortest possible period of time. Currently, this system is used for pulmonary delivery of new antibiotic formulations that are being tested in clinical trials.

4. RECENT ADVANCES IN THE AREA

In order to specifically target innate immune receptors, the exact function of TLRs and their co-receptors needs to be elucidated. A major remaining challenge is the determination of their three-dimensional structures in the presence of bound ligands. Crystal structures of TLR3 and of CD14, both without bound ligands, have been reported [221, 222]. In the case of TLR4, a ternary complex with MD2 and LPS would be especially informative since MD-2 acts as a 'gatekeeper' in endotoxin signaling [223]. Recently, the structural basis of LPS recognition by the TLR4/MD-2 complex has been reported and further illustrates the remarkable versatility of the ligand recognition mechanisms employed by the TLR family [224]. MD-2 has become the main target for pharmacological inhibition of endotoxin responses. If applied prior to or after challenge, a TLR4 decoy receptor could be an effective way to block interaction between the LPS/MD-2 complex and TLR4. Although two research groups have tried to generate the extracellular domain of TLR4 protein as a decoy receptor for MD-2 [225, 226], it proved difficult to generate a substantial amount of the protein. Using the novel 'Hybrid LRR technique', another group recently generated large quantities of soluble fusion proteins capable of binding MD-2, which they termed TLR4 decoy receptor (TOY) [227]. TOY exhibited strong binding to MD-2, but not to the extracellular matrix (ECM), resulting in a favorable pharmacokinetic profile *in vivo*. TOY significantly extended the lifespan, when administered in either preventive or therapeutic manners, in both LPS- and cecal ligation/puncture-induced sepsis models in mice, and markedly attenuated LPS-triggered NF-κB activation, secretion of proinflammatory cytokines, and thrombus formation in multiple organs. These results are of great importance since the strategy used in TOY development can further be applied to the generation of other novel decoy receptor proteins.

The co-receptor CD14 is another target for inhibiting TLR4 activation by endotoxin. Specific high-affinity ligand-receptor interactions involving endotoxin and TLR4 have been characterized using endotoxin-protein complexes [228]. From these results it is evident that CD14 facilitates transfer of endotoxin to MD-2 and hence TLR4 but is not a stable component of the endotoxin-MD-2/TLR4 complex. Recently, new synthetic antisepsis agents interacting with CD14 have been described [229]. These molecules derived from natural sugars with a positively charged amino group or ammonium salt and two lipophilic chains inhibited TLR4 activation by competitively occupying CD14 and thereby reducing the level of delivery of activating endotoxin to MD-2/TLR4.

The TLR adaptor Mal/TIRAP has been reported to be cleaved at position D198 by caspase-1, an event that is indispensable for its function [230]. Interestingly, a recent study using different Mal mutants identified

D198 of Mal as being conserved in MyD88 and TLR4 TIR domains and crucial for the interactions and function of Mal, MyD88 and TLR4 TIR [231]. Therefore, this TIR-domain interaction site might be another possible target for inhibiting TLR4 mediated responses.

In order to reduce the excessive inflammatory response in CF airways, the transcription factor decoy (TFD) strategy might also be of interest [232]. TFD is based on biomolecules mimicking the target sites of transcription factors and thus interfering with transcription factor activity when delivered to target cells. Besides oligodeoxynucleotides (ODNs) that have been shown to inhibit NF-κB-mediated transcription of IL-8 in normal and CF bronchial epithelial cells [233] peptide-nucleic acid-DNA chimeras are such decoy molecules with great potential. They can be complexed with liposomes and microspheres, and unlike ODNs are resistant to DNases, serum and cytoplasmic extracts [234, 235]. This is of great interest for the development of stable decoy molecules that can be used in non-viral gene therapy as inhibitors of proinflammatory activity. Recently, different classes of inhibitory ODNs for TLR7 and 9 have been developed and extensively described [236]. Their specific targeting characteristics are promising regarding their future use as therapeutics.

A novel strategy in developing therapeutics that target TLRs and their signaling intermediates involves microRNAs (miRNAs) and their expression and function in CF. miRNAs have an important role in several biological processes as they regulate gene expression at a post-transcriptional level. Recently, expression of miR-126 has been shown to be downregulated in CF airway epithelial cells [237]. Further results indicate that miR-126 regulates expression of TOM1 (target of Myb1), which might have implications for the airway inflammation in CF. TOM1 interacts with Toll-interacting protein (Tollip), forming a complex to regulate endosomal trafficking of ubiquitinated proteins, and has also been proposed as a negative regulator of IL-1β and TNF-α-induced signaling pathways. This study also reports of an involvement of this protein in the TLR2 and TLR4 signaling pathways suggesting an important role in regulating innate immune responses in the CF lung. The finding of an miRNA involvement in fine-tuning these innate immune responses in CF points to novel therapeutic targets that could be manipulated in the future.

REFERENCES

[1]   Rommens JM, Iannuzzi MC, Kerem B *et al.* Identification of the cystic fibrosis gene: chromosome walking and jumping. Science 1989; 245: 1059-65.

[2]   Welsh MJ, Ramsey BW, Accurso FJ, Cutting GR. Cystic fibrosis. In: Scriver CR, Beaudet AL, Sly WS, Valle D, editors. The metabolic and molecular bases of inherited disease. 8th ed. New York: McGraw Hill; 2001. p. 5121-88.

[3]   Heijerman H. Infection and inflammation in cystic fibrosis: a short review. J Cyst Fibros 2005; 4: 3-5.

[4]   Bobadilla JL, Macek M, Jr., Fine JP, Farrell PM. Cystic fibrosis: a worldwide analysis of CFTR mutations--correlation with incidence data and application to screening. Human Mutation 2002; 19: 575-606.

[5]   Aitken ML. Cystic fibrosis. Curr Op Pulm Med 1995; 1: 425-34.

[6]   Davis PB. Cystic fibrosis since 1938. Am J Respir Crit Care Med. 2006; 173: 475-82.

[7]   Sheppard DN, Welsh MJ. Structure and function of the CFTR chloride channel. Physiol Rev 1999; 79: S23-45.

[8]   Moran O. Model of the cAMP activation of chloride transport by CFTR channel and the mechanism of potentiators. J Theoretical Biol 2010; 262: 73-9.

[9]   Zielenski J. Genotype and phenotype in cystic fibrosis. Respiration 2000; 67: 117-33.

[10]   Tsui LC. The spectrum of cystic fibrosis mutations. Trends Genet 1992; 8: 392-8.

[11]   Welsh MJ, Smith AE. Molecular mechanisms of CFTR chloride channel dysfunction in cystic fibrosis. Cell 1993; 73: 1251-4.

[12]   Zielenski J, Tsui LC. Cystic fibrosis: genotypic and phenotypic variations. Ann Rev Gen 1995; 29: 777-807.

[13]   Haardt M, Benharouga M, Lechardeur D, Kartner N, Lukacs GL. C-terminal truncations destabilize the cystic fibrosis transmembrane conductance regulator without impairing its biogenesis. A novel class of mutation. J Biol Chem 1999 ; 274: 21873-7.

[14]   Kerem B, Rommens JM, Buchanan JA *et al.* Identification of the cystic fibrosis gene: genetic analysis. Science 1989; 245: 1073-80.

[15]   Cheng SH, Gregory RJ, Marshall J *et al.* Defective intracellular transport and processing of CFTR is the molecular basis of most cystic fibrosis. Cell 1990; 63: 827-34.

[16]   Lukacs GL, Mohamed A, Kartner N, Chang XB, Riordan JR, Grinstein S. Conformational maturation of CFTR but not its mutant counterpart (delta F508) occurs in the endoplasmic reticulum and requires ATP. EMBO J 1994; 13: 6076-86.

[17]   Du K, Sharma M, Lukacs GL. The DeltaF508 cystic fibrosis mutation impairs domain-domain interactions and arrests post-translational folding of CFTR. Nat Struct Mol Biol 2005; 12: 17-25.

[18]   Ward CL, Omura S, Kopito RR. Degradation of CFTR by the ubiquitin-proteasome pathway. Cell 1995; 83: 121-7.

[19]   Denning GM, Anderson MP, Amara JF, Marshall J, Smith AE, Welsh MJ. Processing of mutant cystic fibrosis transmembrane conductance regulator is temperature-sensitive. Nature 1992; 358: 761-4.

[20]   Sato S, Ward CL, Krouse ME, Wine JJ, Kopito RR. Glycerol reverses the misfolding phenotype of the most common cystic fibrosis mutation. J Biol Chem 1996 ; 271: 635-8.

[21]   Rubenstein RC, Egan ME, Zeitlin PL. *In vitro* pharmacologic restoration of CFTR-mediated chloride transport with sodium 4-phenylbutyrate in cystic fibrosis epithelial cells containing delta F508-CFTR. J Clin Invest 1997; 100(: 2457-65.

[22]   Sharma M, Benharouga M, Hu W, Lukacs GL. Conformational and temperature-sensitive stability defects of the delta F508 cystic fibrosis transmembrane conductance regulator in post-endoplasmic reticulum compartments. J Biol Chem 2001; 276: 8942-50.

[23]   Gentzsch M, Chang XB, Cui L *et al.* Endocytic trafficking routes of wild type and DeltaF508 cystic fibrosis transmembrane conductance regulator. Mol Biol Cell 2004; 15: 2684-96.

[24]   Dalemans W, Barbry P, Champigny G *et al.* Altered chloride ion channel kinetics associated with the delta F508 cystic fibrosis mutation. Nature 1991; 354: 526-8.

[25]   Haws CM, Nepomuceno IB, Krouse ME *et al.* Delta F508-CFTR channels: kinetics, activation by forskolin, and potentiation by xanthines. Am J Phys 1996; 270: C1544-55.

[26]   Alper OM, Wong LJ, Young S *et al.* Identification of novel and rare mutations in California Hispanic and African American cystic fibrosis patients. Human Mutation 2004; 24: 353.

[27]   Alibakhshi R, Kianishirazi R, Cassiman JJ, Zamani M, Cuppens H. Analysis of the CFTR gene in Iranian cystic fibrosis patients: identification of eight novel mutations. J Cyst Fibros 2008; 7: 102-9.

[28]   Ashavaid TF, Kondkar AA, Dherai AJ *et al.* Application of multiplex ARMS and SSCP/HD analysis in molecular diagnosis of cystic fibrosis in Indian patients. Mol Diagn 2005; 9: 59-66.

[29]   Mutesa L, Azad AK, Verhaeghe C *et al.* Genetic analysis of Rwandan patients with cystic fibrosis-like symptoms: identification of novel cystic fibrosis transmembrane conductance regulator and epithelial sodium channel gene variants. Chest 2009; 135: 1233-42.

[30]   Hamosh A, Rosenstein BJ, Cutting GR. CFTR nonsense mutations G542X and W1282X associated with severe reduction of CFTR mRNA in nasal epithelial cells. Hum Mol Gen 1992; 1: 542-4.

[31]   Fanen P, Ghanem N, Vidaud M *et al.* Molecular characterization of cystic fibrosis: 16 novel mutations identified by analysis of the whole cystic fibrosis conductance transmembrane regulator (CFTR) coding regions and splice site junctions. Genomics. 1992; 13: 770-6.

[32]   Bompadre SG, Sohma Y, Li M, Hwang TC. G551D and G1349D, two CF-associated mutations in the signature sequences of CFTR, exhibit distinct gating defects. J Gen Physiol 2007; 129: 285-98.

[33]   Sheppard DN, Rich DP, Ostedgaard LS, Gregory RJ, Smith AE, Welsh MJ. Mutations in CFTR associated with mild-disease-form Cl- channels with altered pore properties. Nature 1993; 362: 160-4.

[34]   Highsmith WE, Burch LH, Zhou Z *et al.* A novel mutation in the cystic fibrosis gene in patients with pulmonary disease but normal sweat chloride concentrations. N Engl J Med 1994; 331: 974-80.

[35]   Sheppard DN, Ostedgaard LS, Winter MC, Welsh MJ. Mechanism of dysfunction of two nucleotide binding domain mutations in cystic fibrosis transmembrane conductance regulator that are associated with pancreatic sufficiency. EMBO J 1995; 14: 876-83.

[36]   Quinton PM. Cystic fibrosis: a disease in electrolyte transport. Faseb J 1990; 4: 2709-17.

[37]   Stutts MJ, Canessa CM, Olsen JC *et al.* CFTR as a cAMP-dependent regulator of sodium channels. Science 1995; 269: 847-50.

[38]   Boucher RC, Cotton CU, Gatzy JT, Knowles MR, Yankaskas JR. Evidence for reduced Cl- and increased Na+ permeability in cystic fibrosis human primary cell cultures. J Physiol 1988; 405: 77-103.

[39]   Boucher RC, Stutts MJ, Knowles MR, Cantley L, Gatzy JT. Na+ transport in cystic fibrosis respiratory epithelia. Abnormal basal rate and response to adenylate cyclase activation. J Clin Invest 1986; 78: 1245-52.

[40]   Augarten A, Kerem BS, Yahav Y *et al.* Mild cystic fibrosis and normal or borderline sweat test in patients with the 3849 + 10 kb C-->T mutation. Lancet 1993; 342: 25-6.

[41]   Wilschanski M, Zielenski J, Markiewicz D *et al*. Correlation of sweat chloride concentration with classes of the cystic fibrosis transmembrane conductance regulator gene mutations. J Ped 1995; 127: 705-10.

[42]   Anguiano A, Oates RD, Amos JA *et al*. Congenital bilateral absence of the vas deferens. A primarily genital form of cystic fibrosis. Jama 1992; 267: 1794-7.

[43]   Rosenstein BJ, Cutting GR. The diagnosis of cystic fibrosis: a consensus statement. Cystic Fibrosis Foundation Consensus Panel. J Ped 1998; 132: 589-95.

[44]   Riordan JR, Rommens JM, Kerem B *et al*. Identification of the cystic fibrosis gene: cloning and characterization of complementary DNA. Science 1989; 245: 1066-73.

[45]   Wilschanski M, Famini H, Strauss-Liviatan N *et al*. Nasal potential difference measurements in patients with atypical cystic fibrosis. Eur Respir J 2001; 17: 1208-15.

[46]   Knowles M, Gatzy J, Boucher R. Increased bioelectric potential difference across respiratory epithelia in cystic fibrosis. N Engl J Med 1981; 305: 1489-95.

[47]   Standaert TA, Boitano L, Emerson J *et al*. Standardized procedure for measurement of nasal potential difference: an outcome measure in multicenter cystic fibrosis clinical trials. Ped Pulm 2004; 37: 385-92.

[48]   Wilcken B. Newborn screening for cystic fibrosis: techniques and strategies. J Inher Metabol Dis 2007; 30:537-43.

[49]   Romeo G, Devoto M, Galietta LJ. Why is the cystic fibrosis gene so frequent? Hum Gen 1989; 84: 1-5.

[50]   Morral N, Bertranpetit J, Estivill X *et al*. The origin of the major cystic fibrosis mutation (delta F508) in European populations. Nat Gen 1994; 7: 169-75.

[51]   Aidoo M, Terlouw DJ, Kolczak MS *et al*. Protective effects of the sickle cell gene against malaria morbidity and mortality. Lancet 2002; 359: 1311-2.

[52]   Gabriel SE, Brigman KN, Koller BH, Boucher RC, Stutts MJ. Cystic fibrosis heterozygote resistance to cholera toxin in the cystic fibrosis mouse model. Science 1994; 266: 107-9.

[53]   Guggino SE. Gates of Janus: cystic fibrosis and diarrhea. Trends Micro 1994; 2: 91-4.

[54]   Casals T, De-Gracia J, Gallego M *et al*. Bronchiectasis in adult patients: an expression of heterozygosity for CFTR gene mutations? Clin Genet 2004; 65: 490-5.

[55]   Raman V, Clary R, Siegrist KL, Zehnbauer B, Chatila TA. Increased prevalence of mutations in the cystic fibrosis transmembrane conductance regulator in children with chronic rhinosinusitis. Pediatrics. 2002; 109: E13.

[56]   Cohn JA, Friedman KJ, Noone PG, Knowles MR, Silverman LM, Jowell PS. Relation between mutations of the cystic fibrosis gene and idiopathic pancreatitis. N Enlg J Med 1998; 339: 653-8.

[57]   Eaton TE, Weiner Miller P, Garrett JE, Cutting GR. Cystic fibrosis transmembrane conductance regulator gene mutations: do they play a role in the aetiology of allergic bronchopulmonary aspergillosis? Clin Exp Allergy 2002; 32: 756-61.

[58]   Kuningas M, van Bodegom D, May L, Meij JJ, Slagboom PE, Westendorp RG. Common CFTR gene variants influence body composition and survival in rural Ghana. Hum Gen. 2010; 127: 201-6

[59]   Diamond G, Legarda D, Ryan LK. The innate immune response of the respiratory epithelium. Immunol Rev 2000; 173: 27-38.

[60]   Jacquot J, Hayem A, Galabert C. Functions of proteins and lipids in airway secretions. Eur Respir J 1992; 5: 343-58.

[61]   Lillehoj ER, Kim KC. Airway mucus: its components and function. Arch Pharm Res 2002; 25: 770-80.

[62]   Fujiwara N, Kobayashi K. Macrophages in inflammation. Curr Drug Tar 2005; 4: 281-6.

[63]   Luster AD. Chemokines--chemotactic cytokines that mediate inflammation. N Engl J Med 1998; 338: 436-45.

[64]   Curtis JL. Cell-mediated adaptive immune defense of the lungs. Proc Am Thor Soc 2005; 2: 412-6.

[65]   Becker MN, Diamond G, Verghese MW, Randell SH. CD14-dependent lipopolysaccharide-induced beta-defensin-2 expression in human tracheobronchial epithelium. J Biol Chem 2000; 275: 29731-6.

[66]   Greene CM, Carroll TP, Smith SG *et al*. TLR-induced inflammation in cystic fibrosis and non-cystic fibrosis airway epithelial cells. J Immunol 2005; 174: 1638-46.

[67]   Muir A, Soong G, Sokol S *et al*. Toll-like receptors in normal and cystic fibrosis airway epithelial cells. Am J Respir Cell Mol Biol 2004; 30: 777-83.

[68]   Anderson KV, Jurgens G, Nusslein-Volhard C. Establishment of dorsal-ventral polarity in the *Drosophila* embryo: genetic studies on the role of the Toll gene product. Cell 1985; 42: 779-89.

[69]   Lemaitre B, Nicolas E, Michaut L, Reichhart JM, Hoffmann JA. The dorsoventral regulatory gene cassette spatzle/Toll/cactus controls the potent antifungal response in *Drosophila* adults. Cell 1996; 86: 973-83.

[70]   Gay NJ, Keith FJ. *Drosophila* Toll and IL-1 receptor. Nature 1991; 351: 355-6.

[71]   Medzhitov R, Preston-Hurlburt P, Janeway CA, Jr. A human homologue of the *Drosophila* Toll protein signals activation of adaptive immunity. Nature 1997; 388: 394-7.

[72]   Carpenter S, O'Neill LA. How important are Toll-like receptors for antimicrobial responses? Cell Micro 2007; 9: 1891-901.

[73]   Bell JK, Mullen GE, Leifer CA, Mazzoni A, Davies DR, Segal DM. Leucine-rich repeats and pathogen recognition in Toll-like receptors. Trends Immunol 2003; 24: 528-33.

[74]   O'Neill LA. Signal transduction pathways activated by the IL-1 receptor/toll-like receptor superfamily. Curr Top Microbiol Immunol 2002; 270: 47-61.

[75]   Ritter M, Mennerich D, Weith A, Seither P. Characterization of Toll-like receptors in primary lung epithelial cells: strong impact of the TLR3 ligand poly(I:C) on the regulation of Toll-like receptors, adaptor proteins and inflammatory response. J Inflamm 2005; 2: 16.

[76]   Hewson CA, Jardine A, Edwards MR, Laza-Stanca V, Johnston SL. Toll-like receptor 3 is induced by and mediates antiviral activity against rhinovirus infection of human bronchial epithelial cells. J Virol 2005; 79: 12273-9.

[77]   Diebold SS, Kaisho T, Hemmi H, Akira S, Reis e Sousa C. Innate antiviral responses by means of TLR7-mediated recognition of single-stranded RNA. Science 2004; 303: 1529-31.

[78]   Heil F, Hemmi H, Hochrein H *et al.* Species-specific recognition of single-stranded RNA *via* toll-like receptor 7 and 8. Science 2004; 303: 1526-9.

[79]   Hemmi H, Takeuchi O, Kawai T *et al.* A Toll-like receptor recognizes bacterial DNA. Nature 2000; 408: 740-5.

[80]   Chu HW, Jeyaseelan S, Rino JG *et al.* TLR2 signaling is critical for *Mycoplasma pneumoniae*-induced airway mucin expression. J Immunol 2005; 174: 5713-9.

[81]   Schmeck B, Huber S, Moog K *et al.* Pneumococci induced TLR- and Rac1-dependent NF-kappaB-recruitment to the IL-8 promoter in lung epithelial cells. Am J Physiol Lung Cell Mol Physiol 2006 2 90: L730-L7.

[82]   Armstrong L, Medford AR, Uppington KM *et al.* Expression of functional toll-like receptor-2 and -4 on alveolar epithelial cells. Am J Respir Cell Mol Biol 2004 Aug;31(2):241-5.

[83]   Gon Y, Asai Y, Hashimoto S *et al.* A20 inhibits toll-like receptor 2- and 4-mediated interleukin-8 synthesis in airway epithelial cells. Am J Respir Cell Mol Biol. 2004; 31: 330-6.

[84]   Wetzler LM. The role of Toll-like receptor 2 in microbial disease and immunity. Vaccine 2003; 21: S55-60.

[85]   Takeuchi O, Kawai T, Muhlradt PF *et al.* Discrimination of bacterial lipoproteins by Toll-like receptor 6. Int Immunol 2001; 13: 933-40.

[86]   Underhill DM, Ozinsky A, Hajjar AM *et al.* The Toll-like receptor 2 is recruited to macrophage phagosomes and discriminates between pathogens. Nature 1999 ; 401: 811-5.

[87]   Kataoka K, Muta T, Yamazaki S, Takeshige K. Activation of macrophages by linear (1right-arrow3)-beta-D-glucans. Impliations for the recognition of fungi by innate immunity. J Biol Chem 2002; 277: 36825-31.

[88]   Poltorak A, He X, Smirnova I *et al.* Defective LPS signaling in C3H/HeJ and C57BL/10ScCr mice: mutations in Tlr4 gene. Science 1998; 282: 2085-8.

[89]   Nagai Y, Akashi S, Nagafuku M *et al.* Essential role of MD-2 in LPS responsiveness and TLR4 distribution. Nat Immunol 2002; 3: 667-72.

[90]   Chow JC, Young DW, Golenbock DT, Christ WJ, Gusovsky F. Toll-like receptor-4 mediates lipopolysaccharide-induced signal transduction. J Biol Chem 1999; 274: 10689-92.

[91]   da Silva Correia J, Soldau K, Christen U, Tobias PS, Ulevitch RJ. Lipopolysaccharide is in close proximity to each of the proteins in its membrane receptor complex. transfer from CD14 to TLR4 and MD-2. J Biol Chem 2001; 276: 21129-35.

[92]   Sasu S, LaVerda D, Qureshi N, Golenbock DT, Beasley D. *Chlamydia pneumoniae* and chlamydial heat shock protein 60 stimulate proliferation of human vascular smooth muscle cells *via* toll-like receptor 4 and p44/p42 mitogen-activated protein kinase activation. Circ Res 2001; 89: 244-50.

[93]   Malley R, Henneke P, Morse SC *et al.* Recognition of pneumolysin by Toll-like receptor 4 confers resistance to pneumococcal infection. Proc Natl Acad Sci USA 2003; 100: 1966-71.

[94]   Gomi K, Kawasaki K, Kawai Y, Shiozaki M, Nishijima M. Toll-like receptor 4-MD-2 complex mediates the signal transduction induced by flavolipin, an amino acid-containing lipid unique to *Flavobacterium meningosepticum*. J Immunol 2002; 168: 2939-43.

[95]   Kurt-Jones EA, Popova L, Kwinn L *et al.* Pattern recognition receptors TLR4 and CD14 mediate response to respiratory syncytial virus. Nat Immunol 2000; 1: 398-401.

[96]   Rassa JC, Meyers JL, Zhang Y, Kudaravalli R, Ross SR. Murine retroviruses activate B cells *via* interaction with toll-like receptor 4. Proc Natl Acad Sci USA 2002; 99: 2281-6.

[97]   Shoham S, Huang C, Chen JM, Golenbock DT, Levitz SM. Toll-like receptor 4 mediates intracellular signaling without TNF-alpha release in response to *Cryptococcus neoformans* polysaccharide capsule. J Immunol 2001; 166: 4620-6.

[98]   Netea MG, Van der Graaf C, Van der Meer JW, Kullberg BJ. Recognition of fungal pathogens by Toll-like receptors. Eur J Clin Microbiol Infect Dis 2004; 23: 672-6.

[99]   Hayashi F, Smith KD, Ozinsky A *et al.* The innate immune response to bacterial flagellin is mediated by Toll-like receptor 5. Nature 2001; 410: 1099-103.

[100]   Hasan U, Chaffois C, Gaillard C *et al.* Human TLR10 is a functional receptor, expressed by B cells and plasmacytoid dendritic cells, which activates gene transcription through MyD88. J Immunol 2005; 174: 2942-50.

[101]   Biragyn A, Ruffini PA, Leifer CA *et al.* Toll-like receptor 4-dependent activation of dendritic cells by beta-defensin 2. Science 2002; 298: 1025-9.

[102]   Frantz S, Kelly RA, Bourcier T. Role of TLR-2 in the activation of nuclear factor kappaB by oxidative stress in cardiac myocytes. J Biol Chem 2001; 276: 5197-203.

[103]   Guillot L, Balloy V, McCormack FX, Golenbock DT, Chignard M, Si-Tahar M. Cutting edge: the immunostimulatory activity of the lung surfactant protein-A involves Toll-like receptor 4. J Immunol 2002; 168: 5989-92.

[104]   Ohashi K, Burkart V, Flohe S, Kolb H. Cutting edge: heat shock protein 60 is a putative endogenous ligand of the toll-like receptor-4 complex. J Immunol 2000; 164: 558-61.

[105]   Zanin-Zhorov A, Nussbaum G, Franitza S, Cohen IR, Lider O. T cells respond to heat shock protein 60 *via* TLR2: activation of adhesion and inhibition of chemokine receptors. Faseb J 2003; 17: 1567-9.

[106]   Devaney JM, Greene CM, Taggart CC, Carroll TP, O'Neill SJ, McElvaney NG. Neutrophil elastase up-regulates interleukin-8 *via* toll-like receptor 4. FEBS letts 2003; 544: 129-32.

[107]   Okamura Y, Watari M, Jerud ES *et al.* The extra domain A of fibronectin activates Toll-like receptor 4. J Biol Chem 2001; 276: 10229-33.

[108]   Termeer C, Benedix F, Sleeman J *et al.* Oligosaccharides of Hyaluronan activate dendritic cells *via* toll-like receptor 4. J Exp Med 2002; 195: 99-111.

[109]   Akira S, Takeda K. Toll-like receptor signaling. Nat Rev 2004; 4: 499-511.

[110]   Schroder NW, Pfeil D, Opitz B *et al.* Activation of mitogen-activated protein kinases p42/44, p38, and stress-activated protein kinases in myelo-monocytic cells by *Treponema* lipoteichoic acid. J Biol Chem 2001; 276: 9713-9.

[111]   Yamamoto M, Takeda K, Akira S. TIR domain-containing adaptors define the specificity of TLR signaling. Mol Immunol 2004; 40: 861-8.

[112]   Fitzgerald KA, Palsson-McDermott EM, Bowie AG *et al.* Mal (MyD88-adapter-like) is required for Toll-like receptor-4 signal transduction. Nature 2001; 413: 78-83.

[113]   Horng T, Barton GM, Medzhitov R. TIRAP: an adapter molecule in the Toll signaling pathway. Nat Immunol 2001; 2: 835-41.

[114]   Yamamoto M, Sato S, Hemmi H *et al.* Role of adaptor TRIF in the MyD88-independent toll-like receptor signaling pathway. Science 2003; 301: 640-3.

[115]   Yamamoto M, Sato S, Hemmi H *et al.* TRAM is specifically involved in the Toll-like receptor 4-mediated MyD88-independent signaling pathway. Nat Immunol 2003; 4: 1144-50.

[116]   Kawai T, Takeuchi O, Fujita T *et al.* Lipopolysaccharide stimulates the MyD88-independent pathway and results in activation of IFN-regulatory factor 3 and the expression of a subset of lipopolysaccharide-inducible genes. J Immunol 2001; 167: 5887-94.

[117]   Dunne A, O'Neill LA. The interleukin-1 receptor/Toll-like receptor superfamily: signal transduction during inflammation and host defense. Sci STKE. 2003; 2003: re3.

[118]   Becker MN, Sauer MS, Muhlebach MS *et al.* Cytokine secretion by cystic fibrosis airway epithelial cells. Am J Respir Crit Care Med 2004; 169: 645-53.

[119]   Guillot L, Le Goffic R, Bloch S *et al.* Involvement of toll-like receptor 3 in the immune response of lung epithelial cells to double-stranded RNA and influenza A virus. J Biol Chem 2005; 280: 5571-80.

[120]   Monick MM, Yarovinsky TO, Powers LS *et al.* Respiratory syncytial virus up-regulates TLR4 and sensitizes airway epithelial cells to endotoxin. J Biol Chem 2003; 278: 53035-44.

[121]   Hawn TR, Verbon A, Lettinga KD *et al.* A common dominant TLR5 stop codon polymorphism abolishes flagellin signaling and is associated with susceptibility to legionnaires' disease. J Exp Med 2003; 198: 1563-72.

[122]   Lopez-Boado YS, Cobb LM, Deora R. *Bordetella bronchiseptica* flagellin is a proinflammatory determinant for airway epithelial cells. Infect Immun 2005; 73: 7525-34.

[123]   Zhang Z, Louboutin JP, Weiner DJ, Goldberg JB, Wilson JM. Human airway epithelial cells sense *Pseudomonas aeruginosa* infection *via* recognition of flagellin by Toll-like receptor 5. Infect Immun 2005; 73: 7151-60.

[124] Sha Q, Truong-Tran AQ, Plitt JR, Beck LA, Schleimer RP. Activation of airway epithelial cells by toll-like receptor agonists. Am J Respir Cell Mol Biol 2004; 31: 358-64.

[125] Homma T, Kato A, Hashimoto N *et al.* Corticosteroid and cytokines synergistically enhance toll-like receptor 2 expression in respiratory epithelial cells. Am J Respir Cell Mol Biol 2004; 31: 463-9.

[126] Hertz CJ, Wu Q, Porter EM *et al.* Activation of Toll-like receptor 2 on human tracheobronchial epithelial cells induces the antimicrobial peptide human beta defensin-2. J Immunol 2003; 171: 6820-6.

[127] Wang X, Zhang Z, Louboutin JP, Moser C, Weiner DJ, Wilson JM. Airway epithelia regulate expression of human beta-defensin 2 through Toll-like receptor 2. Faseb J 2003; 17: 1727-9.

[128] Jia HP, Kline JN, Penisten A *et al.* Endotoxin responsiveness of human airway epithelia is limited by low expression of MD-2. Am J Physiol Lung Cell Mol Physiol 2004; 287: L428-37.

[129] Jiang D, Liang J, Fan J *et al.* Regulation of lung injury and repair by Toll-like receptors and hyaluronan. Nat Med 2005; 11: 1173-9.

[130] Chaudhuri N, Dower SK, Whyte MK, Sabroe I. Toll-like receptors and chronic lung disease. Clin Sci (Lond) 2005; 109: 125-33.

[131] Syhre M, Scotter JM, Chambers ST. Investigation into the production of 2-Pentylfuran by *Aspergillus fumigatus* and other respiratory pathogens *in vitro* and human breath samples. Med Mycol 2008; 46: 209-15.

[132] Schwartz DA, Quinn TJ, Thorne PS, Sayeed S, Yi AK, Krieg AM. CpG motifs in bacterial DNA cause inflammation in the lower respiratory tract. J Clin Invest 1997; 100: 68-73.

[133] Khan TZ, Wagener JS, Bost T, Martinez J, Accurso FJ, Riches DW. Early pulmonary inflammation in infants with cystic fibrosis. Am J Respir Crit Care Med 1995; 151: 1075-82.

[134] Armstrong DS, Grimwood K, Carlin JB *et al.* Lower airway inflammation in infants and young children with cystic fibrosis. Am J Respir Crit Care Med 1997;156: 1197-204.

[135] Noah TL, Black HR, Cheng PW, Wood RE, Leigh MW. Nasal and bronchoalveolar lavage fluid cytokines in early cystic fibrosis. J Infect Dis 1997; 175: 638-47.

[136] Bonfield TL, Panuska JR, Konstan MW *et al.* Inflammatory cytokines in cystic fibrosis lungs. Am J Respir Crit Care Med 1995; 152: 2111-8.

[137] Wat D, Gelder C, Hibbitts S *et al.* The role of respiratory viruses in cystic fibrosis. J Cyst Fibros 2008; 7: 320-8.

[138] Greene CM, McElvaney NG. Proteases and antiproteases in chronic neutrophilic lung disease - relevance to drug discovery. Br J Pharmacol 2009; 158: 1048-58.

[139] Doring G. The role of neutrophil elastase in chronic inflammation. Am J Respir Crit Care Med 1994; 150: S114-7.

[140] Birrer P, McElvaney NG, Rudeberg A *et al.* Protease-antiprotease imbalance in the lungs of children with cystic fibrosis. Am J Respir Crit Care Med 1994; 150: 207-13.

[141] Brinkmann V, Reichard U, Goosmann C *et al.* Neutrophil extracellular traps kill bacteria. Science 2004; 303: 1532-5.

[142] Geraghty P, Rogan MP, Greene CM *et al.* Neutrophil elastase up-regulates cathepsin B and matrix metalloprotease-2 expression. J Immunol 2007; 178: 5871-8.

[143] Shao MX, Nadel JA. Neutrophil elastase induces MUC5AC mucin production in human airway epithelial cells *via* a cascade involving protein kinase C, reactive oxygen species, and TNF-alpha-converting enzyme. J Immunol 2005; 175: 4009-16.

[144] Bergin DA, Greene CM, Sterchi EE *et al.* Activation of the epidermal growth factor receptor (EGFR) by a novel metalloprotease pathway. J Biol Chem 2008; 283: 31736-44.

[145] Nakamura H, Yoshimura K, McElvaney NG, Crystal RG. Neutrophil elastase in respiratory epithelial lining fluid of individuals with cystic fibrosis induces interleukin-8 gene expression in a human bronchial epithelial cell line. J Clin Invest 1992; 89: 1478-84.

[146] McElvaney NG, Nakamura H, Birrer P *et al.* Modulation of airway inflammation in cystic fibrosis. *In vivo* suppression of interleukin-8 levels on the respiratory epithelial surface by aerosolization of recombinant secretory leukoprotease inhibitor. J Clin Invest 1992; 90: 1296-301.

[147] Walsh DE, Greene CM, Carroll TP *et al.* Interleukin-8 up-regulation by neutrophil elastase is mediated by MyD88/IRAK/TRAF-6 in human bronchial epithelium. J Biol Chem 2001; 276: 35494-9.

[148] Koff JL, Shao MX, Ueki IF, Nadel JA. Multiple TLRs activate EGFR *via* a signaling cascade to produce innate immune responses in airway epithelium. Am J Physiol Lung Cell Mol Physiol 2008; 294: L1068-75.

[149] van Ewijk BE, van der Zalm MM, Wolfs TF, van der Ent CK. Viral respiratory infections in cystic fibrosis. J Cyst Fibros 2005; 4 : 31-6.

[150] Wat D, Doull I. Respiratory virus infections in cystic fibrosis. Paed Resp Rev. 2003; 4: 172-7.

[151] Wang EE, Prober CG, Manson B, Corey M, Levison H. Association of respiratory viral infections with pulmonary deterioration in patients with cystic fibrosis. N Engl J Med 1984; 311: 1653-8.

[152] Abman SH, Ogle JW, Butler-Simon N, Rumack CM, Accurso FJ. Role of respiratory syncytial virus in early hospitalizations for respiratory distress of young infants with cystic fibrosis. J Pediatr 1988; 113: 826-30.

[153] Smyth AR, Smyth RL, Tong CY, Hart CA, Heaf DP. Effect of respiratory virus infections including rhinovirus on clinical status in cystic fibrosis. Arch Dis Child 1995; 73: 117-20.

[154] Hiatt PW, Grace SC, Kozinetz CA, Raboudi SH, Treece DG, Taber LH, *et al.* Effects of viral lower respiratory tract infection on lung function in infants with cystic fibrosis. Pediatrics 1999; 103: 619-26.

[155] Armstrong D, Grimwood K, Carlin JB *et al.* Severe viral respiratory infections in infants with cystic fibrosis. Ped Pulm 1998; 26: 371-9.

[156] van Ewijk BE, Wolfs TF, Fleer A, Kimpen JL, van der Ent CK. High *Pseudomonas aeruginosa* acquisition rate in CF. Thorax 2006 ;61: 641-2.

[157] Paisley JW, Lauer BA, McIntosh K, Glode MP, Schachter J, Rumack C. Pathogens associated with acute lower respiratory tract infection in young children. Ped Infect Dis 1984; 3: 14-9.

[158] Hament JM, Kimpen JL, Fleer A, Wolfs TF. Respiratory viral infection predisposing for bacterial disease: a concise review. FEMS Immunol Med Microbiol 1999; 26: 189-95.

[159] Van Ewijk BE, Wolfs TF, Aerts PC *et al.* RSV mediates *Pseudomonas aeruginosa* binding to cystic fibrosis and normal epithelial cells. Ped Res 2007; 61: 398-403.

[160] Ohrui T, Yamaya M, Sekizawa K *et al.* Effects of rhinovirus infection on hydrogen peroxide- induced alterations of barrier function in the cultured human tracheal epithelium. Am J Respir Crit Care Med 1998; 158: 241-8.

[161] Mastronarde JG, Monick MM, Hunninghake GW. Oxidant tone regulates IL-8 production in epithelium infected with respiratory syncytial virus. Am J Respir Cell Mol Biol 1995; 13: 237-44.

[162] Walsh JJ, Dietlein LF, Low FN, Burch GE, Mogabgab WJ. Bronchotracheal response in human influenza. Type A, Asian strain, as studied by light and electron microscopic examination of bronchoscopic biopsies. Arch Int Med 1961; 108: 376-88.

[163] Winther B, Gwaltney JM, Hendley JO. Respiratory virus infection of monolayer cultures of human nasal epithelial cells. Am Rev Respir Dis 1990; 141: 839-45.

[164] Ramsey BW, Gore EJ, Smith AL, Cooney MK, Redding GJ, Foy H. The effect of respiratory viral infections on patients with cystic fibrosis. Am J Dis Child (1960). 1989; 143: 662-8.

[165] Collinson J, Nicholson KG, Cancio E *et al.* Effects of upper respiratory tract infections in patients with cystic fibrosis. Thorax 1996; 51 :1115-22.

[166] Oliver BG, Lim S, Wark P *et al.* Rhinovirus exposure impairs immune responses to bacterial products in human alveolar macrophages. Thorax 2008; 63: 519-25.

[167] Bonfield TL, Konstan MW, Burfeind P, Panuska JR, Hilliard JB, Berger M. Normal bronchial epithelial cells constitutively produce the anti-inflammatory cytokine interleukin-10, which is downregulated in cystic fibrosis. Am J Respir Cell Mol Biol 1995; 13: 257-61.

[168] Tabary O, Muselet C, Escotte S *et al.* Interleukin-10 inhibits elevated chemokine interleukin-8 and regulated on activation normal T cell expressed and secreted production in cystic fibrosis bronchial epithelial cells by targeting the I(k)B kinase alpha/beta complex. Am J Pathol 2003; 162: 293-302.

[169] Chow CW, Landau LI, Taussig LM. Bronchial mucous glands in the newborn with cystic fibrosis. Eur J Ped 1982; 139: 240-3.

[170] Jiang C, Finkbeiner WE, Widdicombe JH, McCray PB, Jr., Miller SS. Altered fluid transport across airway epithelium in cystic fibrosis. Science 1993; 262: 424-7.

[171] Gilljam H, Ellin A, Strandvik B. Increased bronchial chloride concentration in cystic fibrosis. Scand J Clin Lab Invest 1989; 49: 121-4.

[172] Joris L, Dab I, Quinton PM. Elemental composition of human airway surface fluid in healthy and diseased airways. Am Rev Resp Dis 1993; 148: 1633-7.

[173] Zabner J, Smith JJ, Karp PH, Widdicombe JH, Welsh MJ. Loss of CFTR chloride channels alters salt absorption by cystic fibrosis airway epithelia *in vitro*. Mol Cell 1998; 2: 397-403.

[174] Smith JJ, Travis SM, Greenberg EP, Welsh MJ. Cystic fibrosis airway epithelia fail to kill bacteria because of abnormal airway surface fluid. Cell 1996; 85: 229-36.

[175] Matsui H, Grubb BR, Tarran R *et al.* Evidence for periciliary liquid layer depletion, not abnormal ion composition, in the pathogenesis of cystic fibrosis airways disease. Cell 1998; 95: 1005-15.

[176] Tseng J, Do J, Widdicombe JH, Machen TE. Innate immune responses of human tracheal epithelium to *Pseudomonas aeruginosa* flagellin, TNF-alpha, and IL-1beta. Am J Physiol. 2006; 290: C678-90.

[177] Mayer AK, Muehmer M, Mages J *et al.* Differential recognition of TLR-dependent microbial ligands in human bronchial epithelial cells. J Immunol 2007; 178: 3134-42.

[178] Hemmi H, Kaisho T, Takeuchi O *et al.* Small anti-viral compounds activate immune cells *via* the TLR7 MyD88-dependent signaling pathway. Nat Immunol 2002; 3: 196-200.

[179] Jurk M, Heil F, Vollmer J *et al.* Human TLR7 or TLR8 independently confer responsiveness to the antiviral compound R-848. Nat Immunol 2002; 3: 499.

[180] Guillot L, Medjane S, Le-Barillec K *et al.* Response of human pulmonary epithelial cells to lipopolysaccharide involves Toll-like receptor 4 (TLR4)-dependent signaling pathways: evidence for an intracellular compartmentalization of TLR4. J Biol Chem 2004; 279: 2712-8.

[181] John G, Yildirim AO, Rubin BK, Gruenert DC, Henke MO. Toll-like Receptor (TLR)-4 Mediated Innate Immunity is Reduced in Cystic Fibrosis Airway Cells. Am J Respir Cell Mol Biol 2010; 42: 424-31

[182] Urquhart DS, Allen J, Elrayess M, Fidler K, Klein N, Jaffe A. Modifier effect of the Toll-like receptor 4 D299G polymorphism in children with cystic fibrosis. Archivum Immunologiae et Therap Exp 2006; 54: 271-6.

[183] O'Reilly SM, Moynagh PN. Regulation of Toll-like receptor 4 signaling by A20 zinc finger protein. Biochem Biophys Res Comm 2003; 303: 586-93.

[184] Boone DL, Turer EE, Lee EG, Ahmad RC, Wheeler MT, Tsui C, *et al.* The ubiquitin-modifying enzyme A20 is required for termination of Toll-like receptor responses. Nat Immunol 2004; 5: 1052-60.

[185] Klinkenberg M, Van Huffel S, Heyninck K, Beyaert R. Functional redundancy of the zinc fingers of A20 for inhibition of NF-kappaB activation and protein-protein interactions. FEBS Letts. 2001; 498: 93-7.

[186] Van Huffel S, Delaei F, Heyninck K, De Valck D, Beyaert R. Identification of a novel A20-binding inhibitor of nuclear factor-kappa B activation termed ABIN-2. J Biol Chem 2001; 276: 30216-23.

[187] Yokota S, Okabayashi T, Yokosawa N, Fujii N. Measles virus P protein suppresses Toll-like receptor signal through up-regulation of ubiquitin-modifying enzyme A20. Faseb J 2008; 22: 74-83.

[188] Burns K, Clatworthy J, Martin L, Martinon F, Plumpton C, Maschera B, *et al.* Tollip, a new component of the IL-1RI pathway, links IRAK to the IL-1 receptor. Nat Cell Biol 2000; 2: 346-51.

[189] Zhang G, Ghosh S. Negative regulation of toll-like receptor-mediated signaling by Tollip. J Biol Chem 2002; 277: 7059-65.

[190] Mantovani A, Locati M, Polentarutti N, Vecchi A, Garlanda C. Extracellular and intracellular decoys in the tuning of inflammatory cytokines and Toll-like receptors: the new entry TIR8/SIGIRR. J Leuk Biol 2004; 75: 738-42.

[191] Wald D, Qin J, Zhao Z *et al.* SIGIRR, a negative regulator of Toll-like receptor-interleukin 1 receptor signaling. Nat Immunol 2003; 4: 920-7.

[192] Garlanda C, Riva F, Polentarutti N *et al.* Intestinal inflammation in mice deficient in Tir8, an inhibitory member of the IL-1 receptor family. Proc Natl Acad Sci USA 2004; 101: 3522-6.

[193] Janssens S, Burns K, Tschopp J, Beyaert R. Regulation of interleukin-1- and lipopolysaccharide-induced NF-kappaB activation by alternative splicing of MyD88. Curr Biol 2002; 12: 467-71.

[194] Burns K, Janssens S, Brissoni B, Olivos N, Beyaert R, Tschopp J. Inhibition of interleukin 1 receptor/Toll-like receptor signaling through the alternatively spliced, short form of MyD88 is due to its failure to recruit IRAK-4. J Exp Med 2003; 197: 263-8.

[195] Wesche H, Gao X, Li X, Kirschning CJ, Stark GR, Cao Z. IRAK-M is a novel member of the Pelle/interleukin-1 receptor-associated kinase (IRAK) family. J Biol Chem 1999; 274: 19403-10.

[196] Kobayashi K, Hernandez LD, Galan JE, Janeway CA, Jr., Medzhitov R, Flavell RA. IRAK-M is a negative regulator of Toll-like receptor signaling. Cell 2002; 110: 191-202.

[197] Rothlin CV, Ghosh S, Zuniga EI, Oldstone MB, Lemke G. TAM receptors are pleiotropic inhibitors of the innate immune response. Cell 2007; 131: 1124-36.

[198] Carty M, Goodbody R, Schroder M, Stack J, Moynagh PN, Bowie AG. The human adaptor SARM negatively regulates adaptor protein TRIF-dependent Toll-like receptor signaling. Nat Immunol 2006; 7: 1074-81.

[199] An H, Hou J, Zhou J *et al.* Phosphatase SHP-1 promotes TLR- and RIG-I-activated production of type I interferon by inhibiting the kinase IRAK1. Nat Immunol 2008; 9: 542-50.

[200] Xu H, An H, Hou J *et al.* Phosphatase PTP1B negatively regulates MyD88- and TRIF-dependent proinflammatory cytokine and type I interferon production in TLR-triggered macrophages. Mol Immunol 2008; 45: 3545-52.

[201] Kato K, Lu W, Kai H, Kim KC. Phosphoinositide 3-kinase is activated by MUC1 but not responsible for MUC1-induced suppression of Toll-like receptor 5 signaling. Am J Physiol Lung Cell Mol Physiol 2007; 293: L686-92.

[202] Ueno K, Koga T, Kato K *et al.* MUC1 mucin is a negative regulator of toll-like receptor signaling. Am J Respir Cell Mol Biol 2008; 38: 263-8.

[203] Appel S, Mirakaj V, Bringmann A, Weck MM, Grunebach F, Brossart P. PPAR-gamma agonists inhibit toll-like receptor-mediated activation of dendritic cells *via* the MAP kinase and NF-kappaB pathways. Blood 2005; 106: 3888-94.

[204] Bowie A, Kiss-Toth E, Symons JA, Smith GL, Dower SK, O'Neill LA. A46R and A52R from vaccinia virus are antagonists of host IL-1 and toll-like receptor signaling. Proc Natl Acad Sci USA 2000; 97: 10162-7.

[205] DiPerna G, Stack J, Bowie AG *et al.* Poxvirus protein N1L targets the I-kappaB kinase complex, inhibits signaling to NF-kappaB by the tumor necrosis factor superfamily of receptors, and inhibits NF-kappaB and IRF3 signaling by toll-like receptors. J Biol Chem 2004; 279: 36570-8.

[206] Shingai M, Azuma M, Ebihara T *et al.* Soluble G protein of respiratory syncytial virus inhibits Toll-like receptor 3/4-mediated IFN-beta induction. Int Immunol 2008; 20: 1169-80.

[207] Newman RM, Salunkhe P, Godzik A, Reed JC. Identification and characterization of a novel bacterial virulence factor that shares homology with mammalian Toll/interleukin-1 receptor family proteins. Infect Immun 2006; 74: 594-601.

[208] Salcedo SP, Marchesini MI, Lelouard H *et al.* *Brucella* control of dendritic cell maturation is dependent on the TIR-containing protein Btp1. PLoS Pathog 2008; 4: e21.

[209] Cirl C, Wieser A, Yadav M *et al.* Subversion of Toll-like receptor signaling by a unique family of bacterial Toll/interleukin-1 receptor domain-containing proteins. Nat Med 2008; 14: 399-406.

[210] Bartfai T, Behrens MM, Gaidarova S, Pemberton J, Shivanyuk A, Rebek J, Jr. A low molecular weight mimic of the Toll/IL-1 receptor/resistance domain inhibits IL-1 receptor-mediated responses. Proc Natl Acd Sci USA. 2003; 100: 7971-6.

[211] Davis CN, Mann E, Behrens MM *et al.* MyD88-dependent and -independent signaling by IL-1 in neurons probed by bifunctional Toll/IL-1 receptor domain/BB-loop mimetics. Proc Natl Acad Sci USA 2006; 103: 2953-8.

[212] Toshchakov VY, Vogel SN. Cell-penetrating TIR BB loop decoy peptides a novel class of TLR signaling inhibitors and a tool to study topology of TIR-TIR interactions. Expert Opin Biol Ther 2007; 7: 1035-50.

[213] Greene CM, McElvaney NG, O'Neill SJ, Taggart CC. Secretory leucoprotease inhibitor impairs Toll-like receptor 2- and 4-mediated responses in monocytic cells. Infect Immun. 2004; 72: 3684-7.

[214] Butler MW, Robertson I, Greene CM, O'Neill SJ, Taggart CC, McElvaney NG. Elafin prevents lipopolysaccharide-induced AP-1 and NF-kappaB activation *via* an effect on the ubiquitin-proteasome pathway. J Biol Chem 2006; 281: 34730-5.

[215] Janciauskiene S, Larsson S, Larsson P, Virtala R, Jansson L, Stevens T. Inhibition of lipopolysaccharide-mediated human monocyte activation, *in vitro*, by alpha1-antitrypsin. Biochem Biophys Res Comm 2004; 321: 592-600.

[216] Agu RU, Ugwoke MI, Armand M, Kinget R, Verbeke N. The lung as a route for systemic delivery of therapeutic proteins and peptides. Respir Res 2001; 2: 198-209.

[217] Dawson M, Wirtz D, Hanes J. Enhanced viscoelasticity of human cystic fibrotic sputum correlates with increasing microheterogeneity in particle transport. J Biol Chem 2003; 278: 50393-401.

[218] Fink TL, Klepcyk PJ, Oette SM *et al.* Plasmid size up to 20 kbp does not limit effective *in vivo* lung gene transfer using compacted DNA nanoparticles. Gene Ther 2006; 13: 1048-51.

[219] Li Z, Zhang Y, Wurtz W *et al.* Characterization of nebulized liposomal amikacin (Arikace) as a function of droplet size. J Aerosol Med Pulm Drug Deliv 2008; 21: 245-54.

[220] Anderson P. Emerging therapies in cystic fibrosis. Ther Adv Respir Dis 2010; 4: 177-85.

[221] Choe J, Kelker MS, Wilson IA. Crystal structure of human toll-like receptor 3 (TLR3) ectodomain. Science 2005; 309: 581-5.

[222] Kim JI, Lee CJ, Jin MS *et al.* Crystal structure of CD14 and its implications for lipopolysaccharide signaling. J Biol Chem 2005; 280: 11347-51.

[223] Gangloff M, Gay NJ. MD-2: the Toll 'gatekeeper' in endotoxin signaling. Trends Biochem Sci 2004; 29: 294-300.

[224] Park BS, Song DH, Kim HM, Choi BS, Lee H, Lee JO. The structural basis of lipopolysaccharide recognition by the TLR4-MD-2 complex. Nature 2009; 458: 1191-5.

[225] Hyakushima N, Mitsuzawa H, Nishitani C *et al.* Interaction of soluble form of recombinant extracellular TLR4 domain with MD-2 enables lipopolysaccharide binding and attenuates TLR4-mediated signaling. J Immunol 2004; 173: 6949-54.

[226] Visintin A, Halmen KA, Latz E, Monks BG, Golenbock DT. Pharmacological inhibition of endotoxin responses is achieved by targeting the TLR4 coreceptor, MD-2. J Immunol 2005; 175: 6465-72.

[227] Jung K, Lee JE, Kim HZ *et al.* Toll-like receptor 4 decoy, TOY, attenuates gram-negative bacterial sepsis. PloS One 2009; 4: e7403.

[228] Prohinar P, Re F, Widstrom R *et al.* Specific high affinity interactions of monomeric endotoxin.protein complexes with Toll-like receptor 4 ectodomain. J Biol Chem 2007; 282: 1010-7.

[229] Piazza M, Yu L, Teghanemt A, Gioannini T, Weiss J, Peri F. Evidence of a specific interaction between new synthetic antisepsis agents and CD14. Biochemistry 2009; 48: 12337-44.

[230] Miggin SM, Palsson-McDermott E, Dunne A *et al.* NF-kappaB activation by the Toll-IL-1 receptor domain protein MyD88 adapter-like is regulated by caspase-1. Proc Natl Acad Sci USA 2007; 104: 3372-7.

[231] Ulrichts P, Bovijn C, Lievens S, Beyaert R, Tavernier J, Peelman F. Caspase-1 targets the TLR adaptor Mal at a crucial TIR-domain interaction site. J Cell Sci; 123: 256-65.

[232] Gambari R. New trends in the development of transcription factor decoy (TFD) pharmacotherapy. Curr Drug Targets 2004; 5: 419-30.

[233] Bezzerri V, Borgatti M, Nicolis E *et al.* Transcription factor oligodeoxynucleotides to NF-kappaB inhibit transcription of IL-8 in bronchial cells. Am J Respir Cell Mol Biol 2008; 39: 86-96.

[234] Romanelli A, Pedone C, Saviano M *et al.* Molecular interactions with nuclear factor kappaB (NF-kappaB) transcription factors of a PNA-DNA chimera mimicking NF-kappaB binding sites. Eur J Biochem 2001; 268: 6066-75.

[235] Borgatti M, Finotti A, Romanelli A *et al.* Peptide nucleic acids (PNA)-DNA chimeras targeting transcription factors as a tool to modify gene expression. Curr Drug Targets 2004; 5: 735-44.

[236] Lenert PS. Classification, mechanisms of action, and therapeutic applications of inhibitory oligonucleotides for Toll-like receptors (TLR) 7 and 9. Mediators Inflamm 2010; 2010: 986596.

[237] Oglesby IK, Bray IM, Chotirmall SH *et al.* miR-126 is downregulated in cystic fibrosis airway epithelial cells and regulates TOM1 expression. J Immunol 2010; 184: 1702-9.

CHAPTER 5

COPD: Contribution of TLRs to Disease Pathogenesis

Jeroen van Bergenhenegouwen[1,2,†], Gillina Bezemer[2,†], Johan Garssen[1,2], Gert Folkerts[2,*]

[1]*Danone Research – Centre for Specialised Nutrition, Wageningen, The Netherlands and* [2]*Division of Pharmacology, Utrecht Institute for Pharmaceutical Sciences, Faculty of Science, Utrecht University, Utrecht, The Netherlands*

Abstract: Chronic obstructive pulmonary diseases (COPD) are chronic inflammatory diseases in which exacerbations can be associated with viral or bacterial infections. The innate immune system is the first line of defense against cigarette smoke, pollutants, occupational exposures, pathogens and tissue injury and is responsible for resolving infections and repairing damaged tissues. Initiation of the innate immune response is triggered by recognition of pathogen- or danger-associated molecular patterns (PAMPs and DAMPs) by pathogen recognition receptors (PRRs). The most studied PRRs are the Toll-like receptors (TLRs) which are localized either to the cell surface or within endosomes. Activation of TLRs induces the recruitment of innate immune cells, initiates tissue repair processes, and results in adaptive immune activation; importantly these processes are abnormal in COPD. Understanding the roles of TLRs in the pathogenesis of chronic inflammatory pulmonary disease, may provide novel targets for the prevention and/or treatment of COPD.

Keywords: COPD, TLR stimulation, cigarette smoke, DAMPs.

1. INTRODUCTION

1.1. COPD Prevalence

In 2001 chronic obstructive pulmonary disease (COPD) was the fifth leading cause of death in developed countries and the sixth in lower income countries, as estimated by the global burden of disease and risk factors project [1]. Due to common co-morbidities, COPD might even be underestimated as a contributor to mortality, hospital admission and increased health costs. Moreover, prevalence estimates might be influenced by methods for disease establishment [2]. According to the "international variation in the prevalence of COPD study" (BOLD), COPD remains a growing cause of morbidity and mortality and it is estimated to become the third leading cause of death worldwide by 2020 [3, 4].

1.2. Definitions and Respiratory Pathophysiology

The definition of COPD is "A preventable and treatable disease with some significant extrapulmonary effects that may contribute to the severity in individual patients. Its pulmonary component is characterized by airflow limitation that is not fully reversible. The airflow limitation is usually progressive and is associated with an abnormal inflammatory response of the lungs to noxious particles or gases." [4].

Spirometry is the standard pulmonary function test for the diagnosis of airflow limitation and is a critical measurement for the classification of severity of COPD according to the Global Initiative for Chronic Obstructive Lung Disease (GOLD) stages (Table **1**). The common irreversible nature of COPD can be analyzed by post-bronchodilator spirometry in which COPD patients typically do not show an improvement of the forced expiratory volume in one second (FEV1) compared to pre bronchodilator measurements. Asthma patients usually do respond to bronchodilators, however it should be noted that the classification of the disease is intended to be applicable on a population level, not on the evaluation in individual patients [5]. Due to overlap in disease symptoms, misclassification of airway diseases can occur.

*****Address correspondence to Gert Folkerts:** Division of Pharmacology, Utrecht Institute for Pharmaceutical Sciences, Faculty of Science, Utrecht University, Utrecht, The Netherlands; E-mail: G.Folkerts@uu.nl

[†]Both authors equally contributed to this article.

Catherine M. Greene (Ed)

Table 1: COPD Classification

COPD Severity	Post FEV$_1$/FVC	FEV$_1$ % pred	Symptoms
Stage I: mild	< 0.7	≥ 80%	Chronic cough, sputum production
Stage II: moderate	< 0.7	50-80	Shortness of breath, cough and sputum production
Stage III: severe	< 0.7	30-50	Greater shortness of breath, reduced exercise capacity, fatigue and repeated exacerbations
Stage IV: very severe	< 0.7	<30	Chronic respiratory failure (PaO2 <8 kPa, PaCO2 >6.7kPa at sea level)

FVC = forced vital capacity, which is the volume of air that can forcibly be exhaled after full inhalation, FEV$_1$ = forced expiratory volume in one second, which is the maximum volume of air that can be exhaled during one second, post = post bronchodilator, %pred=% predicted, PaO$_2$ = arterial partial pressure of oxygen, PaCO$_2$ = arterial partial pressure of CO$_2$.

The inflammatory responses which underlie the different conditions, however do differ. By experimental *in vivo* and *in vitro* studies as well as by using patient material such as bronchoalveolar lavage fluid (BALF), sputum and tissue, it has become clear that COPD pathology includes distinct inflammatory patterns [6]. Cell types that play a crucial role in COPD are alveolar macrophages [7], neutrophils, dendritic cells, CD8+ T lymphocytes and B lymphocytes. Eosinophilic infiltration does occur in COPD however in contrast to asthma it makes only a minor contribution to the overall pathology [8]. In patients with severe COPD adaptive immune cells, such as B cells, can form lymphoid follicles in the airway walls however, their pathogenic role is not clear [9]. Both immune cells and epithelial cells secrete mediators that contribute to the disease process. The immune pathology of asthma is defined in part by a deregulated pattern of Th2 cytokine release [10], whereas COPD has a predominant Th1 response.

Important chemokines in COPD are IL-8 (CXCL8) for neutrophilic granulocyte attraction and the mononuclear cell attractants CCL2 and CCL3 (MIP1) [11]. Other key mediators are pro-inflammatory cytokines such as IL-6 and TNF-α. A complete overview of mediators in COPD can be found in Barnes' detailed review [12]. The inflammatory response is usually accompanied by goblet cell hyperplasia and mucus hyper-secretion.

Upon reoccurring irritation of the airway epithelium, the inflammation and mucus accumulation may become chronic leading to chronic bronchitis the progression of which may cause irreversible morphological changes of the peripheral airspaces of the lung. One such change is airway wall thickening of the bronchi and the bronchiole, initiated by repair and remodeling processes [11]. Persistent inflammation in the adjacent air spaces of the respiratory bronchioles, alveolar ducts, and alveoli may cause destruction of airway walls which results in a permanent increase in the size of the air spaces, also known as emphysema. This is a feature that is typically seen in severe COPD patients with alpha-1 antitrypsin deficiency [13]. Alpha-1 antitrypsin is a protease inhibitor which is important in maintaining the lung parenchymal integrity. This finding has led to the hypothesis that an imbalance between extracellular matrix (ECM) degrading enzymes and proteins that oppose this activity underlies the early development of emphysema [14, 15]. This theory is also known as the protease:anti-protease hypothesis.

Although COPD affects the lungs, significant systemic effects do occur. There is abundant evidence that COPD is correlated with cardiovascular disease, skeletal muscle dysfunction, systemic inflammation, nutritional abnormalities and weight loss [16-18].

2. TOLL-LIKE RECEPTORS

In this chapter we aim to discuss the role of Toll like receptors (TLRs) in COPD. The TLR family is a member of the Pattern Recognition Receptors (PRRs). TLRs are involved in both innate and adaptive immunity, both of which are implicated in COPD pathology [19-21]. The contribution of TLRs to fungal defense was first described in *Drosophila melanogaster*. Later, a family of mammalian proteins was discovered, sharing structural similarities with *Drosophila* Toll and these were named Toll "like" receptors. So far, thirteen TLRs have been identified in humans and mice. TLRs are characterized by a diverse extracellular, leucine rich repeat (LRR) domain and a less diverse intracellular Toll/IL-1R (TIR) domain [19]. The various LRR domains are involved in the recognition of exogenous compounds such as viral and bacterial products as well as endogenous derived materials (Tables **2** and **3**). TLR2 and TLR4 can be classified as lipid recognizing receptors (LPS and lipoproteins respectively) whereas TLR5 primarily recognizes the protein component of bacterial flagellae. Nucleic acids derived from viruses or bacteria can be recognized by TLR3 and TLR7-9 [21]. Most TLRs are localized on the cell surface of various types of cells however some TLRs such as TLR3, TLR7, TLR8 and TLR9 are localized in the cellular endosome.

Table 2: Exogenous TLRs Agonists

TLR	Exogenous Agonists
TLR2	Bacterial lipoproteins and glycolipids Cigarette smoke Air pollutants
TLR2/TLR1	Diacyl lipopeptides
TLR2/TLR6	Triacyl lipopeptides
TLR3	Double stranded viral RNA
TLR4	Lipopolysaccharides (LPS) Cigarette smoke Diesel exhaust particles
TLR5	Bacterial flagellin
TLR7	Single stranded viral RNA Imidazoquinoline (anti-viral compounds)
TLR8	Single stranded viral RNA
TLR9	Unmethylated bacterial CpG-DNA Cigarette smoke
TLR10	Unknown
TLR11	Profilin

Upon stimulation by an agonist, TLRs activate different sets of downstream signaling pathways. Detailed overviews of TLR signaling can be found in various reviews [19, 21-23]. Briefly, downstream signaling depends on the adaptor molecule that is recruited to the intracellular TLR-TIR domain [19]. All TLRs except TLR3 signal *via* the shared MyD88 adaptor molecule followed by subsequent association with the tumor necrosis factor receptor associated factors (TRAFs) or with kinases such as the IL-1RI-associated protein kinases (IRAKs) and the transforming growth factor β activated kinase (TAK). TLR3 signals *via* the TIR-domain-containing adapter-inducing interferon-β (TRIF) adaptor molecule, which is shared with TLR4. The downstream TLR signaling cascade leads to pro-inflammatory gene transcription and the production of various cytokines which results in a specific cellular response (Fig. **1**).

Table 3: Endogenous TLRs Agonists

TLR	Endogenous Agonists
TLR2	HMGB1, HSP70, EDN, HA, HS
TLR4	HMGB1, HSP60, HSP70, EDN, HA, HS, Fibrinogen, S100 protein

HMGB1, High-mobility group protein B1; HSP, Heat shock protein; EDN, Eosinophil-derived neurotoxin; HA, Hyaluronan; HS, Heparan-sulphate.

Due to the gas exchange function of the lungs, the respiratory tract is constantly exposed to the external environment. Alveolar macrophages (AMs) and pulmonary epithelium form the first line of defense in the lung, and are thus directly exposed to environmental factors including microbes. Airway epithelial cells and alveolar macrophages as well as neutrophils and dendritic cells express functional active TLRs [24-26]; these cell types play a role in COPD. Here we will focus on the TLRs and TLR agonists that specifically contribute to COPD disease pathology. Moreover, TLR polymorphisms and TLR expression will be discussed.

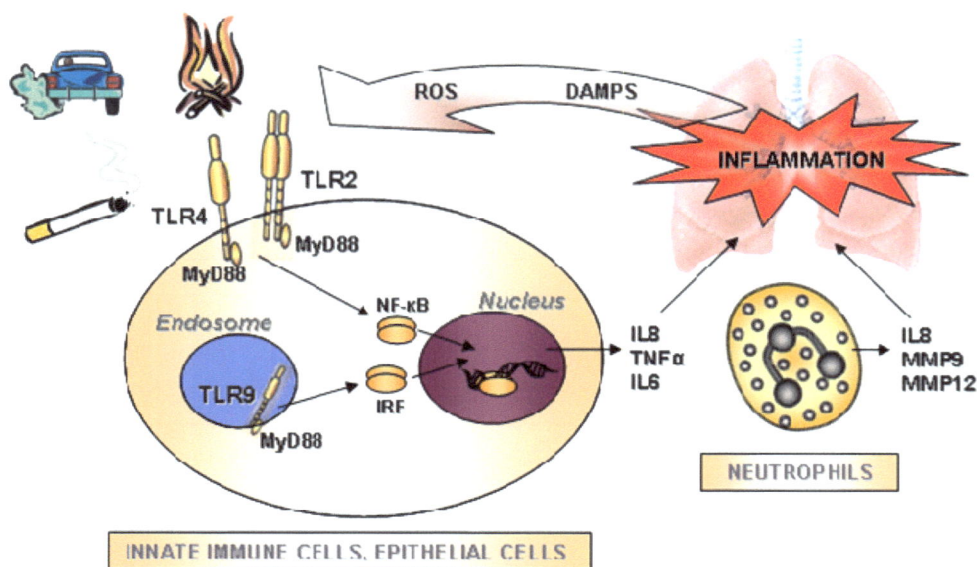

Figure 1: Mechanisms regulating pulmonary inflammation in COPD.

3. EXOGENOUS TLR STIMULI

3.1. Cigarette Smoke

According to the COPD definition, noxious particles and gases are the trigger for the abnormal inflammatory response seen in COPD patients. COPD risk factors are listed in Table **4**. Cigarette smoking is the best studied risk factor for COPD. Cigarette smoke (CS) contains over 4,500 components in its gaseous and particulate phases which encompass a major source of particles, free radicals and reactive chemicals. Many of these components have been shown to modulate the function of immune cells both *in vivo* and *in vitro*. CS components activate and increase the numbers of AMs [27]. In concert with activated epithelium, this will lead to an inflammatory response and subsequent tissue damage. The CS-induced inflammatory response encompasses neutrophil, monocyte, dendritic cell and T-lymphocyte attracting factors, and the secretion of pro-inflammatory mediators, reactive oxygen species (ROS) and proteolytic enzymes all of which are important in COPD [28, 29].

Tobacco leaves contain bacterial residue components such as LPS and CpG-DNA known as TLR4 and TLR9 agonists, respectively [30-32]. Studies from Hasday and colleagues have shown that LPS is present in the mainstream and to a lesser extend in the sidestream of cigarette smoke [30]. Karimi *et al.* demonstrated for the first time that TLR4 is involved in CS induced cytokine production [33]. Later Sarir *et al.* showed that TLR4 surface expression is downregulated upon short term CS medium (CSM) exposure, which could be explained by internalization of TLR4. The subsequent intracellular TLR4 pool might be further up-regulated due to an increase in TLR4 mRNA. CSM furthermore increased IL-8 mRNA and protein *via* TLR4 in a ROS-dependent matter [34]. Maes and colleagues have studied the role of TLR4 in cigarette smoke induced pulmonary inflammation using TLR4 knockout mice. They showed that bronchoalveolar neutrophil, dendritic cell and lymphocyte levels were decreased in TLR4-deficient mice compared to wild type mice upon subacute cigarette smoke exposure [35]. Pace *et al.* also concluded from their studies that cigarette smoke alters the expression and the activation of TLR4 *via* the preferential release of IL-8, which may contribute to the accumulation of neutrophils within the airways of smokers

[36]. More evidence for a role of TLR4 in smoking-related COPD comes from a study by Speletas and coworkers in which they investigated the association between common TLR polymorphisms (TLR2-R753Q, TLR4-D299G, and TLR4-T399I) and the development of COPD in a group of 240 heavy smokers [37]. They reported that dysfunctional polymorphisms of innate immune genes such as TLR4-T399I can affect the development of COPD in smokers, whilst a study by Sabroe confirms a possible effect of the Asp299Gly TLR4 polymorphism on the severity of COPD. At population level however it is unlikely that this polymorphism has a major impact on the severity of COPD. Experimental data has shown that TLR4 deficiency in mice results in the spontaneous development of lung emphysema, indicating an involvement of TLR4 in normal tissue homeostasis [38].

TLR2 expression is also influenced by cigarette smoke. Droemann's group showed decreased TLR2 expression on macrophages derived from cigarette smokers and COPD patients [39]. Furthermore, TLR2 mRNA and protein expression was not increased after LPS stimulation of the macrophages of smokers and COPD patients in contrast to nonsmokers. However, Pons *et al.* reported an up-regulation of TLR2 in monocytes from COPD patients [40]. This might seem conflicting with Droemann's findings, however, the cells used in the latter study were peripheral blood-derived monocytes, suggesting a difference between alveolar and systemic effects in terms of TLR expression.

More recently Mortaz and colleagues focused on the effect that cigarette smoke has on human TLR9 signaling [31, 41, 42]. Their *in vitro* work points to the possible involvement of TLR9 in cigarette smoke induced IL-8 production by neutrophils and plasmacytoid DCs. This is currently being investigated *in vivo*.

Table 4: COPD risk factors

Cigarette smoke
Indoor air pollutants as a consequence of the burning of biomass fuel derived from plant or animal sources.
Outdoor air pollutants from traffic and industry.
Occupational exposures: (in)organic dusts in crop and animal farming; coal, rock, concrete, brick, gold, iron, steel dusts and fumes exposure during construction work, mining and manufacturing; chemical exposures in amongst others plastic, leather, food and rubber industry
Repeated respiratory tract infections and a history of respiratory diseases such as tuberculosis and chronic asthma
Genetic susceptibility: alpha-1 antitrypsin deficiency, ECM homeostasis genes, ROS genes, TLR4-T399I Polymorphism
Poor nutrition and low socioeconomic status.

3.2. TLR Stimuli in Non-Smokers with COPD

The prevalence of COPD amongst non-smokers is also considerable, especially in developing countries [43]. Amongst the worldwide COPD patient population, 25-45% of patients have never smoked, which confirms the finding that smoking does not fully explain the variations in disease prevalence. There is growing evidence for the association between the burning of biomass fuel and the development or aggravation of COPD [44-47]. Biomass fuels have a low combustion efficiency resulting in higher pollution when compared with kerosene, coal or gas fuel. Moreover biomass fuel is especially hazardous because half of the world's population is exposed to its smoke [43]. Other pollutants that have been associated with COPD originate from traffic and industry but also on the work floor various particulates can be found that have been linked to COPD [43, 48-50] (Table **4**).

There is still limited data available on the possible role of pollutants other than cigarette smoke on TLR signaling. Some associations have been made between organic dust exposure and TLR expression and/or signaling. A study of Bailey and colleagues, for example, shows that TLR2 gene and protein expression is up regulated in cultured bronchial epithelial cells derived from hog confinement workers who are at risk of developing COPD [51]. Inoue and colleagues studied the effect of diesel exhaust particles (DEP) on TLR4 signaling in the airways of TLR4-deficient and wild-type mice [52]. Total cell levels and neutrophil influx into the bronchoalveolar lavage fluid of DEP exposed mice was significantly decreased in the TLR4 mutant mice compared to the wild-type animals. Inhaled ozone also alters the distribution of TLR4 on alveolar macrophages and it increases the functional response of alveolar macrophages to endotoxin [53]. Ozone is thus able to modulate innate immune responses *via* TLR4. A study from Shoenfelt and coworkers indicates the involvement of TLR2 and TLR4 in the immune response against fine and coarse air pollution particles [54]. This study demonstrated a shared use of MyD88 by fine and coarse air pollution particles. It can however not be excluded, that the responses induced by particulate matter of different sizes collected at different locations, may be triggered by other TLRs or even by other PRRs. Becker and colleagues reported an indirect effect of particulate air pollutants on TLR2 and 4 expression and signaling in human primary epithelial cell cultures *via* endogenous TLR ligands [55].

3.3. Pathogen-Associated Molecular Patterns (PAMPs)

Acute viral infection in childhood is a risk factor for the development of COPD in later life [56]. Also, the majority of COPD exacerbations are associated with viral and/or bacterial respiratory tract infections [57-60]. Exacerbations are episodes of disease worsening and are common among COPD patients. Symptoms include increased sputum production, increased cough and wheeze. Lung function and quality of life of COPD patients significantly declines as a result of frequent exacerbations [60, 61].

Molecules derived from microbes and viruses are often referred to as pathogen associated molecular patterns (PAMPs). TLRs are involved in the defense against bacterial and viral pathogens by sensing these PAMPs and it can thus be hypothesized that TLRs play an important role during disease exacerbations. To date, only a few studies have addressed this question. Stowell and colleagues investigated the role of TLR3 in virus induced pulmonary disease exacerbations [62]. They found that compared to wild-type animals, TLR3 knockout animals had a milder lung inflammation and reduced epithelial cell hypertrophy following intranasal administration of the TLR3 ligand poly (I:C), a synthetic double stranded RNA analogue. The hypothesis that TLR3 activation is involved in virally-induced COPD exacerbations, is also supported by Sajjan and colleagues [63]. They additionally gave insight into mechanisms by which existing infections in COPD patients can aggravate viral susceptibility. They showed that *Haemophilus influenza* infection increases lung cell TLR3 and ICAM-1 expression which helps explain the enhanced binding and potentiation of a subsequently administered rhinovirus.

TLR2 and TLR4 have also been linked to bacterial exacerbations in COPD. Tokairin and colleagues showed that animals with elastase-induced lung emphysema had a significantly increased inflammatory response to streptococcal infection, compared to non emphysematous animals [64]. They related enhanced TLR2 and 4 expression on alveolar macrophages from emphysematous lungs to the fact that these animals showed an enhanced response upon infection.

TLR7 and 8 are known to play a role in virus-induced neutrophil activation and IL-8 production, thus possibly having some part to play in COPD exacerbations [65]. Triggering of TLR8 during viral-induced disease exacerbations, has been reported to be potentiated by oxidative stress [66].

Although CS has many pro-inflammatory effects, it can also act as an immunosuppressive and anti-inflammatory agents in some contexts [67, 68] leading to compromised sensing of bacterial or viral components [69-72], or ineffective phagocytosis of bacteria [73, 74] and apoptotic cells [75, 76]. CS may therefore aggravate exacerbations during viral or bacterial infections. Mortaz and co workers gave mechanistic insight into how CS can augment virally-induced COPD pathogenesis. CS extract down regulates the release of IFN-α and other pro-inflammatory cytokines by plasmacytoid dendritic cells which might explain why smokers are more susceptible for viral infections [41].

3.4. Reactive Oxygen Species (ROS)

A common feature of the different particulate, viral and bacterial exposures that have been linked to COPD is that they induce oxidative stress, which is a key feature of the disease pathology [77]. Local oxidative stress originates either directly from free radicals containing particulates or indirectly from oxygen species that are released from cells. Cigarette smoke contains high amounts of ROS which can mainly be found in the gaseous phase (14.3-39.0 nmol H_2O_2/l) and originates from the combustion process [78]. ROS cannot be eliminated by filters and will thus be inhaled upon cigarette smoking. The exogenous derived oxidant burden on the lungs can induce damage through multiple mechanisms. It can directly oxidize cellular lipids and DNA and it can inactivate important proteins such as alpha-1 antitrypsin. Subsequently it can lead to immune cell activation thereby inducing an additional oxidative potential. Oxidative stress regulates specific signal transduction pathways and histone modifications that are involved in lung inflammation [79]. Although the lung epithelium and lung lining fluid are equipped to cope with oxidative stress *via* the excretion and presence of non-enzymatic and enzymatic antioxidants, in susceptible individuals these defenses might be overwhelmed leading to a compromised epithelial barrier, impaired mucociliary clearance, cell death and possibly a permanently altered epithelium [68, 80, 81]. Polymorphisms in detoxifying enzymes such as glutathione S-transferase, heme oxygenase 1, superoxide dismutase and possibly others are thus likely to be involved in the disease pathology [15].

TLR signaling pathways are dependent on ROS [82-84]. Lipid-recognizing TLR2 and TLR4 receptors as well as the protein sensing TLR5 and nucleic-acid sensing TLR3 and TLR7-9 are all oxidative stress sensitive. TLR2 has recently even been reported to be essential for oxidant sensing during inflammation [85] (Fig. **1**).

4. ENDOGENOUS TLR STIMULI

Patients suffering from a variety of chronic lung diseases show enhanced numbers of apoptotic cells and fragmented extracellular matrix components (ECM) in their lungs. This might be due to increased apoptosis as well as to impaired clearance by alveolar macrophages [75, 76, 86-89]. Apoptotic cells, when not cleared quickly enough, will undergo a process called secondary necrosis and lose cell wall integrity resulting in the release of immunogenic intracellular content [90]. Moreover, anti-inflammatory processes which are normally associated with the clearance of apoptotic cells are not initiated [91]. In sum, COPD patients are prone to undergo secondary inflammation due to impaired efferocytosis [87, 91, 92]. Polly Matzinger was the first to suggest that the immune system might become activated by self-generated alarm signals [93]. In a normal situation, cells die by controlled mechanisms, in the case of abnormal cell death or distressed cells, alarm signals are generated. These alarm signals might be generated by intracellular content in the case of necrotic cells, or any molecule made or modified by stressed cells [94]. All in all, it can be reasoned that damage communication is not based upon how the cell dies, but more on whether or not the released intracellular content is able to start an inflammatory chain of events, which might lead to tissue-repair or exaggeration of the inflammatory response.

Damage associated molecular patterns or DAMPs were originally described as any molecule that is not normally exposed during, after, or because of injury or damage [95]. DAMPs can be subdivided into molecules from microbial origin, as the aforementioned PAMPs, and endogenous DAMPs, in some cases also referred to as alarmins [93]. Since DAMPs cannot be synthesized or replenished by dead cells the pro-inflammatory activity of dead cells decays over time. Furthermore, the biologic activities of DAMPs are temporally and spatially controlled due to the fact that most are derived from intracellular content and are redox-sensitive. Inside cells and nuclei there is a highly reducing environment, while outside the cell it is highly oxidative. This difference means that DAMPs that were protected from oxidation inside the cells become oxidized very rapidly in the extracellular milieu. In most cases the DAMP will have lost its biological activity, while in some cases the DAMP will gain biological activity. If the balance tips toward exacerbation instead of resolution, more cells undergo necrosis. Molecules like oxidoreductases and non-protein thiols, responsible inside the cells for maintaining the reducing environment, will start to reduce the oxidative extracellular content and therefore increase the biological activity of DAMPs [96, 97]. DAMPs that are not classical cytokines but have adjuvant activity should fulfill certain criteria. First, they should be rapidly released in response to infection or injury and they should be active as a highly purified molecule. Second, they should have chemotactic and activating properties on cells of the innate immune system at physiological levels. Third, inhibiting the DAMP should modulate the biological activity of the dead or injured cell [93, 98, 99]. Below we will describe those DAMPs that contribute to the pathogenesis of COPD and are reported to utilize TLR signaling to mediate their biological activity. For a more complete overview regarding DAMPs and receptors involved, see references [96-99].

4.1. Intracellular DAMPS

HMGB1

One of the best known DAMPs released by cells that die in a traumatic way is High-mobility group protein B1 (HMGB1), also known as amphoterin [98-100].

In COPD patients HMGB1 expression is correlated with inflammatory and clinical parameters. Bronchoalveolar lavage levels of HMGB1 positively correlate with IL-1β and negatively with FEV_1 [101]. HMGB1 is both a nuclear factor and an excreted protein. Inside the nucleus it is loosely bound to chromatin, outside it is bound with high affinity to the receptor for advanced glycation end-products (RAGE) and functions as a potent mediator of inflammation and cell migration [102, 103]. When cells undergo apoptosis HMGB1 becomes tightly bound to chromatin. In contrast, when cells undergo trauma-induced necrosis HMGB1 is released from binding chromatin and leaks into the extracellular space [104]. In addition, HMGB1 is actively secreted by immuno-stimulated macrophages [105, 106] and natural killer (NK) cells [107, 108]. Highly purified HMGB1 reveals that HMGB1 by itself is not proinflammatory [109-111] but is able to recruit cells and promote tissue regeneration requiring activation of RAGE [112, 113]. HMGB proteins function as carrier proteins in a way that they have not only been found to be complexed with intracellular DNA, RNA, transcriptional factors, steroid receptors and viral proteins [114], but are also reported to bind with high affinity to extracellular proteins, such as cytokines and DNA-containing immune complexes [110, 111]. Furthermore, HMGB1 is found to bind LPS [115], nucleosomes [116], phosphatidylserine [117] and sulfoglycolipids [118].

It seems unlikely that only one receptor is capable of discriminating between such varieties of HMGB1 complexes. If we regard HMGB1 as a carrier protein the different actions of HMGB1 might therefore be regulated at the receptor level. Indeed, many reports have suggested different receptors for HMGB1 and this might be the reason for the apparent dichotomy between two sets of activities (inflammation *versus* regeneration) [98, 102, 119].

With regard to enhancing inflammatory conditions:

TLR2 and TLR4 have been suggested as receptors for HMGB1 and mediate its inflammatory action *via* stimulating neutrophils, monocytes and macrophages to secrete pro-inflammatory mediators [120, 121]. When added intraperitoneally to mice, HMGB1 elicits an inflammatory response which was ameliorated in TLR4 knockout mice but enhanced in TLR2 knockout mice [122]. In contrast to the response in primary cells, when HMGB1 was added to human embryonic kidney (HEK) TLR transfected cells, only TLR2 transfected cells responded to HMGB1 with increased IL-8 production [123]. Some conflicting data was reported by Park *et al.*, as they could find increased NFκB activity in TLR2 as well as TLR4 transfected HEK cells. In addition, by using fluorescent resonance energy transfer techniques and immunoprecipitation they showed that HMGB1 was bound to TLR2 and TLR4 [124]. HMGB1 nucleosome complexes have been found to have inflammatory activities *via* its interaction with TLR2 [116]. Binding of HMGB1 to phophatidylserine is found to play a role in platelet activation [117], and inhibiting phagocytosis of apoptotic neutrophils adding to the inflammatory condition [125]. Complexes of IL-1 and HMGB1 proteins are found to be more potent in stimulating cells as IL-1 signaling alone, enhancing inflammatory conditions [110].

Furthermore, with regard to its function as a carrier protein for nucleic acids, HMGB1 facilitates binding to the more specific nucleic acid sensing PRRs which results in enhanced immune activation [126].

With regard to regenerative signaling:

Proteoglycans and glycolipids are found to bind to HMGB1, and thought to play a role in cell motility regulation and cell migration control [127-129]. When no ligands bind to HMGB1, and HGMB1 subsequently binds RAGE this has been shown to enhance migration and proliferation of smooth muscle cells [130] and stem cell migration, homing and development [131-133].

Heat Shock Proteins (HSPs)

HSPs are a family of proteins that are essential for maintaining normal cell function by assisting in folding, assembly and translocation of newly synthesized proteins. Furthermore, HSPs are involved in antigen presentation and cross-presentation *via* chaperoned delivery of antigenic peptides to MHC class I and class II molecules which involves the HSP-receptor, CD91[134, 135]. HSP family members share at least two common domains: (i) an ATP binding domain and (ii) a peptide binding domain that binds exposed hydrophobic residues. Under normal physiological condition HSPs are expressed at low levels, upon cellular stress their expression is markedly increased [136, 137]. In accordance, patients suffering from COPD were found to have elevated HSP serum levels [138]. Necrotic cell death, in contrast to apoptotic cell death, results in the release of HSPs in the extracellular milieu [139]. In addition, HSPs might be actively released as part of the protein content of exosomes [140, 141]. TLR4 and TLR2 have both been implicated as receptors for endogenous HSPs [142]. HSP60 was able to induce inflammatory reactions in macrophages from C57BL/6 and C3H/HeN mice but not from C3H/HeJ mice which have a non-functional TLR4 mutant receptor [143]. In addition, TLR2 and TLR4 mediated endocytosis of HSP60, or recognition of extracellular HSP70 was found to be needed to initiate TLR signaling cascades [144-146]. In contrast, although the above suggests TLRs as receptors for HSPs, bacterial PAMPs or ATP contaminants of HSP preparations were found to be the actual mediators of effect [147, 148]. Moreover, highly purified preparations of HSP60 and HSP70 were found to have no cytokine effects and were unable to induce cell activation [149, 150].

S100 Proteins

The S100 protein family encompasses multifunctional signaling proteins that are involved in the regulation of diverse cellular processes such as contraction, motility, cell growth, differentiation, cell cycle progression, transcription, and secretion. An excellent overview of the diversity of S100 family members and their functions is described by Marenholz *et al.* [151]. Here we will focus on just two family members in particular that are specifically linked to immune function and TLR-signaling; S100A8 (calgranulin A) and S100A9 (calgranulin B) [152, 153].

Clinical data from BAL fluid obtained from patients with lung disorders revealed that concentrations of S100A8 and S100A9 were elevated in smokers with COPD *versus* asymptomatic smokers. Moreover, S100A8 protein levels were increased when asymptomatic smokers were compared to non-smokers. In contrast, no difference in S100A8, S100A9 levels were detected when induced sputum of COPD patients was compared to healthy subjects [154]

S100A8 is the active component in the S100A8-S100A9 complex, whereas S100A9 functions as a modulator of the activity of S100A8. TLR4 has been identified as the receptor for either S100A8 and the S100A8-S100A9 complex [155]. Both proteins are specifically released during the activation of phagocytes and the subsequent formation of S100A8 and S100A9 complexes is correlated to disease activity in many inflammatory disorders [156]. In addition, S100A8-S100A9 proteins are not only involved in amplifying the inflammatory responses of antigen presenting cells, but are also capable of activating endothelial cells, chondrocytes and tumor cells [153].

Eosinophil-Derived Neurotoxin

The RNase A super-family consists of members that all have ribonuclease activity, and have been found to be involved in host defense. More than one of the members of the RNase A family have some documented bactericidal or anti-viral activity [157]. Eosinophil-derived neurotoxin (EDN; RNase2) is produced by eosinophils and placental epithelial cells. In addition to its release by degranulation of eosinophils, stimulated neutrophils and macrophages can be induced to express EDN. COPD patients show a substantial degree of eosinophilic inflammation, even in patients without a history of allergy or asthma [158]. In addition, markers for eosinophilic inflammation are found to be predictive for COPD disease progression [159]. Based on the findings that EDN can act as a chemo-attractant for, and stimulator of immature DCs, Yang *et al.* have classified EDN as a DAMP [160-163]. In addition, they found that EDN signaling was

TLR2 mediated. However, the precise role and mode of action of EDN in inflammation still remains obscure [164].

4.2. Extracellular DAMPs

Extracellular Matrix Components

Extracellular matrix (ECM) components are significantly involved in the structure and function of the lung. They mainly consist of glycosaminoglycan (GAG) molecules which form highly charged 3D structures. In addition to maintaining tissue structure they also play a significant role in lung function by means of regulation of hydration and water homeostasis. Furthermore, GAGs are involved in modulation of inflammatory responses, lung tissue repair and remodeling. There are two main types of GAGs: Hyaluronic acid or hyaluronan (HA) a non-sulphated GAG that remains non-covalently attached to cells, and the sulphated GAGs (heparin, heparan sulphate, chondrotin sulphate, dermatan sulphate and keratin sulphate) that remain attached to cells *via* their covalent binding to a protein core which protrudes from the cell membrane.

A hallmark of tissue injury is increased turnover of ECM. Asthma, pulmonary fibrosis and emphysema are three chronic lung diseases that are associated with abnormal ECM turnover [92]. The inflammatory milieu, by means of oxidants and other mechanisms, creates an imbalance in ECM degradation and synthesis. A subsequent failure to clear ECM degradation products will result in an unremitting inflammation [165]. The role of ECM in health and disease has received a lot of attention in recent years and has been reviewed by Jiang *et al.* [166], and Papakonstantinou *et al.* [167]. Here we will focus on the described interactions of ECM components with TLRs.

Hyaluronan

HA is the most abundant non-sulphated GAG in the lung ECM. It is synthesized from the cell membrane by hyaluronan synthases which extrude HA into the extracellular space by polymerization at the reducing intracellular end.

In patients with mild to severe COPD enhanced levels of HA were detected in the sputum and found to be correlated to disease severity and markers of inflammation. In addition, lungs of patients with severe COPD show an increased expression of hyaluronidase which suggests an enhanced HA turnover [168]. Animals exposed to CS display an acute increased deposition of HA in the alveolar and bronchial walls, further CS exposure results in an increased accumulation of HA fragments which correlate with CS-induced changes in genes associated with HA modulation [169]. Turnover of high molecular weight HA (HMW-HA) into low molecular weight HA (LMW-HA) is mediated by hyaluronidases present in various tissues, including the lung. Upon inflammation a shift in the balance between HMW-HA and LWM-HA occurs which adds to the inflammatory cycle [166, 170-172]. CD44 is the major cell receptor for HA and is present on both hematopoietic cells as well as parenchymal cells such as epithelial cells and fibroblasts [173].

In normal physiological situations the majority of LMW-HA product is cleared *via* lymphatic transport to the liver where it is degraded; left over LMW-HA is cleared by alveolar macrophages. Under inflammatory conditions the removal of LMW-HA is critically dependant on CD44 present on hematopoietic cells [165]. Conflicting evidence is to be found in the literature regarding the critical receptors for mediating the response to HA and HA fragments.

Although CD44-TLR2 receptor complexes have been found to play a protective role in TLR-mediated inflammation, this was not dependent on HA binding [174]. Receptor complexes formed by CD44-MD2-TLR4 are functionally involved in the biological activity of LMW-HA, but the presence of CD44 was not critical and may function more to enhance or stabilize the interaction of HA with TLR4 [175]. In addition, TLR4 but not TLR2 or CD44 binding of HA fragments was able to induce dendritic cell (DC) maturation and initiate a inflammatory response [176]. In contrast, Scheibner *et al.* found that the inflammatory response by DCs to LWM-HA was critically dependent on TLR2 and this could be blocked by the addition of HMW-HA [177]. Moreover, data obtained by Jiang *et al.* implicates both TLR2 and TLR4 to be necessary for the recognition of HA and HA fragments in the regulation of lung injury and repair [178].

Overall, it can be noted that the more work on HA recognition that appears, the more complicated it gets. Differences found in the literature might be related to the purity, source and structure of HA, fragment size of HA and the type of cells used in the various experiments. Future work should address these issues to clarify the role of the different receptors in HA signaling.

Heparan Sulphate

Heparan sulphate (HS) is the most abundantly expressed sulphated GAG within the lung ECM. It is commonly found on virtually every cell of the body in a cell-surface bound manner, but it can also be excreted as a soluble GAG. HS chains at the cell surface can be attached to transmembrane proteins like syndecans and glypicans, among others, and act as co-receptors for or signal *via* G-protein coupled receptors or glycosylphosphatidylinositol-linked proteins. The HS chains, due to their vast structural diversity, are able to bind and interact with a wide variety of proteins, such as growth factors, chemokines, morphogens, extracellular matrix components, and enzymes [179]. Neutrophils, upon activation, release heparanases which are able to degrade HS in the ECM [180]. In accordance, COPD patients were found to have elevated levels of cleaved HS products at the epithelium [181]. Binding of soluble HS to murine DCs was able to induce DC maturation mediated *via* TLR4 [182]. In addition, when soluble HS was intraperitoneally-injected into mice they developed systemic inflammatory response syndrome, which was dependent on TLR4 [183].

4.3. Extracellur DAMPs (not ECM)

Fibrinogen

Fibrinogen (FBG) is a well-characterized acute phase reactant (APR) that is up-regulated as part of the innate immune response to inflammation [184].

A population based study on the systemic inflammation of COPD reports a correlation between C-reactive protein and IL-6, IL-8, alpha-1 antitrypsin and fibrinogen as systemic inflammation biomarkers [185]. Although the liver is the main producer of APR proteins, several reports have found that under inflammatory conditions several different types of epithelial cells are able to synthesize and release fibrinogen in a polarized manner [186-189]. The appearance of fibrinogen in the ECM is thought to be beneficial to tissue repair processes [190]. Recognition of extra-vascular FBG by TLR4 has been found to stimulate monocytes and macrophages to release inflammatory markers, which are thought to increase immune surveillance at sites of inflammation [191-193].

5. COPD TREATMENT

The first step in COPD management is the reduction of risk factors [4]: smoking cessation, minimizing occupational exposures and to lessen exposure to other indoor and outdoor pollutants. Risk reduction such as smoking cessation, is currently the only effective therapy for reduction of COPD progression [194].

The control of stable COPD is the second component of disease management. There are several pharmacologic treatments available that can help to decrease symptoms or complications; however, none of the existing medications for COPD have proven to diminish the long term reduction in lung function. The main symptomatic COPD treatment is the administration of one or more aerosolized bronchodilators such as β2-agonists, anti-cholinergics or methylxanthines. Depending on disease severity, bronchodilators can be supplemented with inhaled glucocorticosteroid therapy upon GOLD stage III and stage IV (Table **1**). Long term oral glucocorticosteroid therapy does cause significant side effects such as muscle weakness and a decrease in muscle functionality. Other treatments include influenza vaccine and pneumococcal polysaccharide vaccine, exercise training and oxygen therapy.

As described previously, COPD patients often experience disease exacerbations, which form the third component of disease management [4]. Inhaled bronchodilators in combination with glucocorticosteroids are the most effective treatment for exacerbations. If there are clear signs that the exacerbation is caused by an infection, antibiotic treatment can be beneficial.

The inflammatory response used in the defense against microbes, such as generation of reactive oxygen species and elaboration of proteases also damages surrounding cells and extracellular matrix components. During microbial infection, the damage to the surrounding tissues might be a small price to pay. However, in situations of sterile tissue injury, inflammation might be more costly and do more harm than good. In addition, when the body is not allowed enough recovery time from the sterile insult (*e.g.* smoking), acute inflammatory processes might become a major factor in the development of a chronic inflammatory status.

It would be interesting therapeutically if it were possible to block these responses to sterile inflammation. However, this should be done without affecting the inflammatory response against microbes, or interfering with the healing and repair processes. This might be achieved if it were possible to inhibit the inflammatory response to dead cells or ECM fragments.

5.1. Targetting TLRs in COPD

TLRs might be considered as therapeutic targets for COPD given that they are implicated in mediating the biological activity of components released by necrotic or dying cells and ECM fragments.

TLR specific treatment can be classified in three clusters [195]: agonists (induce protective immunity), agonist adjuvancy (antitumor treatment, Th1/Th2 balance and vaccination) and antagonists (down regulation of excessive inflammation). Targetting TLRs could be useful because the primary function of TLRs is to induce cytokines which lead to an inflammatory response. In this view TLRs offer a set of targets that are involved in the onset (CS, airpollution and DAMPs), during exarcebations (bacterial and/or viral infection) and throughout the chronic low grade systemic inflammation often seen in COPD patients. Different approaches can be undertaken to target them. Neutralizing antibodies might be possible for surface TLRs. Other TLRs might be targetable by small molecule antagonists although the efficacy and specificity is still under investigation. Kinases involved in the TLR signal transduction might also be inhibited, but care should be taken to avoid unwanted immunosupression due to blocking multiple TLRs and other receptor mediated responses [196].

It is well established that TLRs play a crucial role as a first line of defense against microbial infection [197]. Triggering of TLRs using agonists may boost the protective inflammatory response that destroys pathogens and protects the host. Such therapeutic approaches could thus be favorable during microbial-induced COPD exacerbations. Agonist therapy such as CpG-mediated activation of TLR9 might help to drive the inflammatory response away from Th2 towards a Th1 response an ultimatley be beneficial in allergic diseases such as asthma; in COPD where there is already an established Th1 response it could cause disease worsening.

Due to the involvement of TLR signaling as a part of the maintenance of homeostasis between damage and repair mechanisms [172, 198], caution is needed when designing TLR-based therapies. Whilst TLR agonists might enhance the protective inflammatory response needed to help clear invaded pathogens, on the other hand such therapies may amplify unwanted destructive inflammation. In that respect TLR antagonists might reduce or inhibit unwanted inflammation. Antagonists may however, also impair healing processes and local immune defenses [199]. Proper understanding of disease conditions and timing of TLR based therapies should thus be tightly controlled.

In designing TLR-directed therapies for COPD, one should also carefully consider the impact on established homeostatic systems elsewhere in the body especially when TLRs are targeted systemically. Here we have focused on COPD however, TLRs are strongly implicated in many diseases that involve innate and adaptive immunity. In particular, TLR signaling has been implicated in autoimmune diseases and several other immune-mediated inflammatory diseases [200-203]. In a healthy person there is a balance between the protective inflammatory host response and inhibition of an overzealous autoimmune response which might be disturbed during disease. This is another reason for the need of a good understanding of the molecular mechanisms regarding TLR activation [204].

6. CONCLUSIONS

There is growing evidence for the involvement of various TLRs in COPD disease pathology. COPD-specific risk factors such as CS and air pollutants are clearly linked to TLR signaling. TLRs that have so far been suggested to play a role in COPD during sterile inflammation are TLR2, TLR4 and TLR9. Receptors that have been linked to bacterial induced disease exacerbations are TLR2 and TLR4, whereas TLR3, TLR7 and TLR8 are implicated in viral induced disease exacerbations. There is also strong evidence for endogenous derived TLR stimuli during the COPD disease process such as ECM components as well as intracellular derived HMGB1, HSPs, S100 proteins and eosinophil derived neurotoxin. It seems unlikely however that the different molecules (*e.g.* proteins, sugar moieties, lipoproteins, *etc.*) are recognized by the same extracellular LRR domain. Many of the proposed TLR binding molecules failed to demonstrate biological activity in subsequent studies wherein the molecule was rigorously purified. Further research is necessary to unravel the true importance of the various described ligands. Intrinsic to the function of many of those endogenous ligands (*i.e.* in their normal physiological state) it could be argued that these molecules are very 'sticky', and therefore themselves do not directly interact with TLRs but facilitate TLR interaction of a contaminating PAMP [95, 119, 147]. In theory, as suggested by Clett Erridge, upon sterile tissue damage the released endogenous molecules could bind and trap circulating PAMPs and lower the threshold of cellular responsiveness, adding to the inflammatory status. That would indicate that PAMPs are the actual mediators of inflammation, whereby DAMPs function as initiators and facilitators of inflammation [147]. Targeting TLR in COPD might be a valuable therapeutic implication; however caution is needed when designing TLR-based therapies.

REFERENCES

[1]   Lopez AD, Mathers CD, Ezzati M, Jamison DT, Murray CJL. Global and regional burden of disease and risk factors, 2001: systematic analysis of population health data. Lancet 2006; 367: 1747-57.

[2]   Mannino DM, Buist AS. Global burden of COPD: risk factors, prevalence, and future trends. Lancet 2007; 370: 765-73.

[3]   Buist AS, McBurnie MA, Vollmer WM *et al.* International variation in the prevalence of COPD (The BOLD Study): a population-based prevalence study. Lancet 2007; 370: 741-50.

[4]   Rabe KF, Hurd S, Anzueto A *et al.* Global strategy for the diagnosis, management, and prevention of chronic obstructive pulmonary disease - GOLD executive summary. Am J Respir Crit Care Med 2007; 176: 532-55.

[5]   Celli BR, MacNee W, Agusti A *et al.* Standards for the diagnosis and treatment of patients with COPD: a summary of the ATS/ERS position paper. Eur Resp J 2004; 23: 932-46.

[6]   Larsson K. Inflammatory markers in COPD. Clinical Respiratory Journal 2008; 2: 84-7.

[7]   Tetley TD. Macrophages and the Pathogenesis of COPD. Chest 2002; 121: 156S.

[8]   Lacoste JY, Bousquet J, Chanez P *et al.* Eosinophilic and Neutrophilic Inflammation in Asthma, Chronic-Bronchitis, and Chronic Obstructive Pulmonary-Disease. J Allergy Clin Immunol 1993; 92: 537-48.

[9]   Brusselle GG, Demoor T, Bracke KR, Brandsma CA, Timens W. Lymphoid follicles in (very) severe COPD: beneficial or harmful? Eur Resp J 2009; 34: 219-30.

[10] Robinson DS, Hamid Q, Ying S *et al.* Predominant Th2-Like Bronchoalveolar Lymphocyte-T Population in Atopic Asthma. N Engl J Med 1992; 326: 298-304.

[11] Hogg JC, Chu F, Utokaparch S *et al.* The nature of small-airway obstruction in chronic obstructive pulmonary disease. N Engl J Med 2004; 350: 2645-53.

[12] Barnes PJ. Mediators of chronic obstructive pulmonary disease. Pharmacological Reviews 2004; 56: 515-48.

[13] Snider GL, Kleinerman JL, Thurlbeck WM, Bengali ZH. The Definition of Emphysema - Report of a National-Heart-Lung-and-Blood-Institute, Division of Lung-Diseases Workshop. Am Rev Respir Dis 1985; 132: 182-5.

[14] Gooptu B, Ekeowa UI, Lomas DA. Mechanisms of emphysema in alpha(1)-antitrypsin deficiency: molecular and cellular insights. Eur Resp J 2009; 34: 475-88.

[15]   Marciniak SJ, Lomas DA. What can naturally occurring mutations tell us about the pathogenesis of COPD? Thorax 2009; 64: 359-64.

[16]   Agusti AGN, Noguera A, Sauleda J, Sala E, Pons J, Busquets X. Systemic effects of chronic obstructive pulmonary disease. Eur Resp J 2003; 21: 347-60.

[17]   Barnes PJ, Celli BR. Systemic manifestations and comorbidities of COPD. Eur Resp J 2009; 33: 1165-85.

[18]   Gan WQ, Man SFP, Senthilselvan A, Sin DD. Association between chronic obstructive pulmonary disease and systemic inflammation: a systematic review and a meta-analysis. Thorax 2004; 59: 574-80.

[19]   Akira S. Toll-like receptor signaling. J Biol Chem 2003; 278: 38105-8.

[20]   Pandey S, Agrawal DK. Immunobiology of Toll-like receptors: Emerging trends. Immunology and Cell Biology 2006; 84: 333-41.

[21]   Takeda K, Kaisho T, Akira S. Toll-like receptors. Annual Review of Immunology 2003; 21: 335-76.

[22]   Kaisho T, Akira S. Toll-like receptor function and signaling. J Allergy Clin Immunol 2006; 117: 979-87.

[23]   Takeda K, Akira S. TLR signaling pathways. Seminars in Immunology 2004; 16:3-9.

[24]   Sha Q, Truong-Tran AQ, Plitt JR, Beck LA, Schleimer RP. Activation of airway epithelial cells by toll-like receptor agonists. Am J Respir Cell Mol Biol 2004; 31: 358-64.

[25]   Hertz CJ, Wu Q, Porter EM *et al.* Activation of toll-like receptor 2 on human tracheobronchial epithelial cells induces the antimicrobial peptide human beta defensin-2. J Immunol 2003; 171: 6820-6.

[26]   Koller B, Bals R, Roos D, Korting HC, Griese M, Hartl D. Innate immune receptors on neutrophils and their role in chronic lung disease. European Journal of Clinical Investigation 2009; 39: 535-47.

[27]   Sarir H, Mortaz E, Janse WT, Givi ME, Nijkamp FP, Folkerts G. IL-8 production by macrophages is synergistically enhanced when cigarette smoke is combined with TNF-alpha. Biochem Pharmacol 2010; 79: 698-705.

[28]   Xu X, Wang H, Wang Z, Xiao W. Plasminogen activator inhibitor-1 promotes inflammatory process induced by cigarette smoke extraction or lipopolysaccharides in alveolar epithelial cells. Exp Lung Res 2009; 35: 795-805.

[29]   Reynolds PR, Cosio MG, Hoidal JR. Cigarette smoke-induced Egr-1 upregulates proinflammatory cytokines in pulmonary epithelial cells. Am J Respir Cell Mol Biol 2006; 35: 314-9.

[30]   Hasday JD, Bascom R, Costa JJ, Fitzgerald T, Dubin W. Bacterial endotoxin is an active component of cigarette smoke. Chest 1999; 115: 829-35.

[31]   Mortaz E, Adcock IM, Ito K, Kraneveld AD, Nijkamp FP, Folkerts G. Cigarette smoke induces CXCL8 production by human neutrophils *via* activation of TLR9 receptor. Eur Respir J 2010; 36: 1143-54.

[32]   Pauly JL, Smith LA, Rickert MH, Hutson A, Paszkiewicz GM. Review: Is lung inflammation associated with microbes and microbial toxins in cigarette tobacco smoke? Immunol Res 2010; 46: 127-36.

[33]   Karimi K, Sarir H, Mortaz E *et al.* Toll-like receptor-4 mediates cigarette smoke-induced cytokine production by human macrophages. Respir Res 2006; 7: 66

[34]   Sarir H, Mortaz E, Karimi K *et al.* Cigarette smoke regulates the expression of TLR4 and IL-8 production by human macrophages. J Inflamm-Lond. 2009; 1: 12.

[35]   Maes T, Bracke KR, Vermaelen KY *et al.* Murine TLR4 is implicated in cigarette smoke-induced pulmonary inflammation. International Archives of Allergy and Immunology 2006; 141: 354-68.

[36]   Pace E, Ferraro M, Siena L *et al.* Cigarette smoke increases Toll-like receptor 4 and modifies lipopolysaccharide-mediated responses in airway epithelial cells. Immunology 2008; 124: 401-11.

[37]   Speletas M, Merentiti V, Kostikas K *et al.* Association of TLR4-T399I Polymorphism with Chronic Obstructive Pulmonary Disease in Smokers. Clin Dev Immunol 2009; 260286.

[38]   Zhang XC, Shan PY, Jiang G, Cohn L, Lee PJ. Toll-like receptor 4 deficiency causes pulmonary emphysema. J Clin Invest 2006; 116: 3050-9.

[39]   Droemann D, Goldmann T, Tiedje, Zabel P, Dalhoff K, Schaaf B. Toll-like receptor 2 expression is decreased on alveolar macrophages in cigarette smokers and COPD patients. Respir Res 2005; 6: 68.

[40]   Pons J, Sauleda J, Regueiro V *et al.* Expression of Toll-like receptor 2 is up-regulated in monocytes from patients with chronic obstructive pulmonary disease. Respir Res 2006; 7: 64.

[41]   Mortaz E, Lazar Z, Koenderman L, Kraneveld AD, Nijkamp FP, Folkerts G. Cigarette smoke attenuates the production of cytokines by human plasmacytoid dendritic cells and enhances the release of IL-8 in response to TLR-9 stimulation. Respir Res 2009; 10: 47.

[42]   Mortaz E, Raats D, Vader P, Adcock I *et al.* CpG Potentiates the Effects of Cigarette Smoke on Releases of IL-8 in Neutrophils. Naunyn-Schmiedebergs Arch Pharmacol 2009; 379:27.

[43]   Salvi SS, Barnes PJ. Chronic obstructive pulmonary disease in non-smokers. Lancet 2009; 374: 733-43.

[44]   Liu SM, Zhou YM, Wang XP *et al.* Biomass fuels are the probable risk factor for chronic obstructive pulmonary disease in rural South China. Thorax 2007; 62: 889-97.

[45]   Mattson J, Haus B, Desai B *et al.* Enhanced Acute Responses in an Experimental Exposure Model to Biomass Smoke Inhalation in Chronic Obstructive Pulmonary Disease. Exp Lung Res 2008; 34: 631-62.

[46]   Orozco-Levi M, Garcia-Aymerich J, Villar J, Ramirez-Sarmiento A, Anto JM, Gea J. Wood smoke exposure and risk of chronic obstructive pulmonary disease. Eur Resp J 2006; 27: 542-6.

[47]   Shrestha IL, Shrestha SL. Indoor air pollution from biomass fuels and respiratory health of the exposed population in Nepalese households. Int J Occup Environ Health 2005; 11: 150-60.

[48]   Schikowski T, Sugiri D, Ranft U *et al.* Long-term air pollution exposure and living close to busy roads are associated with COPD in women. Respir Res 2005; 6: 152.

[49]   Trupin L, Earnest G, San Pedro M *et al.* The occupational burden of chronic obstructive pulmonary disease. Eur Resp J 2003; 22: 462-9.

[50]   MacNee W, Donaldson K. Exacerbations of COPD - Environmental mechanisms. Chest 2000; 117: 390S-7S.

[51]   Bailey KL, Poole JA, Mathisen TL, Wyatt TA, Von Essen SG, Romberger DJ. Toll-like receptor 2 is upregulated by hog confinement dust in an IL-6-dependent manner in the airway epithelium. American Journal of Physiology-Lung Cellular and Molecular Physiology 2008; 294: L1049-L54.

[52]   Inoue K, Takano H, Yanagisawa R *et al.* The role of Toll-like receptor 4 in airway inflammation induced by diesel exhaust particles. Arch Toxicol 2006; 80: 275-9.

[53]   Hollingsworth JW, Maruoka S, Li ZW *et al.* Ambient ozone primes pulmonary innate immunity in mice. J Immunol 2007; 179: 4367-75.

[54]   Shoenfelt J, Mitkus RJ, Zeisler R *et al.* Involvement of TLR2 and TLR4 in inflammatory immune responses induced by fine and coarse ambient air particulate matter. J Leukoc Biol 2009; 86: 303-12.

[55]   Becker S, Dailey L, Soukup JM, Silbajoris R, Devlin RB. TLR-2 is involved in airway epithelial cell response to air pollution particles. Toxicol Appl Pharmacol 2005; 203: 45-52.

[56]   Kim EY, Battaile JT, Patel AC *et al.* Persistent activation of an innate immune response translates respiratory viral infection into chronic lung disease. Nat Med 2008; 14: 633-40.

[57]   Papi A, Bellettato CM, Braccioni F *et al.* Infections and airway inflammation in chronic obstructive pulmonary disease severe exacerbations. Am J Respir Crit Care Med. 2006; 173: 1114-21.

[58]   Patel IS, Seemungal TAR, Wilks M, Lloyd-Owen SJ, Donaldson GC, Wedzicha JA. Relationship between bacterial colonisation and the frequency, character, and severity of COPD exacerbations. Thorax 2002; 57: 759-64.

[59]   Seemungal T, Harper-Owen R, Bhowmik A *et al.* Respiratory viruses, symptoms, and inflammatory markers in acute exacerbations and stable chronic obstructive pulmonary disease. Am J Respir Crit Care Med 2001; 164: 1618-23.

[60]   Seemungal TAR, Donaldson GC, Paul EA, Bestall JC, Jeffries DJ, Wedzicha JA. Effect of exacerbation on quality of life in patients with chronic obstructive pulmonary disease. Am J Respir Crit Care Med 1998; 157: 1418-22.

[61]   Donaldson GC, Seemungal TAR, Bhowmik A, Wedzicha JA. Relationship between exacerbation frequency and lung function decline in chronic obstructive pulmonary disease. Thorax 2002; 57: 847-52.

[62]   Stowell NC, Seideman J, Raymond HA *et al.* Long-term activation of TLR3 by Poly(I:C) induces inflammation and impairs lung function in mice. Respir Res.2009; 10: 43.

[63]   Sajjan US, Jia Y, Newcomb DC *et al.* *H. influenzae* potentiates airway epithelial cell responses to rhinovirus by increasing ICAM-1 and TLR3 expression. Faseb J 2006; 20: 2121-3.

[64]   Tokairin Y, Shibata Y, Sata M *et al.* Enhanced immediate inflammatory response to *Streptococcus pneumonia*e in the lungs of mice with pulmonary emphysema. Respirology 2008; 13: 324-32.

[65]   Wang JP, Bowen GN, Padden C *et al.* Toll-like receptor-mediated activation of neutrophils by influenza A virus. Blood 2008; 112: 2028-34.

[66]   Yanagisawa S, Koarai A, Sugiura H *et al.* Oxidative stress augments toll-like receptor 8 mediated neutrophilic responses in healthy subjects. Respir Res 2009; 10: 50.

[67]   Barnes PJ. Alveolar macrophages as orchestrators of COPD. COPD 2004; 1: 59-70.

[68]   Stampfli MR, Anderson GP. How cigarette smoke skews immune responses to promote infection, lung disease and cancer. Nat Rev Immunol 2009; 9: 377-84.

[69]   Laan M, Bozinovski S, Anderson GP. Cigarette smoke inhibits lipopolysaccharide-induced production of inflammatory cytokines by suppressing the activation of activator protein-1 in bronchial epithelial cells. J Immunol 2004; 173: 4164-70.

[70]   Manzel LJ, Shi L, O'Shaughnessy PT, Thorne PS, Look DC. Inhibition by cigarette smoke of nuclear factor-κB-dependent response to bacteria in the airway. Am J Respir Cell Mol Biol 2011; 44: 155-65.

[71] Eddleston J, Lee RU, Doerner AM, Herschbach J, Zuraw BL. Cigarette smoke decreases the innate responses of epithelial cells to rhinovirus infection. Am J Respir Cell Mol Biol 2011; 44: 118-26.

[72] Kulkarni R, Rampersaud R, Aguilar JL, Randis TM, Kreindler JL, Ratner AJ. Cigarette smoke inhibits airway epithelial innate immune responses to bacteria. Infect Immun 2010; 78: 2146-52.

[73] Phipps JC, Aronoff DM, Curtis JL, Goel D, O'Brien E, Mancuso P. Cigarette smoke exposure impairs pulmonary bacterial clearance and alveolar macrophage complement-mediated phagocytosis of *Streptococcus pneumoniae*. Infect Immun 2010; 78: 1214-20.

[74] Hodge S, Hodge G, Ahern J, Jersmann H, Holmes M, Reynolds PN. Smoking alters alveolar macrophage recognition and phagocytic ability: implications in chronic obstructive pulmonary disease. Am J Respir Cell Mol Biol 2007; 37: 748-55.

[75] Richens TR, Linderman DJ, Horstmann SA *et al.* Cigarette smoke impairs clearance of apoptotic cells through oxidant-dependent activation of RhoA. Am J Respir Crit Care Med 2009; 179: 1011-21.

[76] Hodge S, Hodge G, Scicchitano R, Reynolds PN, Holmes M. Alveolar macrophages from subjects with chronic obstructive pulmonary disease are deficient in their ability to phagocytose apoptotic airway epithelial cells. Immunol Cell Biol 2003; 81: 289-96.

[77] MacNee W, Rahman I. Is oxidative stress central to the pathogenesis of chronic obstructive pulmonary disease? Trends in Molecular Medicine 2001; 7: 55-62.

[78] Huang MF, Lin WL, Ma YC. A study of reactive oxygen species in mainstream of cigarette. Indoor Air 2005; 15: 135-40.

[79] Rahman I, Adcock IM. Oxidative stress and redox regulation of lung inflammation in COPD. Eur Resp J 2006; 28: 219-42.

[80] Tzortzaki EG, Siafakas NM. A hypothesis for the initiation of COPD. Eur Respir J 2009; 34: 310-5.

[81] Thorley AJ, Tetley TD. Pulmonary epithelium, cigarette smoke, and chronic obstructive pulmonary disease. Int J Chron Obstruct Pulmon Dis. 2007; 2: 409-28.

[82] Ryan KA, Smith MF, Sanders MK, Ernst PB. Reactive oxygen and nitrogen species differentially regulate toll-like receptor 4-mediated activation of NF-kappa B and interleukin-8 expression. Infect Immun 2004; 72: 2123-30.

[83] Asehnoune K, Strassheim D, Mitra S, Kim JY, Abraham E. Involvement of reactive oxygen species in Toll-like receptor 4-dependent activation of NF-kappa B. J Immunol 2004; 172: 2522-9.

[84] Matsuzawa A, Saegusa K, Noguchi T *et al.* ROS-dependent activation of the TRAF6-ASK1-p38 pathway is selectively required for TLR4-mediated innate immunity. Nat Immunol 2005; 6: 587-92.

[85] Paul-Clark MJ, McMaster SK, Sorrentino R *et al.* Toll-like Receptor 2 Is Essential for the Sensing of Oxidants during Inflammation. Am J Respir Crit Care Med 2009; 179: 299-306.

[86] Kasahara Y, Tuder RM, Cool CD, Lynch DA, Flores SC, Voelkel NF. Endothelial cell death and decreased expression of vascular endothelial growth factor and vascular endothelial growth factor receptor 2 in emphysema. Am J Respir Crit Care Med 2001; 163: 737-44.

[87] Vandivier RW, Henson PM, Douglas IS. Burying the dead: the impact of failed apoptotic cell removal (efferocytosis) on chronic inflammatory lung disease. Chest 2006; 129: 1673-82.

[88] Vandivier RW, Fadok VA, Hoffmann PR *et al.* Elastase-mediated phosphatidylserine receptor cleavage impairs apoptotic cell clearance in cystic fibrosis and bronchiectasis. J Clin Invest 2002; 109: 661-70.

[89] Hodge S, Hodge G, Ahern, Jersmann H, Holmes M, Reynolds PN. Smoking alters alveolar macrophage recognition and phagocytic ability. Am J Respir Cell Mol Biol 2007; 37: 748-55.

[90] Rock KL, Kono H. The inflammatory response to cell death. Annu Rev Pathol 2008; 3: 99-126.

[91] Voll RE, Herrmann M, Roth EA, Stach C, Kalden JR, Girkontaite I. Immunosuppressive effects of apoptotic cells. Nature. 1997; 390:350-1.

[92] Noble PW, Jiang D. Matrix regulation of lung injury, inflammation, and repair: the role of innate immunity. Proc Am Thorac Soc. 2006; 3: 401-4.

[93] Oppenheim JJ, Yang D. Alarmins: chemotactic activators of immune responses. Curr Opin Immunol 2005; 17: 359-65.

[94] Matzinger P. The danger model: a renewed sense of self. Science 2002; 296: 301-5.

[95] Seong SY, Matzinger P. Hydrophobicity: an ancient damage-associated molecular pattern that initiates innate immune responses. Nat Rev Immunol 2004; 4: 469-78.

[95] Carta S, Castellani P, Delfino L, Tassi S, Vene R, Rubartelli A. DAMPs and inflammatory processes: the role of redox in the different outcomes. J Leukoc Biol 2009; 86: 549-55.

[97] Rubartelli A, Lotze MT. Inside, outside, upside down: damage-associated molecular-pattern molecules (DAMPs) and redox. Trends Immunol 2007; 28: 429-36.

[98]   Bianchi ME. DAMPs, PAMPs and alarmins: all we need to know about danger. J Leukoc Biol 2007; 81: 1-5.

[99]   Kono H, Rock KL. How dying cells alert the immune system to danger. Nat Rev Immunol 2008; 8: 279-89.

[100]   Lotze MT, Zeh HJ, Rubartelli A *et al.* The grateful dead: damage-associated molecular pattern molecules and reduction/oxidation regulate immunity. Immunol Rev 2007; 220: 60-81.

[101]   Ferhani N, Letuve S, Kozhich A *et al.* Expression of High-Mobility Group Box 1 and of Receptor for Advanced Glycation End Products in Chronic Obstructive Pulmonary Disease. Am J Respir Crit Care Med 2010; 181: 917-27.

[102]   Rauvala H, Rouhiainen A. Physiological and Pathophysiological outcomes of the interactions of HMGB1 with cell surface receptors. Biochim Biophys Acta 2009; 1799:164-70.

[103]   Yang H, Wang H, Czura CJ, Tracey KJ. The cytokine activity of HMGB1. J Leukoc Biol 2005; 78: 1-8.

[104]   Scaffidi P, Misteli T, Bianchi ME. Release of chromatin protein HMGB1 by necrotic cells triggers inflammation. Nature 2002; 418: 191-5.

[105]   Bonaldi T, Talamo F, Scaffidi P *et al.* Monocytic cells hyperacetylate chromatin protein HMGB1 to redirect it towards secretion. EMBO J. 2003; 22: 5551-60.

[106]   Gardella S, Andrei C, Ferrera D *et al.* The nuclear protein HMGB1 is secreted by monocytes *via* a non-classical, vesicle-mediated secretory pathway. EMBO Rep 2002; 3: 995-1001.

[107]   Semino C, Ceccarelli J, Lotti LV, Torrisi MR, Angelini G, Rubartelli A. The maturation potential of NK cell clones toward autologous dendritic cells correlates with HMGB1 secretion. J Leukoc Biol 2007; 81:92-9.

[108]   Semino C, Angelini G, Poggi A, Rubartelli A. NK/iDC interaction results in IL-18 secretion by DCs at the synaptic cleft followed by NK cell activation and release of the DC maturation factor HMGB1. Blood 2005; 106: 609-16.

[109]   Rouhiainen A, Tumova S, Valmu L, Kalkkinen N, Rauvala H. Pivotal advance: analysis of proinflammatory activity of highly purified eukaryotic recombinant HMGB1 (amphoterin). J Leukoc Biol 2007; 81: 49-58.

[110]   Sha Y, Zmijewski J, Xu Z, Abraham E. HMGB1 develops enhanced proinflammatory activity by binding to cytokines. J Immunol 2008; 180: 2531-7.

[111]   Tian J, Avalos AM, Mao SY *et al.* Toll-like receptor 9-dependent activation by DNA-containing immune complexes is mediated by HMGB1 and RAGE. Nat Immunol 2007; 8: 487-96.

[112]   Klune JR, Dhupar R, Cardinal, Billiar TR, Tsung A. HMGB1: endogenous danger signaling. Mol Med 2008; 14: 476-84.

[113]   Ulloa L, Messmer D. High-mobility group box 1 (HMGB1) protein: friend and foe. Cytokine Growth Factor Rev 2006; 17: 189-201.

[114]   Dintilhac A, Bernues J. HMGB1 interacts with many apparently unrelated proteins by recognizing short amino acid sequences. J Biol Chem 2002; 277: 7021-8.

[115]   Youn JH, Oh YJ, Kim ES, Choi JE, Shin JS. High mobility group box 1 protein binding to lipopolysaccharide facilitates transfer of lipopolysaccharide to CD14 and enhances lipopolysaccharide-mediated TNF-alpha production in human monocytes. J Immunol 2008; 180: 5067-74.

[116]   Urbonaviciute V, Furnrohr BG, Meister S *et al.* Induction of inflammatory and immune responses by HMGB1-nucleosome complexes: implications for the pathogenesis of SLE. J Exp Med 2008; 205: 3007-18.

[117]   Rouhiainen A, Imai S, Rauvala H, Parkkinen J. Occurrence of amphoterin (HMG1) as an endogenous protein of human platelets that is exported to the cell surface upon platelet activation. Thromb Haemost. 2000; 84: 1087-94.

[118]   Mohan PS, Laitinen J, Merenmies J, Rauvala H, Jungalwala FB. Sulfoglycolipids bind to adhesive protein amphoterin (P30) in the nervous system. Biochem Biophys Res Commun 1992; 182: 689-96.

[119]   Bianchi ME. HMGB1 loves company. J Leukoc Biol 2009; 86: 573-6.

[120]   Park JS, Svetkauskaite D, He Q *et al.* Involvement of toll-like receptors 2 and 4 in cellular activation by high mobility group box 1 protein. J Biol Chem 2004; 279: 7370-7.

[121]   Yang H, Tracey KJ. Targeting HMGB1 in inflammation. Biochim Biophys Acta 2010; 1799: 149-56.

[122]   van Zoelen MA, Yang H, Florquin S *et al.* Role of toll-like receptors 2 and 4, and the receptor for advanced glycation end products in high-mobility group box 1-induced inflammation *in vivo*. Shock 2009; 31: 280-4.

[123]   Yu M, Wang H, Ding A *et al.* HMGB1 signals through toll-like receptor (TLR) 4 and TLR2. Shock 2006; 26: 174-9.

[124]   Park JS, Gamboni-Robertson F, He Q *et al.* High mobility group box 1 protein interacts with multiple Toll-like receptors. Am J Physiol Cell Physiol 2006; 290: C917-24.

[125]   Liu G, Wang J, Park YJ *et al.* High mobility group protein-1 inhibits phagocytosis of apoptotic neutrophils through binding to phosphatidylserine. J Immunol 2008; 181: 4240-6.

[126]   Yanai H, Ban T, Wang Z *et al.* HMGB proteins function as universal sentinels for nucleic-acid-mediated innate immune responses. Nature 2009; 462: 99-103.

[127] Orlova VV, Choi EY, Xie C *et al.* A novel pathway of HMGB1-mediated inflammatory cell recruitment that requires Mac-1-integrin. EMBO J. 2007; 26: 1129-39.

[128] Chavakis E, Hain A, Vinci M *et al.* High-mobility group box 1 activates integrin-dependent homing of endothelial progenitor cells. Circ Res 2007; 100: 204-12.

[129] Chavakis T, Bierhaus A, Al-Fakhri N *et al.* The pattern recognition receptor (RAGE) is a counterreceptor for leukocyte integrins: a novel pathway for inflammatory cell recruitment. J Exp Med 2003; 198: 1507-15.

[130] Porto A, Palumbo R, Pieroni M *et al.* Smooth muscle cells in human atherosclerotic plaques secrete and proliferate in response to high mobility group box 1 protein. Faseb J 2006; 20: 2565-6.

[131] Palumbo R, Sampaolesi M, De Marchis F *et al.* Extracellular HMGB1, a signal of tissue damage, induces mesoangioblast migration and proliferation. J Cell Biol 2004; 164: 441-9.

[132] Germani A, Limana F, Capogrossi MC. Pivotal advances: high-mobility group box 1 protein--a cytokine with a role in cardiac repair. J Leukoc Biol 2007; 81: 41-5.

[133] Limana F, Germani A, Zacheo A *et al.* Exogenous high-mobility group box 1 protein induces myocardial regeneration after infarction *via* enhanced cardiac C-kit+ cell proliferation and differentiation. Circ Res 2005; 97: e73-83.

[134] Li Z, Menoret A, Srivastava P. Roles of heat-shock proteins in antigen presentation and cross-presentation. Curr Opin Immunol 2002 ; 14: 45-51.

[135] Basu S, Binder RJ, Ramalingam T, Srivastava PK. CD91 is a common receptor for heat shock proteins gp96, hsp90, hsp70, and calreticulin. Immunity. 2001; 14: 303-13.

[136] Lindquist S. The heat-shock response. Annu Rev Biochem 1986; 55: 1151-91.

[137] Hartl FU, Hayer-Hartl M. Molecular chaperones in the cytosol: from nascent chain to folded protein. Science 2002; 295: 1852-8.

[138] Hacker S, Lambers C, Hoetzenecker K *et al.* Elevated HSP27, HSP70 and HSP90 alpha in Chronic Obstructive Pulmonary Disease: Markers for Immune Activation and Tissue Destruction. Clin Lab. 2009; 55: 31-40.

[139] Basu S, Binder RJ, Suto R, Anderson KM, Srivastava PK. Necrotic but not apoptotic cell death releases heat shock proteins, which deliver a partial maturation signal to dendritic cells and activate the NF-kappa B pathway. Int Immunol 2000; 12: 1539-46.

[140] Bausero MA, Gastpar R, Multhoff G, Asea A. Alternative mechanism by which IFN-gamma enhances tumor recognition: active release of heat shock protein 72. J Immunol 2005; 175: 2900-12.

[141] Clayton A, Turkes A, Navabi H, Mason MD, Tabi Z. Induction of heat shock proteins in B-cell exosomes. J Cell Sci 2005; 118: 3631-8.

[142] Asea A. Heat shock proteins and toll-like receptors. Handb Exp Pharmacol. 2008; 183: 111-27.

[143] Ohashi K, Burkart V, Flohe S, Kolb H. Cutting edge: heat shock protein 60 is a putative endogenous ligand of the toll-like receptor-4 complex. J Immunol 2000; 164: 558-61.

[144] Vabulas RM, Ahmad-Nejad P, Ghose S, Kirschning CJ, Issels RD, Wagner H. HSP70 as endogenous stimulus of the Toll/interleukin-1 receptor signal pathway. J Biol Chem 2002; 277: 15107-12.

[145] Vabulas RM, Ahmad-Nejad P, da Costa C *et al.* Endocytosed HSP60s use toll-like receptor 2 (TLR2) and TLR4 to activate the toll/interleukin-1 receptor signaling pathway in innate immune cells. J Biol Chem 2001; 276: 31332-9.

[146] Asea A, Rehli M, Kabingu E, Boch JA *et al.* Novel signal transduction pathway utilized by extracellular HSP70: role of toll-like receptor (TLR) 2 and TLR4. J Biol Chem 2002; 277: 15028-34.

[147] Erridge C. Endogenous ligands of TLR2 and TLR4: agonists or assistants? J Leukoc Biol 2010; 87: 989-9.

[148] Tsan MF, Gao B. Heat shock proteins and immune system. J Leukoc Biol 2009; 85: 905-10.

[149] Gao B, Tsan MF. Recombinant human heat shock protein 60 does not induce the release of tumor necrosis factor alpha from murine macrophages. J Biol Chem. 2003 Jun 20;278(25):22523-9.

[150] Bausinger H, Lipsker D, Ziylan U *et al.* Endotoxin-free heat-shock protein 70 fails to induce APC activation. Eur J Immunol 2002; 32: 3708-13.

[151] Marenholz I, Heizmann CW, Fritz G. S100 proteins in mouse and man: from evolution to function and pathology (including an update of the nomenclature). Biochem Biophys Res Commun. 2004; 322: 1111-22.

[152] Foell D, Wittkowski H, Vogl T, Roth J. S100 proteins expressed in phagocytes: a novel group of damage-associated molecular pattern molecules. J Leukoc Biol 2007; 81: 28-37.

[153] Ehrchen JM, Sunderkotter C, Foell D, Vogl T, Roth J. The endogenous Toll-like receptor 4 agonist S100A8/S100A9 (calprotectin) as innate amplifier of infection, autoimmunity, and cancer. J Leukoc Biol 2009; 86: 557-66.

[154] Lorenz E, Muhlebach MS, Tessier PA *et al.* Different expression ratio of S100A8/A9 and S100A12 in acute and chronic lung diseases. Respir Med 2008; 102: 567-73.

[155] Vogl T, Tenbrock K, Ludwig S, Leukert N *et al.* Mrp8 and Mrp14 are endogenous activators of Toll-like receptor 4, promoting lethal, endotoxin-induced shock. Nat Med 2007; 13: 1042-9.

[156] Foell D, Roth J. Proinflammatory S100 proteins in arthritis and autoimmune disease. Arthritis Rheum 2004; 50: 3762-71.

[157] Rosenberg HF. RNase A ribonucleases and host defense: an evolving story. J Leukoc Biol 2008; 83: 1079-87.

[158] Perng DW, Huang HY, Chen HM, Lee YC, Perng RP. Characteristics of airway inflammation and bronchodilator reversibility in COPD - A potential guide to treatment. Chest 2004; 126: 375-81.

[159] D'Armiento JM, Scharf SM, Roth MD *et al.* Eosinophil and T cell markers predict functional decline in COPD patients. Respir Res 2009; 10: 113.

[160] Yang D, Chen Q, Rosenberg HF *et al.* Human ribonuclease A superfamily members, eosinophil-derived neurotoxin and pancreatic ribonuclease, induce dendritic cell maturation and activation. J Immunol 2004; 173: 6134-42.

[161] Yang D, Chen Q, Su SB *et al.* Eosinophil-derived neurotoxin acts as an alarmin to activate the TLR2-MyD88 signal pathway in dendritic cells and enhances Th2 immune responses. J Exp Med 2008; 205: 79-90.

[162] Yang D, Rosenberg HF, Chen Q, Dyer KD, Kurosaka K, Oppenheim JJ. Eosinophil-derived neurotoxin (EDN), an antimicrobial protein with chemotactic activities for dendritic cells. Blood 2003; 102: 3396-403.

[163] Sur S, Glitz DG, Kita H *et al.* Localization of eosinophil-derived neurotoxin and eosinophil cationic protein in neutrophilic leukocytes. J Leukoc Biol 1998; 63: 715-22.

[164] Rosenberg HF. Eosinophil-derived neurotoxin / RNase 2: connecting the past, the present and the future. Curr Pharm Biotechnol. 2008; 9: 135-40.

[165] Teder P, Vandivier RW, Jiang D *et al.* Resolution of lung inflammation by CD44. Science 2002; 296: 155-8.

[166] Jiang D, Liang J, Noble PW. Hyaluronan in tissue injury and repair. Annu Rev Cell Dev Biol 2007; 23: 435-61.

[167] Papakonstantinou E, Karakiulakis G. The 'sweet' and 'bitter' involvement of glycosaminoglycans in lung diseases: pharmacotherapeutic relevance. Br J Pharmacol 2009; 157: 1111-27.

[168] Dentener MA, Vernooy JHJ, Hendriks S, Wouters EFM. Enhanced levels of hyaluronan in lungs of patients with COPD: relationship with lung function and local inflammation. Thorax 2005; 60: 114-9.

[169] Bracke KR, Dentener MA, Papakonstantinou E *et al.* Enhanced Deposition of Low-Molecular-Weight Hyaluronan in Lungs of Cigarette Smoke-Exposed Mice. Am J Respir Cell Mol Biol; 42: 753-61.

[170] Bollyky PL, Falk BA, Wu RP, Buckner JH, Wight TN, Nepom GT. Intact extracellular matrix and the maintenance of immune tolerance: high molecular weight hyaluronan promotes persistence of induced CD4+CD25+ regulatory T cells. J Leukoc Biol 2009; 86: 567-72.

[171] Bollyky PL, Lord JD, Masewicz SA *et al.* Cutting edge: high molecular weight hyaluronan promotes the suppressive effects of CD4+CD25+ regulatory T cells. J Immunol 2007; 179: 744-7.

[172] O'Neill LA. TLRs play good cop, bad cop in the lung. Nat Med 2005; 11: 1161-2.

[173] Aruffo A, Stamenkovic I, Melnick M, Underhill CB, Seed B. CD44 is the principal cell surface receptor for hyaluronate. Cell 1990; 61: 1303-13.

[174] Kawana H, Karaki H, Higashi M *et al.* CD44 suppresses TLR-mediated inflammation. J Immunol 2008; 180: 4235-45.

[175] Taylor KR, Yamasaki K, Radek KA *et al.* Recognition of hyaluronan released in sterile injury involves a unique receptor complex dependent on Toll-like receptor 4, CD44, and MD-2. J Biol Chem 2007; 282: 18265-75.

[176] Termeer C, Benedix F, Sleeman J *et al.* Oligosaccharides of Hyaluronan activate dendritic cells *via* toll-like receptor 4. J Exp Med 2002; 195: 99-111.

[177] Scheibner KA, Lutz MA, Boodoo S, Fenton MJ, Powell JD, Horton MR. Hyaluronan fragments act as an endogenous danger signal by engaging TLR2. J Immunol 200; 177: 1272-81.

[178] Jiang D, Liang J, Fan J *et al.* Regulation of lung injury and repair by Toll-like receptors and hyaluronan. Nat Med 2005; 11: 1173-9.

[179] Dreyfuss JL, Regatieri CV, Jarrouge TR, Cavalheiro RP, Sampaio LO, Nader HB. Heparan sulfate proteoglycans: structure, protein interactions and cell signaling. An Acad Bras Cienc 2009; 81: 409-29.

[180] Matzner Y, Barner M, Yahalom J, Ishaimichaeli R, Fuks Z, Vlodavsky I. Degradation of Heparan-Sulfate in the Subendothelial Extracellular-Matrix by a Readily Released Heparinase from Human-Neutrophils - Possible Role in Invasion through Basement-Membranes. J Clin Invest 1985; 76: 1306-13.

[181] Solic N, Wilson J, Wilson SJ, Shute JK. Endothelial activation and increased heparan sulfate expression in cystic fibrosis. Am J Respir Crit Care Med 2005; 172: 892-8.

[182] Johnson GB, Brunn GJ, Kodaira Y, Platt JL. Receptor-mediated monitoring of tissue well-being *via* detection of soluble heparan sulfate by Toll-like receptor 4. J Immunol 2002; 168: 5233-9.

[183] Johnson GB, Brunn GJ, Platt JL. Cutting edge: an endogenous pathway to systemic inflammatory response syndrome (SIRS)-like reactions through Toll-like receptor 4. J Immunol 2004; 172: 20-4.

[184] Baumann H, Gauldie J. The acute phase response. Immunol Today 1994; 15: 74-80.

[185] Garcia-Rio F, Miravitlles M, Soriano JB *et al.* Systemic inflammation in chronic obstructive pulmonary disease: a population-based study. Respir Res 2010;11; 53.

[186] Molmenti EP, Ziambaras T, Perlmutter DH. Evidence for an acute phase response in human intestinal epithelial cells. J Biol Chem 1993; 268: 14116-24.

[187] Lee SY, Lee KP, Lim JW. Identification and biosynthesis of fibrinogen in human uterine cervix carcinoma cells. Thromb Haemost 1996; 75: 466-70.

[188] Haidaris PJ. Induction of fibrinogen biosynthesis and secretion from cultured pulmonary epithelial cells. Blood 1997; 89: 873-82.

[189] Simpson-Haidaris PJ, Courtney MA, Goss R, Harmsen A, Gigliotti F. Induction of fibrinogen expression in the lung epithelium during *Pneumocystis carinii* pneumonia. Infect Immun 1998; 66: 4431-9.

[190] Rybarczyk BJ, Lawrence SO, Simpson-Haidaris PJ. Matrix-fibrinogen enhances wound closure by increasing both cell proliferation and migration. Blood 2003; 102: 4035-43.

[191] Hodgkinson CP, Patel K, Ye S. Functional Toll-like receptor 4 mutations modulate the response to fibrinogen. Thromb Haemost 2008; 100: 301-7.

[192] Smiley ST, King JA, Hancock WW. Fibrinogen stimulates macrophage chemokine secretion through toll-like receptor 4. J Immunol 2001; 167: 2887-94.

[193] Kuhns DB, Priel DA, Gallin JI. Induction of human monocyte interleukin (IL)-8 by fibrinogen through the toll-like receptor pathway. Inflammation 2007; 30: 178-88.

[194] Donnelly LE, Rogers DF. Therapy for chronic obstructive pulmonary disease in the 21st century. Drugs 2003; 63: 1973-98.

[195] Chaudhuri N, Whyte MKB, Sabroe I. Reducing the toll of inflammatory lung disease. Chest 2007; 131: 1550-6.

[196] O'Neill LA, Bryant CE, Doyle SL. Therapeutic targeting of Toll-like receptors for infectious and inflammatory diseases and cancer. Pharmacol Rev 2009; 61: 177-97.

[197] Akira S, Takeda K. Toll-like receptor signaling. Nat Rev Immunol 2004; 4: 499-511.

[198] Zhang Z, Schluesener HJ. Mammalian toll-like receptors: from endogenous ligands to tissue regeneration. Cell Mol Life Sci 2006; 63: 2901-7.

[199] Sabroe I, Parker LC, Dower SK, Whyte MK. The role of TLR activation in inflammation. J Pathol 2008 ;214: 126-35.

[200] Rifkin IR, Leadbetter EA, Busconi L, Viglianti G, Marshak-Rothstein A. Toll-like receptors, endogenous ligands, and systemic autoimmune disease. Immunol Rev 2005; 204: 27-42.

[201] Drexler SK, Foxwell BM. The role of Toll-like receptors in chronic inflammation. Int J Biochem Cell Biol 2009; 42: 506-18.

[202] Ospelt C, Gay S. TLRs and chronic inflammation. Int J Biochem Cell Biol 2009; 42; 495-505.

[203] Marshak-Rothstein A. Toll-like receptors in systemic autoimmune disease. Nat Rev Immunol 2006; 6: 823-35.

[204] Liew FY, Xu D, Brint EK, O'Neill LA. Negative regulation of toll-like receptor-mediated immune responses. Nat Rev Immunol 2005; 5: 446-58.

CHAPTER 6

Pulmonary Mycobacterial Infections and TLRs

Valerie F.J. Quesniaux[*]

University of Orleans and CNRS UMR6218 Molecular Immunology and Embryology, 3B rue de la Ferollerie, 45071 Orleans, France

Abstract: *Mycobacterium tuberculosis* expresses molecular motifs that are potent TLR agonists, targeting especially TLR2, and resulting in rapid activation of cells of the innate immune system. The control of experimental acute *M. tuberculosis* infection seems rather independent of the presence of TLRs, as is the induction of adaptive immunity to mycobacteria, while long term control of chronic infection might be more TLR dependent. Conversely, some molecules produced by *M. tuberculosis* can modulate the host innate TLR mediated responses. Control of *M. tuberculosis* infection depends on a balance between the host recognition of the pathogen and activation of both innate and adaptive immune responses, and immune evasion strategies developed by the bacteria.

Keywords: TLRs, tuberculosis, mycobacterial cell wall, PAMPS, macrophages, dendritic cells.

1. INTRODUCTION

Tuberculosis (TB) is still a major health problem, with about one-third of the global population considered to be infected with *Mycobacterium tuberculosis*. Only 5% to 10% of infected individuals develop an active disease, suggesting that the host immune system can usually efficiently deal with the bacterium and the majority of healthy individuals are asymptomatic. However, the infection is not cleared and it can remain in a latent form for many years [1]. A recent quantification of bacterial growth and death rates showed that *M. tuberculosis* replicates throughout the course of chronic TB infection in mice and is restrained by the host immune system [2]. Depression of the host immune system by different causes such as immunodeficiency due to HIV, malnutrition, complications of aging and some genetic factors can favor a reactivation of latent tuberculosis infection. The neutralization of TNF for treatment of severe inflammatory diseases such as rheumatoid arthritis, Crohn's disease, and ulcerative colitis has been associated with reactivation of latent tuberculosis and increased susceptibility to primary tuberculosis infection [3-6].

M. tuberculosis is an intracellular pathogen capable of surviving within host mononuclear cells through inhibition of phagosome maturation and fusion with lysosomes [7]. For the control of infection a coordinated response of cells of the innate and adaptive immune system is required [8, 9]. Control and resolution of the infection involves the sequestration of the surviving pathogens in macrophages within a granuloma, a dynamic structure containing activated lymphocytes and continuously stimulated macrophages. Host mechanisms leading to protective immunity controlling tuberculosis and reactivation of infection are associated with T cells, macrophages, interferon-γ (IFNγ), TNF, interleukin-12 (IL-12), nitric oxide (NO), reactive oxygen and reactive nitrogen intermediates (RNI), as reviewed [8-10]. While IL-23 and IL-17 contribute to host resistance [11], they do not seem essential to control acute TB infection [12, 13].

Upon phagocytosis by macrophages, *M. tuberculosis* activates various pattern recognition receptors and stimulates the production TNF, IL-12, RNI as well as the expression of costimulatory molecules, leading to T and NK cell activation, IFNγ production, and increased microbiocidal activity of the phagocytes [8, 10]. The IL-1 pathway also seems essential for the control of acute *M. tuberculosis* infection [14, 15], indicating that several pro-inflammatory cytokines produced during tuberculosis are non-redundant. Therefore, a continuous, smouldering activation of the phagocytes, in concert with activated T cells, may be required to exert an active immunological pressure.

[*]**Address correspondence to Valerie Quesniaux:** University of Orleans and CNRS UMR6218 Molecular Immunology and Embryology, 3B rue de la Ferollerie, 45071 Orleans Cedex 2, France; E-mail:quesniaux@cnrs-orleans.fr

TLRs are believed to represent key receptors for the recognition of mycobacterial antigens and activation of macrophages and dendritic cells, as well as other cells of the innate immune system, thereby likely modulating the adaptive immune response [16, 17]. This chapter is aimed at discussing current knowledge about the interaction between TLRs and mycobacteria such as *M. tuberculosis*, with special emphasis on the biological implications *in vitro* and *in vivo*. We will first review the mycobacterial PAMPs recognized by TLRs, then ask whether TLR pathways are essential for the control of experimental or clinical *M. tuberculosis* infection. We will also see briefly how *M. tuberculosis* subverts the host inflammatory response to TLR trigger.

2. EXPRESSION OF TLRs DURING MYCOBACTERIAL INFECTION

A variety of microbial products are able to recognize and activate mammalian TLRs, facilitating the transcription of genes that regulate the adaptive immune response, including chemokines, cytokines and costimulatory molecules [18-21]. The greatest variety of TLR mRNAs is found in professional phagocytes suggesting a major role of TLRs in innate immunity. TLRs are also broadly expressed in tissues and the complete panel of TLR mRNA is expressed in spleen and peripheral blood [22, 23], but also airway epithelia [24, 25]. The expression of TLRs seems to be modulated during mycobacterial infections. mRNA encoding TLR1, TLR2, TLR4 and TLR6 are increased in blood from patients with active pulmonary tuberculosis but not in bronchoalveolar lavage [26]. An increased level of a human splice variant of TLR1 mRNA has been found in both CD3- and CD4+ cells, likely through mRNA stabilization [26] whilst TLR2 is up-regulated on monocytes from tuberculous pleural fluid [27]. Both TLR2 and TLR4 expression can also be enhanced on IFNγ secreting CD4+ T cells. However, TLR2 and TLR4 expression is down-regulated on natural regulatory T cells despite their higher number at sites of infection. *M. tuberculosis* heat shock protein (hsp) 60 preferentially induces TLR2, without affecting TLR4 expression, and reduces PPD-induced IL-12 p40 release by macrophages [28]. Further, lipid fractions from the *M. tuberculosis* hypervirulent Beijing genotype downregulate TLR2, TLR4 and MHC class II expression on human macrophages whilst inducing the secretion of high amounts of TNF and IL-10 [29].

3. TLR IMPLICATION IN WHOLE MYCOBACTERIA RECOGNITION

Viable and killed *M. tuberculosis* bacilli (virulent and attenuated) can activate CHO cells and murine macrophages that express either TLR2 or TLR4 [30]. Macrophages expressing a dominant negative mutant of MyD88 cannot react to mycobacteria, underlining the requirement of TLRs mediating the downstream signaling cascade responsible for the transcription of TNF. Neither membrane bound nor soluble CD14 are required for cellular activation. As opposed to LPS-induced macrophage activation, the overexpression of MD-2, a protein that is associated with TLR4, does not augment TNF production induced by viable mycobacteria [31]. Using macrophages from TLR2 and/or TLR4 deficient mice, we have confirmed some TLR2- and to a lesser extent TLR4-dependent activation of TNF and IL-12 production occurs after infection with live *M. bovis* BCG [32], an effect which is abrogated in MyD88 deficient macrophages [33]. However, recognition of heat-killed *M. bovis* BCG, extensive-freeze-dried *M. bovis* BCG, or a soluble fraction of *M. bovis* BCG culture supernatant, was found to be mediated predominantly through TLR2, as essentially no response remained in TLR2-deficient macrophages or dendritic cells [34]. TLR1- or TLR6-deficient macrophages respond normally to these complex mycobacterial preparations suggesting a double implication or potential compensation of TLR1/6 [34].

Furthermore, we showed that mycobacteria induce production of nitric oxide, a potent antimycobacterial effector molecule, in primary macrophages in a TLR2-dependent way, in contrast with previous reports [31]. However, intracellular pathogens also induce expression of arginase 1 (Arg1) in mouse macrophages through TLR independently of the STAT6 pathway. This may be beneficial to the pathogen since specific elimination of Arg1 in macrophages decreases lung bacterial load during tuberculosis infection [35]. Thus, infection with whole bacilli evokes a complex activation pattern involving at least TLR2 and TLR4 and leads to differential activation of antibacterial effector pathways.

4. TLR LIGANDS OF MYCOBACTERIAL ORIGIN

The initial recognition of mycobacterial components by the innate immune system through TLRs, and likely other PRRs, contributes to triggering the host immune response. TLRs 1, 2, 4 or 6 acting in heterodimers with

TLR2 and TLR9 have been implicated in the recognition of mycobacterial antigens [17, 36-38]. Over-expression of either TLR2 or TLR4 in CHO cells confers cellular activation by viable *M. tuberculosis* [30]. Soluble heat-stable mycobacterial fractions distinct from the mycobacterial cell wall lipoarabinomannan (LAM) signal through TLR2, whereas heat-labile cell-associated agonists signal through TLR4 [30]. *M. tuberculosis*-induced TNF production by macrophages can be blocked by a TLR4 antagonist [31].

The mycobacterial cell wall comprises different glyocolipids including LAM, mycolic acid, lipopeptides and peptidoglycan as shown schematically in Fig. **1**.

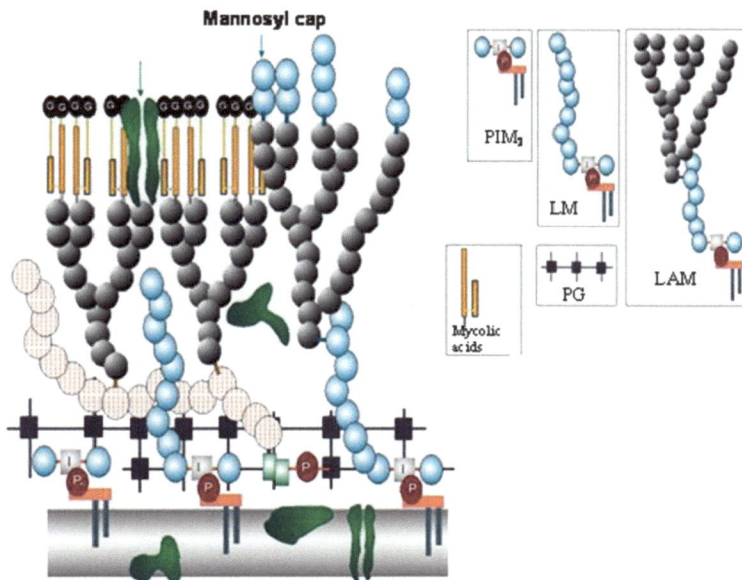

Figure 1: Model of mycobacterial cell wall showing several molecular motifs recognized by pattern recognition receptors, including TLRs, such as phosphatidyl-myoinositol mannosides (PIM), lipomannan (LM) and lipoarabinomannan (LAM), modified after Chatterjee [149].

Most purified mycobacterial antigens tested so far signal through TLR2 (Table **1**), although some molecularly defined TLR4 agonists have been reported [39]. TLR2-dependent cell activation has been described for LAM from rapidly growing mycobacteria, lipomannan (LM), PIM (phosphatidyl-myo-inositol mannoside), or the 19kDa mycobacterial lipoprotein [40-47]. A more detailed discussion of mycobacterial ligands, their receptor specificity and biological properties is given below.

Table 1: Mycobacterial PAMPs Recognized by TLRs

• **TLR2**: PIM, *M. bovis* BCG tri-acylated LM, AraLAM, 19kDa, 38kDa, lipoprotein LprA, LprG, LpqH, Hsp65, PhoS1, Hsp70, PE_PGRS33, ESAT-6
• **TLR4**: *M. tuberculosis* LM, *M. bovis* BCG tetra-acylated LM, 38kDa, Hsp70
• **TLR9**: DNA

4.1. LAM, LM, PIMs

LAMs are lipoglycans ubiquitously found in the envelope of mycobacteria. They are composed of a carbohydrate backbone made of a mannosyl-phosphatidylinositol anchor (MPI), a D-mannan core and a D-arabinan domain, and some capping motifs (Fig. **1**) [48, 49]. The arabinan domain is either uncapped (AraLAM), or capped by mannosyl (ManLAM) or phosphoinositide residues (PILAM). Uncapped LAM has been described in *M. chelonae* [50], while ManLAMs have been found in the slow-growing mycobacteria, including *M. tuberculosis* [51], *M. bovis* BCG [52, 53], *M. avium* [54] and *M. kansasii* [55]. PILAMs have been identified in fast-growing species such as *M. smegmatis* [56]. LAMs are heterogeneous in composition, depending on the number of arabinosyl or mannosyl units composing the homopolysaccharides, or the structure of the MPI anchor and the capping motifs [57].

PILAMs from rapidly growing mycobacteria strains are pro-inflammatory molecules stimulating the production of TNF and IL-12, while ManLAMs are rather anti-inflammatory as they do not trigger the production of pro-inflammatory cytokines but rather stimulate IL-10 production and inhibit the production of IL-12 and TNF by dendritic cells or monocytic cell lines [58-60]. ManLAM has also been found to induce TGFβ [61]. As summarized in Table **2** PILAMs from avirulent, fast-growing mycobacteria activate macrophages in a TLR2-dependent manner by activating the NFκB signaling pathway [42] whereas the anti-inflammatory effects of ManLAMs have been attributed to their binding to the mannose receptor [58] or to DC-specific intercellular adhesion molecule-3 grabbing nonintegrin (DC-SIGN) [60, 62]. This suggests a correlation between LAM capping structures and their immunomodulatory effect.

LMs, the biosynthetic precursors of LAMs, represent another class of abundant pro-inflammatory molecules of the mycobacterial cell wall. LM from various mycobacterial origins, including *M. tuberculosis*, *M. bovis*, *M. chelonae*, *M. kansasii*, but none of the corresponding LAM, have been shown to induce macrophage activation. LM induction of CD40 and CD86 cell surface expression, abundant cytokine expression such as TNF, IL-8 or IL-12 and secretion of the antimycobacterial effector molecule nitric oxide has been reported [46, 47].

Activation by unseparated LM preparations is dependent on the presence of TLR2 and is mediated through the adaptor protein MyD88 [47]. The fact that the stimulatory effects of the different LM are absent for their respective LAM, supports the hypothesis that steric hindrance by the arabinan moiety blocks the TLR2 agonist activity of the LM moieties. Indeed, chemical degradation of the arabinan domain of *M. kansasii* LAM can restore the cytokine-inducing activity to a level similar to that seen with *M. kansasii* LM [46].

Further studies of the TLR agonist properties of isolated LM acylated isoforms of *M. bovis* have established that the pro-inflammatory activity is attributable to tri- and tetra-acylated forms of *M. bovis* BCG LM [39]. Tri-acyl-LM, an agonist of TLR2/TLR1, promotes interleukin-12 p40 and NO secretion through the adaptor proteins MyD88 and TIRAP, whereas the fraction containing tetra-acylated LM activates macrophages in a MyD88-dependent fashion, mostly through TLR4 [39]. TLR4-dependent pro-inflammatory activity was also seen with *M. tuberculosis* LM, composed mostly of tri-acylated LM, suggesting that the degree of acylation *per se* might not be sufficient to determine TLR2 *versus* TLR4 usage [39].

Table 2: TLR Usage of Mycobacterial Glycolipids

Glycolipid	TLR Usage	Species	References
PIM$_2$	TLR2, MyD88	*M. bovis*	[43]
PIM$_6$	TLR2, MyD88	*M. bovis*	[44]
LM	TLR2, TLR1, TLR4	*M. bovis*	[39, 64]
LM	TLR4, MyD88	*M. tuberculosis*	[39, 47]
ManLAM	--	*M. tuberculosis, M. bovis,*	[47]
PILAM	TLR2, MyD88	*M.smegmatis*	[42, 43]
AraLAM	TLR2, MyD88	*M.chelonae*	[46]

PIMs, the GPI anchor motifs of LM and LAM, have slight pro-inflammatory activities [63]. Dimannoside (PIM2) and hexa-mannoside (PIM6), the two most abundant classes of PIM found in *M. bovis* BCG and *M. tuberculosis* H37Rv, activate macrophages to secrete low levels of TNF through TLR2 and MyD88 [43, 44].

Therefore, the balance between PIM, LM and LAM synthesis by pathogenic mycobacteria, together with their acylation degree might provide different immunomodulatory signals during primary infection but also during latent infection.

4.2. Lipoproteins

Recognition of mycobacterial lipoproteins modulates the functions of both innate and acquired immunity. The *M. tuberculosis* glycolipoprotein 19kDa is both cell wall-associated and secreted and is a candidate virulence factor. It is a potent inducer of T-cell responses and it activates murine and human macrophages to secrete TNF and nitric oxide *via* interaction with TLR2, but not TLR4 [40, 41]. Further, *M. tuberculosis* lipoproteins LpqH, LprA, LprG and PhoS1 are TLR2 agonists, in combination with TLR1 for LpqH, LprG, and PhoS1. LprA does not require TLR1 and none require TLR6 [65]. CD14 contributes to detection of LpqH, LprA, and LprG whereas CD36 contributes only to detection of LprA [65]. However, definitive evidence for a physical interaction between these lipoproteins and TLRs is still lacking.

4.3. Soluble Tuberculosis Factor (STF)

STF is a component of a short term culture filtrate of *M. tuberculosis* purified by proteinase K digestion and triton extraction. Similar to 19kDa lipoprotein, STF interacts with TLR2, but not TLR4. Biochemical studies revealed PIMs as critical components of STF for the activation of NFκB, activator protein-1 and mitogen-activated protein kinases in murine macrophages [43]. Interestingly, dominant negative constructs of TLR2 or TLR6 inhibit the cellular responses induced by STF, suggesting a functional interaction between TLR2 and TLR6 [37], although no definitive involvement of TLR6 in the response to PIM2 or PIM6 could be demonstrated in TLR6-deficient macrophages [44]. The combined ligation of TLRs may potentially increase the diversity of responses to microbial antigens and enhance the spectrum of pathogen-associated molecular patterns which can be detected by the innate immune system.

5. TLR SIGNALING, PHAGOSOME MATURATION AND APOPTOSIS

Several pathogens induce apoptosis of infected cells [66], which may serve to sequester and increase killing of the pathogen. TLR2 is a molecular link between microbial products and host cell apoptosis, and bacterial lipoprotein-induced apoptosis could be important for generating the signals required to initiate adaptive immune responses. Macrophages infected with *M. tuberculosis* undergo increased rates of apoptosis. The 19kDa *M. tuberculosis* glycolipoprotein can induce apoptosis through TLR2 [40, 67] in a caspase-8-dependent and caspase-9-independent way, consistent with a transmembrane pathway signaling cell death through TLR2. Furthermore, *M. tuberculosis* LM can induce the synthesis of IL-12 and apoptosis in macrophages [68]. The viability of *M. tuberculosis* in cells undergoing apoptosis induced by 19kDa and possibly by other components is reduced, suggesting the possibility that this may favour containment of infection [67]. TLR pathways seem to contribute to mycobacteria internalisation [33, 34], and TLRs have been shown to induce a phagocytic gene program through p38 MAPK [69]. A role for TLR2 in survival strategies of *M. tuberculosis* in macrophage phagosomes has been proposed [70]. *M. tuberculosis* is phagocytosed by alveolar macrophages but is not digested and eventually survives and proliferates. Although TLR2 fulfills and important role in the host in multiple steps related to *M. tuberculosis*-macrophage association including macrophage activation during the early stage of the immune response, suppression of *M. tuberculosis* proliferation, direct bactericidal effect and also induction of apoptosis, TLR2 signaling also appears to play a key role in the *M. tuberculosis* strategy to escape immune responses by macrophages.

6. TLR MEDIATED DC MATURATION AND T CELL POLARIZATION

Dendritic cells (DC) have a key role in linking innate and adaptive immunity. Maturation of DC, which is a prerequisite for efficient activation of T-cells, is induced by infection with numerous pathogens, including *M. tuberculosis* [71]. The maturation *in vivo* is likely to be driven by mycobacterial PAMPs such as the 19kDa lipoprotein [72] or cell wall components [73] and is mediated by TLR2 or TLR4. Therefore lipopeptides can promote DC maturation, thus providing a mechanism by which products of mycobacteria can participate in the initiation of an adaptive immune response.

However, *M. tuberculosis* derived 19kDa lipoprotein actually inhibits antigen (Ag) processing by murine macrophages *via* a mechanism involving decreased synthesis of MHC class II molecules, which is dependent on TLR2 and independent of TLR4 [74-76]. Microarray gene expression analysis indicated that *M. tuberculosis* and 19kDa lipoprotein inhibited macrophage induction of 42 and 36% of 347 IFNγ-induced genes, including genes involved in MHC Class II Ag processing, Ag presentation, and recruitment of T cells, and that these effects were largely dependent on MyD88 [77]. Furthermore, *M. tuberculosis* and the 19kDa lipoprotein inhibits MHC class I expression and antigen processing [78]. Therefore, mycobacteria are capable of escaping efficient recognition by CD4 and CD8 T cells. In addition, transfection of fast-growing mycobacteria with the 19kDa lipoprotein reduces their ability to induce TNF and IL-12 release by human macrophages [79] and induces a Th2 polarised response [80, 81]. These observations may explain why vaccination with recombinant *M. vaccae* or *M. smegmatis* expressing 19kDa lipoprotein results in less protection than vaccination with non-recombinant strains [82, 83]. Similarly, Pam3Cys, a synthetic TLR2 agonist results in a predominant Th2 response, whilst TLR9 ligation with CpG induces a distinct Th1 response [84].

M. tuberculosis was shown to regulate CD1 antigen presentation pathways through TLR2 [85]. Infection with *M. tuberculosis* or exposure to mycobacterial cell wall products converts CD1- myeloid precursors into competent APCs that expressed CD1a, CD1b, and CD1c while CD1d expression is down-regulated. This process involves polar lipids that signal through TLR2 [85]. Thus, mycobacterial cell wall lipids provide two distinct signals for the activation of lipid-reactive T cells: lipid antigens that activate T cell receptors and lipid adjuvants that activate APCs through TLR2.

Infection of macrophages with a variety of bacteria, including *M. tuberculosis*, results in the upregulation of several genes required to mount an efficient immune response against pathogens [86]. The activation of these genes is similarly induced by bacterial components that are agonists for TLR2 or TLR4, suggesting that TLRs are responsible for triggering the adaptive immune response. TLRs were first seen as key molecules for shaping the quality of the immune response against microbes since mice lacking MyD88 were reportedly incapable of developing antigen-specific Th1 responses after immunization with ovalbumin mixed with complete Freunds adjuvant (containing heat-killed *M. tuberculosis* H37Ra as active component) [87]. However, this concept was challenged by the finding that a Th1 responses to *Listeria* and *Mycobacteria* can be induced in the absence of MyD88 signaling [88-90].

7. PATTERN RECOGNITION RECEPTOR INTERPLAY FOR MYCOBACTERIAL RECOGNITION

Although macrophages respond to several products of *M. tuberculosis* through TLR2 or TLR4, their transcriptional response to viable, virulent *M. tuberculosis* has been shown to be mediated by pathways largely independent of TLR2, TLR4, and MyD88, but requiring IFN$\alpha\beta$R and STAT1 [91]. Release of IL-1β, which plays an important role in the anti-mycobacterial host defense mechanisms was recently reported to be induced by *M. tuberculosis* through pathways involving TLR2/TLR6 and NOD2 receptors, but not TLR4, TLR9 and TLR1 [92]. Recognition of *M. tuberculosis* by TLRs and NOD2 led to transcription of proIL-1β through mechanisms involving ERK, p38 MAPK and Rip2, but not JNK. In addition secretion of IL-1β was dependent on the activation of P2X7-induced pathways by endogenously released ATP [92].

Receptors other than TLRs such as CD14, scavenger and complement receptors, pulmonary surfactant protein A, C-type lectins including the mannose receptor and DC-SIGN, CD40 and CD44, have all been implicated in mycobacteria binding, recognition of mycobacterial antigens, or coupling to a cellular response. The C-type lectin β-glucan receptor, Dectin-1 functions together with TLR2 to mediate macrophage activation by mycobacteria [93] and induction of Dectin-1 by *M. tuberculosis* in type II airway epithelial cells, *via* TLR2 and Src kinases, has been shown to be involved in bacillus internalization, pro-inflammatory cytokine release and antimicrobial effects on intracellular mycobacterial growth [94]. *M. tuberculosis* cell wall glycolipid, trehalose 6,6'-dimycolate (TDM or cord factor) was shown to mediate NFκB activation and potent inflammatory responses *via* the macrophage receptor with collagenous structure (MARCO), a class A scavenger receptor, in addition to TLR2 and CD14. MARCO was used preferentially over scavenger receptor class A (SRA), which required TLR2 and TLR4, as well as their respective accessory molecules [95]. Complement receptors play an important role for the binding and phagocytosis of many pathogens, including mycobacteria [96]. In addition, mannose receptors bind *M. tuberculosis* through LAM, and might be required for phagocytosis [97]. Binding of *M. tuberculosis* to human macrophages is dependent on the terminal mannosyl residues of LAM and is competed by excess mannan [98]. By contrast, complement receptor 3 and mannose receptor, which are major *M. tuberculosis* receptors on macrophages, appear to play a minor role for binding to DCs [96]. *M. tuberculosis* has been shown to bind to human DCs through DC-SIGN [62, 99] with LAM being identified as a key ligand of DC-SIGN [99]. DC-SIGN-mediated entry of *M. tuberculosis* into DCs *in vivo* might influence bacterial persistence and host immunity. The murine DC-SIGN homologue SIGNR3 was recently shown to be expressed in lung phagocytes during infection, and to interact with *M. tuberculosis* and mycobacterial surface glycoconjugates to induce secretion of critical host defense inflammatory cytokines such as TNF [100]. Also, CD44, an adhesion molecule upregulated in inflammatory responses and involved in phagocytosis, has been shown to be a macrophage receptor capable of binding to *M. tuberculosis* [101]. In summary, several receptors other than TLRs are involved in mycobacteria recognition. The contribution of single, but more likely a combination of different PRRs may be required for optimal mycobacteria recognition, binding and downstream signal transduction and cell activation [102].

8. INHIBITION OF INFLAMMATORY RESPONSES BY MYCOBACTERIA MOTIFS

The immune evasion of mycobacteria may be the result of complex interactions between molecular motifs of the mycobacteria and several levels of the immune response. As mentioned, 19kD lipoprotein down-modulates host MHC Class I and II expression through TLR2 [74-76, 78]. Expression of 19kDa lipoprotein inhibits *M. smegmatis*-induced cytokine production in human macrophages [79]. Further, 19kDa inhibits macrophage responses to IFNγ at a transcriptional level, in a TLR2-dependent and MyD88-dependent fashion [103]. Cell wall peptidoglycan (mAGP) also inhibits macrophage responses to IFNγ, but independently of TLR2, TLR4, and MyD88, and both 19kDa and mAGP can inhibit the ability of IFNγ to activate murine macrophages to kill *M. tuberculosis* without inhibiting production of NO [103]. Other negative regulators have been well characterised. Direct binding of the early secreted antigen ESAT-6 to TLR2 has been shown to inhibit TLR4 signaling in macrophages by activating Akt and preventing interaction between MyD88 and the downstream kinase IRAK4, thus abrogating NFκB activation [104].

A strong inhibition of TNF and IL-12 release by ManLAM from *M. bovis* BCG and *M. tuberculosis* in human dendritic or THP-1 cells stimulated with LPS was shown, and ManLAM's anti-inflammatory effects were attributed to binding to the mannose receptor or DC-SIGN [58-60]. Mannose receptor ligation inhibits IL-12 production by human dendritic cells [58] and DC-SIGN has been shown to be involved in ManLAM inhibition of mycobacteria- or LPS-induced DC maturation [60]. ManLAM, but not PILAM, inhibits *M. tuberculosis* binding to DC-SIGN [62]. *M. tuberculosis* interacts with DC-SIGN to activate the Raf-1-acetylation-dependent signaling pathway to modulate signaling by different TLRs, leading to NFκB p65 subunit acetylation, and prolonged and increased IL-10 transcription [105]. On the other hand, ManLAM inhibition of TLR4-induced IL-12 p40 expression was reported to be independent of IL-10 expression and mediated by induction of IRAK-M, a negative regulator of TLR signaling [106].

A dual function has been described for LMs, the biosynthetic precursors of LAMs. Although LM from several mycobacterial species stimulate cytokine synthesis, di-acylated forms of *M. bovis* BCG LM can exert a potent inhibitory effect on TNF, IL-12p40 and nitric oxide production by LPS-activated macrophages, independent of TLR2, TLR6 and MyD88 [47]. Therefore, mycobacterial LM bear structural motifs that can interact with different pattern recognition receptors with pro- or anti-inflammatory effects. ManLAM, predominantly anti-inflammatory, may be viewed as an "attenuated" form of LM. LM's inhibitory effects on macrophages are presumably mediated through other PRRs such as the mannose receptor or DC-SIGN, as proposed for ManLAM on DC [58, 60]. While earlier studies using coated polystyrene beads indicated that neither PILAM nor LM bound to mannose receptor [97], LM was recently shown to bind to the DC-SIGN murine homologues SIGNR1 and SIGNR3, but not SIGNR5 [100].

Therefore, mycobacteria may influence the cytokine environment by favouring LAM *versus* LM synthesis, its expression in the cell wall, and release out of the mycobacterial phagosome to the medium and bystander cells, as previously shown for LAM and PIM [107]. Indeed, the LM/LAM ratio seems variable in different mycobacteria, from 9:1 (mol:mol) in *M. chelonae* [50], 3:1 in *M. kansasii* [55] and 1:1 in *M. bovis* BCG [108]. Thus, regulation of the arabinosyltransferases involved in the synthesis of the arabinan domain of LAM may lead to important changes regarding to the LM/LAM balance, which may be a critical step for directing the outcome of innate immunity against mycobacteria. Inactivation of the *embC* gene in *M.*

smegmatis affected LAM arabinosylation and resulted in complete cessation of LAM biosynthesis although LM and PIMs were still synthesized [109]. Further, the degree of LM acylation may favour pro-inflammatory (in tri- or tetra-acylated forms) *versus* anti-inflammatory (in di-acylated forms) effects. The biological significance of the LM/LAM balance and LM acylation pattern in the establishment and the persistence of the host immune response during tuberculosis infection remain to be investigated.

9. ROLE OF TLR PATHWAYS DURING *IN VIVO* INFECTION BY *M. TUBERCULOSIS*

The role of TLR signaling in controlling mycobacterial infection has been addressed in a series of *in vivo* infectious studies in gene deficient mice [16, 110, 111]. The recent results for *M. bovis* BCG and *M. tuberculosis* are summarized in Table 3 and below.

After chronic aerosol infection with virulent *M. tuberculosis*, TLR4 deficient mice have a slightly reduced bacterial clearance, develop a chronic pneumonia and die within 6 months [112, 113]. Further, TLR4 deficient mice displayed increased susceptibility at an early stage of *M. tuberculosis* by aerosol, which was overcome at a later stage [114]. However, other have reported no significant differences in the inflammatory response or the bacterial burden in infected organs during acute and long-term infection of TLR4 deficient mice [115-117]. CD14, a coreceptor of TLR4, appears not to be involved in host resistance, as CD14 deficient mice normally clear the infection [115].

TLR2 deficient mice infected by aerosol using 500 CFU had reduced bacterial clearance, a defective granulomatous response and developed chronic pneumonia [118]. Analysis of pulmonary immune responses in TLR2 deficient mice showed increased levels of IFNγ, TNF, and IL-12p40 as well as increased numbers of CD4+ and CD8+ cells. Furthermore, TLR2 deficient mice mounted an elevated antigen-specific type 1 T cell response that was not protective as all deficient mice succumbed to infection within 5 months, suggesting that TLR2 may function as a regulator of inflammation, and in its absence an exaggerated immune-inflammatory response develops [118].

Table 3: Redundancy of TLRs in Controlling *M.tuberculosis* Infection

Susceptibility of TLR Deficient Mice to *M. Tuberculosis* Infection *in vivo*	References
TLR4	
- Some control of chronic infection	[112-114]
- No role in control of infection	[115-117]
TLR2	
- Discrete effect at 100 cfu	[118]
- Role only at high *M. tuterculosis* dose	[114, 115, 119]
TLR6	
No effect	[119]
TLR2 + TLR9	
More effect than either alone	[120]
TLR2 + TLR4 + TLR9	
No effect of triple TLR2+4+9 ko on acute TB	[121]

Increased susceptibility of TLR2 deficient mice was reported at an early stage of *M. tuberculosis* aerosol infection, correlated to reduced induction of anti-bacterial activity by infected TLR2-deficient macrophages, and resumed thereafter [114]. A limited role for TLR2 in the control of *M. tuberculosis* infection was also found, most visible at high dose infection [115, 119]. TLR2 forms heterodimers with either TLR6 or TLR1, and the role of these receptors in mycobacterial responses was questioned. TLR6 deficient mice are resistant to high *M. tuberculosis* aerosol infection [119], however no data has so far been reported on the role of TLR1 signaling in the *in vivo* host response.

The question of TLR redundancy was addressed when TLR9 was reported to cooperate with TLR2 in mediating optimal resistance to *M. tuberculosis* [120]. Mice deficient for both TLR2 and TLR9 displayed markedly enhanced susceptibility to *M. tuberculosis* infection and altered pulmonary pathology, as compared to single TLR-deficient animals [120]. However, it was reported recently that mice triple deficient for TLR2, TLR4 and TLR9 survive acute *M. tuberculosis* infection and control *M. tuberculosis* replication essentially as well as wild-type mice [121], questioning the overall role of TLRs in the control of acute *M. tuberculosis* infection.

The implication of the TLR/IL-1R common adaptor protein MyD88, in host resistance to *M. tuberculosis* was addressed. Either only minor effects [122] or a profound loss of resistance [90, 121, 123, 124] were reported in MyD88 deficient mice, as summarized in Table **4**. We found that a low dose aerosol infection with *M. tuberculosis* caused acute necrotic pneumonia with uncontrolled bacterial growth in the lung [90], ressembling the phenotype of TNF deficiency [125, 126]. Interestingly MyD88 deficient mice developed an antigen specific response with IFNγ production, and BCG vaccination conferred a partial immune protection [90]. However, examination of other pathways which also use MyD88 as an adaptor demonstrated that although IL-18R signaling seem dispensable for the control of acute TB infection, IL-1R was essential for host resistance [14]. Aerogenic *M. tuberculosis* infection of IL-1R1-deficient mice was lethal within 4 weeks with uncontrolled bacterial growth in the lung and necrotic pneumonia but efficient pulmonary CD4 and CD8 T cell responses, as seen in MyD88-deficient mice [14]. Thus, IL-1R, together with IL-1-induced innate responses, might account for most of MyD88-dependent host response to control acute *M. tuberculosis* infection. Indeed, the side-by-side study of mice deficient for MyD88 or triple deficient for TLR2, TLR4 plus TLR9 clearly demonstrated that MyD88 deficient mice rapidly succumbed to unrestrained mycobacterial growth while triple TLR2/TLR4/ TLR9 deficient mice controlled *M. tuberculosis* replication [121].

Table 4: Implication of MyD88 in the Responses to *M.tuberculosis* Infection

Profound Defect of Innate Immunity Despite Adaptive Response in MyD88 KO:	
- Low cytokine, chemokine response to mycobacteria *in vitro*	
- Reduced internalization of mycobacteria	
- Uncontrolled infection, extracellular *M. tuberculosis*	
- No granuloma formation, necrosis	
but	
- Induction of mycobacteria specific adaptive response	
- Recruitment of primed activated CD4+ and CD8+ T cells,	
- Partial protection after BCG vaccination	
Phenotype Reported for MyD88 KO Upon *M. tuberculosis* Infection	**References**
- Uncontrolled infection	[90, 121, 123, 124]
- Limited effect	[122]

In conclusion, TLR signaling seems to play only a modest role in the control of acute mycobacterial infection and generation of adaptive immunity, and the role of MyD88 may be largely due to its implication in IL-1R signaling. In addition, the role of MyD88 signaling is dependent on mycobacteria virulence since MyD88-deficient mice survived 8 months *M. bovis* BCG infection, although they had a reduced capacity to clear mycobacteria from the lung and developed large, confluent pulmonary granulomata [33]. This is in contrast with TNF deficient mice which are also unable to control infection with the attenuated *M. bovis* BCG and succumb within 3 months [127]. Thus, MyD88 is crucial for the immediate innate response to virulent *M. tuberculosis* while a less virulent mycobacteria may be handled by MyD88 independent innate responses in the first weeks needed to establish an efficient adaptive response.

10. PRR INTERPLAY IN THE CONTROL OF *M. TUBERCULOSIS* INFECTION

As mentioned, beyond TLRs several receptor families such as C-type lectins, scavenger and complement receptors, have been implicated in mycobacteria recognition. There are 7 murine orthologues of DCSIGN,

SIGNR1-5 and SIGNR7-8, and mice singly deficient for some of these receptors have been studied. Deficiency in SIGNR1 did not alter the control of acute or chronic *M. tuberculosis* infection [102, 128]. In a comparative study of mice lacking SIGNR1, SIGNR3 or SIGNR5, only SIGNR3-deficient animals had an impaired resistance to acute *M. tuberculosis*, with a less effective control of bacterial load 3-6 weeks post-infection [100]. SIGNR3 was expressed in lung phagocytes during infection, and interacted with *M. tuberculosis* bacilli and mycobacterial surface glycoconjugates to induce TNF secretion through a tyrosine kinase Syk dependent signaling [100]. Another elegant approach was undertaken to explore the role of DC-SIGN in the control of *M. tuberculosis* infection *in vivo* using transgenic mice expressing the human DC-SIGN/CD209 under the control of the murine CD11c promoter (hSIGN). Upon mycobacterial infection, DCs from hSIGN mice produced significantly less IL-12p40 but similar levels of IL-10 relative to wild-type DCs. After high dose *M. tuberculosis* aerosol infection hSIGN mice showed massive accumulation of DC-SIGN+ cells in infected lungs, with reduced tissue damage and prolonged survival, suggesting that instead of favoring mycobacteria immune evasion, DC-SIGN promoted protection by limiting tuberculosis-induced pathology [129].

A systematic study of several C-type lectins or scavenger receptors documented that single deficiency in either SR-A, MARCO, CD36, mannose receptor, SIGNR1, or the seven transmembrane receptor, EGF-module-containing mucin-like hormone receptor 1 (EMR1) murine ortholog F4/80 did not impair the host resistance to acute or chronic *M. tuberculosis* infection in terms of survival, control of bacterial clearance, lung inflammation, granuloma formation and cytokine expression [102]. Double deficiency for the scavenger receptors SR-A plus CD36 or for the C-type lectins mannose receptor plus SIGNR1 had a limited effect on macrophage uptake of mycobacteria, on TNF response and on the long-term control of *M. tuberculosis* infection [102]. By contrast, mice deficient in TNF, IL-1 or IFNγ pathways were unable to control acute *M. tuberculosis* infection. Thus, there seem to be a functional redundancy in the pattern recognition receptors, which might cooperate in a coordinated response to sustain the full immune control of *M. tuberculosis* infection. This is in sharp contrast with the non-redundant, essential role of TNF, IL-1 or IFNγ pathways for host resistance to *M. tuberculosis*.

11. TLR POLYMORPHISMS AND MYCOBACTERIAL INFECTION

The functional relevance of the experimental data may be confirmed in humans through genetic studies of mutations or epidemiological studies of common single nucleotide polymorphism. The fact that only 5-10% of individuals infected with *M. tuberculosis* develop active tuberculosis disease suggests a significant role for genetic variation in the human immune response to this infection and has prompted numerous studies of associations between TLR polymorphisms and mycobacterial infection.

The screening of the TLR2 intracellular domain in the peripheral blood from leprosy patients demonstrated a band variant that was detected by single-stranded conformational polymorphism in 10 of 45 subjects with severe disease. The Arg677Trp mutation in one of the conserved regions of TLR2's intracellular signaling domain was associated with decreased IL-12, IL-2, IFNγ and TNF release by *M. leprae*-stimulated PBMCs, together with increased production of IL-10 [130-132]. Analysis of polymorphisms in intron II of the TLR2 gene showed that the development of tuberculosis in Koreans was associated with shorter GT repeats in TLR2 intron II and correlated with the lower expression of TLR2 through weaker promoter activity [133]. The influence of host and bacterial genotype on the development of disseminated disease with *M. tuberculosis* was studied in Vietnamese patients with tuberculous meningitis or uncomplicated pulmonary tuberculosis [134] and a significant protective association between the Euro-American lineage of *M. tuberculosis* and pulmonary rather than meningeal tuberculosis was found, suggesting these strains are less capable of extra-pulmonary dissemination than others in the study population. Further, individuals with a TLR2 T597C allele were more likely to have tuberculosis caused by the East-Asian/Beijing genotype than other individuals [134].

Recently, 71 polymorphisms in TLR1, TLR2, TLR4, TLR6, and TLR9 were examined and variants in TLR2 and TLR9 were found to influence susceptibility to pulmonary tuberculosis in Caucasians, African-Americans, and West Africans, with the strongest evidence for association at an insertion (I)/deletion (D) polymorphism (-196 to -174) in TLR2 that associated with tuberculosis in both Caucasians and Africans [135]. The Arg753Gln polymorphism in TLR2 led to a weaker response against *M. tuberculosis* [136].

Variation in the inflammatory response to bacterial lipopeptides was associated with a TLR1 transmembrane domain, non-synonymous polymorphism, I602S, with the I variant mediating substantially greater NFκB signaling than the S variant in response to lipopeptide or *M. tuberculosis* extracts [137]. The TLR1 I602S common polymorphism impaired trafficking of the receptor to the cell surface and diminished responses of blood monocytes to bacterial agonists but it was associated with a decreased incidence of leprosy [138]. Also consistent with disease association, rare TLR6 variants were defective in their ability to mediate NFκB signal transduction in transfected human cells [139]. A large population-based case-control study with full-exon resequencing revealed common nonsynonymous polymorphisms in TLR6-TLR1-TLR10 significantly associated with tuberculosis disease in certain ethnic groups, with African Americans homozygotes for the common-variant haplotype TLR1-248S, TLR1-602I, and TLR6-249S at significantly increased tuberculosis disease risk [139].

A role for the TLR8 gene in susceptibility to tuberculosis was revealed through analysis of association of 18 genes involved in the TLR pathways [140]: genotyping of 149 sequence polymorphisms in pulmonary tuberculosis patients from Indonesia revealed four polymorphisms in the TLR8 gene on chromosome X with association with tuberculosis susceptibility in males, including a non-synonymous polymorphism Met1Val; these four TLR8 polymorphisms were analyzed in pulmonary tuberculosis patients from Russia and evidence of association confirmed in males. TLR8 transcript levels were significantly up-regulated in patients during the acute phase of disease and a marked increase in TLR8 protein expression was also observed in macrophages upon *M. bovis* BCG infection [140]. Taken together, the data suggest that variant TLRs contribute to human susceptibility to tuberculosis disease.

A single-nucleotide polymorphism, C558T, in TIRAP, the adaptor common to TLR2 and TLR4, was associated with increased susceptibility to tuberculosis and furthermore to the meningeal rather than pulmonary form of tuberculosis [141, 142]. In comparison to the 558CC genotype, the 558TT genotype was associated with decreased whole-blood IL-6 production, which suggested that TIRAP influenced disease susceptibility by modulating the inflammatory response. A large case-control study of individuals from the UK, Vietnam and several African countries revealed a protective effect of TIRAP S180L heterozygosity against invasive pneumococcal disease, bacteremia, malaria and tuberculosis, and the TIRAPS180L variant was found to attenuate TLR2 signal transduction [143, 144]. Another TIRAP allele, Leu180, was also found to be a common protective factor against developing tuberculosis and systemic lupus erythematosus in a case-control and family based association study of 1325 Colombian individuals [145]. A further study indicated that the TIRAP S180L polymorphism was virtually absent in Ghana, and no significant association of TIRAP S180L heterozygous genotype with sepsis or leprosy was found, while those homozygous for TIRAP 180L tended to increase the risk of sepsis in a German study [146].

Interestingly, children with autosomal recessive MyD88 deficiency or children lacking IL-1 receptor–associated kinase 4 (IRAK-4), recruited by MyD88 to TLRs and IL-1Rs, presented with a life-threatening but narrow and transient predisposition to infection, apparently restricted to pyogenic bacterial infections [147, 148]. These patients were otherwise healthy, with normal resistance to other microbes, including most common bacteria, viruses, fungi, and parasites, and it was suggested that the MyD88-dependent TLRs and IL-1Rs, although essential for protective immunity to a small number of pyogenic bacteria, may be redundant for host defense to most natural infections in these patients [148].

12. CONCLUSIONS AND PERSPECTIVES

Mycobacteria express a series of molecular motifs capable of triggering different pattern recognition receptors, including TLR2 in association with TLR1 or TLR6, but also TLR4 or TLR9, that trigger innate immune responses with induction of proinflammatory cytokines. They also express several peptides or glycolipids able to downregulate host inflammatory responses, that may contribute to immune evasion [149]. *In vivo* however, single or combined TLR2, TLR4 and/or TLR9 are not essential for the control of acute tuberculosis infection in mice but these receptors may interfere in the control of chronic infection. The lack of control of acute tuberculosis infection in the absence of MyD88 in mice, may be attributed to IL-1R signaling, rather than TLRs. There seem to be a functional redundancy of different pattern recognition receptors, in sharp contrast to the pro-inflammatory cytokine TNF, IL-1 and IFNγ pathways, which are each essential and cannot compensate for each other in the control of *M. tuberculosis* infection. While most pathogens are recognized by a unique or a limited set of receptors, mycobacteria express multiple molecular motifs recognized by multiple receptors and can trigger the activation of different signaling pathways that might cooperate in a coordinated response to sustain the full immune control of *M. tuberculosis* infection.

REFERENCES

[1] Dye C, Watt CJ, Bleed DM, Hosseini SM, Raviglione MC. Evolution of tuberculosis control and prospects for reducing tuberculosis incidence, prevalence, and deaths globally. Jama 2005; 293: 2767-75.

[2] Gill WP, Harik NS, Whiddon MR, Liao RP, Mittler JE, Sherman DR. A replication clock for *Mycobacterium tuberculosis*. Nat Med 2009; 15: 211-4.

[3] Keane J. TNF-blocking agents and tuberculosis: new drugs illuminate an old topic. Rheumatology (Oxford) 2005; 44: 714-20

[4] Keane J, Gershon S, Wise RP *et al.* Tuberculosis associated with infliximab, a tumor necrosis factor alpha-neutralizing agent. N Engl J Med 2001; 345: 1098-104.

[5] Mohan AK, Cote TR, Siegel JN, Braun MM. Infectious complications of biologic treatments of rheumatoid arthritis. Curr Opin Rheumatol 2003; 15: 179-84.

[6] Mohan VP, Scanga CA, Yu K *et al.* Effects of tumor necrosis factor alpha on host immune response in chronic persistent tuberculosis: possible role for limiting pathology. Infect Immun 2001; 69: 1847-55.

[7] Mwandumba HC, Russell DG, Nyirenda MH *et al. Mycobacterium tuberculosis* resides in nonacidified vacuoles in endocytically competent alveolar macrophages from patients with tuberculosis and HIV infection. J Immunol 2004; 172: 4592-8.

[8] Flynn JL, Chan J. Immunology of tuberculosis. Annu Rev Immunol 2001; 19: 93-129.

[9] Flynn JL. Immunology of tuberculosis and implications in vaccine development. Tuberculosis (Edinb) 2004; 84: 93-101.

[10] North RJ, Jung YJ. Immunity to tuberculosis. Annu Rev Immunol 2004;22:599-623.

[11] Umemura M, Yahagi A, Hamada S *et al.* IL-17-mediated regulation of innate and acquired immune response against pulmonary *Mycobacterium bovis* bacille Calmette-Guerin infection. J Immunol 2007; 178: 3786-96.

[12] Khader SA, Cooper AM. IL-23 and IL-17 in tuberculosis. Cytokine 2008; 41: 79-83.

[13] Khader SA, Bell GK, Pearl JE *et al.* IL-23 and IL-17 in the establishment of protective pulmonary CD4+ T cell responses after vaccination and during *Mycobacterium tuberculosis* challenge. Nat Immunol 2007; 8: 369-77.

[14] Fremond CM, Togbe D, Doz E *et al.* IL-1 receptor-mediated signal is an essential component of MyD88-dependent innate response to *Mycobacterium tuberculosis* infection. J Immunol 2007; 179: 1178-89.

[15] Master SS, Rampini SK, Davis AS *et al. Mycobacterium tuberculosis* prevents inflammasome activation. Cell Host Microbe 2008; 3: 224-32.

[16] Stenger S, Modlin RL. Control of *Mycobacterium tuberculosis* through mammalian Toll-like receptors. Curr Opin Immunol 2002; 14: 452-7.

[17] Heldwein KA, Fenton MJ. The role of Toll-like receptors in immunity against mycobacterial infection. Microbes Infect 2002; 4: 937-44.

[18] Medzhitov R, Biron CA. Innate immunity. Curr Opin Immunol 2003; 15: 2-4.

[19] Takeda K, Kaisho T, Akira S. Toll-like receptors. Annu Rev Immunol 2003; 21: 335-76.

[20] Akira S. Mammalian Toll-like receptors. Curr Opin Immunol 2003; 15: 5-11.

[21] O'Neill LA. The interleukin-1 receptor/Toll-like receptor superfamily: 10 years of progress. Immunol Rev 2008; 226: 10-8.

[22] Zarember KA, Godowski PJ. Tissue expression of human Toll-like receptors and differential regulation of Toll-like receptor mRNAs in leukocytes in response to microbes, their products, and cytokines. J Immunol 2002; 168: 554-61.

[23] O'Neill LA. Immunology. After the toll rush. Science 2004; 303: 1481-2.

[24] Droemann D, Goldmann T, Branscheid D *et al.* Toll-like receptor 2 is expressed by alveolar epithelial cells type II and macrophages in the human lung. Histochem Cell Biol 2003; 119: 103-8.

[25]   Hertz CJ, Wu Q, Porter EM *et al.* Activation of Toll-like receptor 2 on human tracheobronchial epithelial cells induces the antimicrobial peptide human beta defensin-2. J Immunol 2003; 171: 6820-6.

[26]   Chang JS, Huggett JF, Dheda K, Kim LU, Zumla A, Rook GA. Myobacterium tuberculosis induces selective up-regulation of TLRs in the mononuclear leukocytes of patients with active pulmonary tuberculosis. J Immunol 2006; 176: 3010-8.

[27]   Pompei L, Jang S, Zamlynny B *et al.* Disparity in IL-12 Release in Dendritic Cells and Macrophages in Response to *Mycobacterium tuberculosis* Is Due to Use of Distinct TLRs. J Immunol 2007; 178: 5192-9.

[28]   Khan N, Alam K, Mande SC, Valluri VL, Hasnain SE, Mukhopadhyay S. *Mycobacterium tuberculosis* heat shock protein 60 modulates immune response to PPD by manipulating the surface expression of TLR2 on macrophages. Cell Microbiol 2008; 10: 1711-22.

[29]   Rocha-Ramirez LM, Estrada-Garcia I, Lopez-Marin LM *et al. Mycobacterium tuberculosis* lipids regulate cytokines, TLR-2/4 and MHC class II expression in human macrophages. Tuberculosis (Edinb) 2008; 88: 212-20.

[30]   Means TK, Wang S, Lien E, Yoshimura A, Golenbock DT, Fenton MJ. Human toll-like receptors mediate cellular activation by *Mycobacterium tuberculosis*. J Immunol 1999; 163: 3920-7.

[31]   Means TK, Jones BW, Schromm AB *et al.* Differential effects of a Toll-like receptor antagonist on *Mycobacterium tuberculosis*-induced macrophage responses. J Immunol 2001; 166: 4074-82.

[32]   Fremond CMC, Nicolle, D.M.M., Torres, D.S., Quesniaux, V.F.J. Control of *Mycobacterium bovis* BCG infection with increased inflammation in TLR4-deficient mice. Microbes Infect 2003; 5: 1070.

[33]   Nicolle DM, Pichon X, Bouchot A *et al.* Chronic pneumonia despite adaptive immune response to *Mycobacterium bovis* BCG in MyD88-deficient mice. Lab Invest 2004; 84: 1305-21.

[34]   Nicolle D, Fremond C, Pichon X *et al.* Long-term control of *Mycobacterium bovis* BCG infection in the absence of Toll-like receptors (TLRs): investigation of TLR2-, TLR6-, or TLR2-TLR4-deficient mice. Infect Immun 2004; 72: 6994-7004.

[35]   El Kasmi KC, Qualls JE, Pesce JT *et al.* Toll-like receptor-induced arginase 1 in macrophages thwarts effective immunity against intracellular pathogens. Nat Immunol 2008; 9: 1399-406.

[36]   Heldwein KA, Liang MD, Andresen TK *et al.* TLR2 and TLR4 serve distinct roles in the host immune response against *Mycobacterium bovis* BCG. J Leukoc Biol 2003; 74: 277-86.

[37]   Bulut Y, Faure E, Thomas L, Equils O, Arditi M. Cooperation of Toll-like receptor 2 and 6 for cellular activation by soluble tuberculosis factor and *Borrelia burgdorferi* outer surface protein A lipoprotein: role of Toll-interacting protein and IL-1 receptor signaling molecules in Toll-like receptor 2 signaling. J Immunol 2001; 167: 987-94.

[38]   Hajjar AM, O'Mahony DS, Ozinsky A *et al.* Cutting edge: functional interactions between toll-like receptor (TLR) 2 and TLR1 or TLR6 in response to phenol-soluble modulin. J Immunol 2001; 166: 15-9.

[39]   Doz E, Rose S, Nigou J *et al.* Acylation determines the toll-like receptor (TLR)-dependent positive versus TLR2-, mannose receptor-, and SIGNR1-independent negative regulation of pro-inflammatory cytokines by mycobacterial lipomannan. J Biol Chem 2007; 282: 26014-25.

[40]   Aliprantis AO, Yang RB, Mark MR *et al.* Cell activation and apoptosis by bacterial lipoproteins through toll-like receptor-2. Science 1999; 285: 736-9.

[41]   Brightbill HD, Libraty DH, Krutzik SR *et al.* Host defense mechanisms triggered by microbial lipoproteins through toll-like receptors. Science 1999; 285: 732-6.

[42]   Means TK, Lien E, Yoshimura A, Wang S, Golenbock DT, Fenton MJ. The CD14 ligands lipoarabinomannan and lipopolysaccharide differ in their requirement for Toll-like receptors. J Immunol 1999; 163: 6748-55.

[43]   Jones BW, Means TK, Heldwein KA *et al.* Different Toll-like receptor agonists induce distinct macrophage responses. J Leukoc Biol 2001;69:1036-44.

[44]   Gilleron M, Quesniaux VF, Puzo G. Acylation state of the phosphatidylinositol hexamannosides from *Mycobacterium bovis* bacillus Calmette Guerin and *Mycobacterium tuberculosis* H37Rv and its implication in Toll-like receptor response. J Biol Chem 2003; 278: 29880-9.

[45]   Barnes PF, Chatterjee D, Abrams JS *et al.* Cytokine production induced by *Mycobacterium tuberculosis* lipoarabinomannan. Relationship to chemical structure. J Immunol 1992; 149: 541-7.

[46]   Vignal C, Guerardel Y, Kremer L *et al.* Lipomannans, but not lipoarabinomannans, purified from *Mycobacterium chelonae* and *Mycobacterium kansasii* induce TNF-alpha and IL-8 secretion by a CD14-toll-like receptor 2-dependent mechanism. J Immunol 2003; 171: 2014-23.

[47]   Quesniaux VJ, Nicolle DM, Torres D *et al.* Toll-like receptor 2 (TLR2)-dependent-positive and TLR2-independent-negative regulation of proinflammatory cytokines by mycobacterial lipomannans. J Immunol 2004; 172: 4425-34.

[48]   Besra GS, Morehouse CB, Rittner CM, Waechter CJ, Brennan PJ. Biosynthesis of mycobacterial lipoarabinomannan. J Biol Chem 1997; 272: 18460-6.

[49]   Nigou J, Gilleron M, Puzo G. Lipoarabinomannans: characterization of the multiacylated forms of the phosphatidyl-myo-inositol anchor by NMR spectroscopy. Biochem J 1999; 337: 453-60.

[50]   Guerardel Y, Maes E, Elass E *et al.* Structural study of lipomannan and lipoarabinomannan from *Mycobacterium chelonae.* Presence of unusual components with alpha 1,3-mannopyranose side chains. J Biol Chem 2002; 277: 30635-48.

[51]   Chatterjee D, Roberts AD, Lowell K, Brennan PJ, Orme IM. Structural basis of capacity of lipoarabinomannan to induce secretion of tumor necrosis factor. Infect Immun 1992; 60: 1249-53.

[52]   Prinzis S, Chatterjee D, Brennan PJ. Structure and antigenicity of lipoarabinomannan from *Mycobacterium bovis* BCG. J Gen Microbiol 1993; 139: 2649-58.

[53]   Venisse A, Riviere M, Vercauteren J, Puzo G. Structural analysis of the mannan region of lipoarabinomannan from *Mycobacterium bovis* BCG. Heterogeneity in phosphorylation state. J Biol Chem 1995; 270: 15012-21.

[54]   Khoo KH, Tang JB, Chatterjee D. Variation in mannose-capped terminal arabinan motifs of lipoarabinomannans from clinical isolates of *Mycobacterium tuberculosis* and *Mycobacterium avium* complex. J Biol Chem 2001;276:3863-71.

[55]   Guerardel Y, Maes E, Briken V *et al.* Lipomannan and lipoarabinomannan from a clinical isolate of *Mycobacterium kansasii:* novel structural features and apoptosis-inducing properties. J Biol Chem 2003; 278: 36637-51.

[56]   Khoo KH, Dell A, Morris HR, Brennan PJ, Chatterjee D. Inositol phosphate capping of the nonreducing termini of lipoarabinomannan from rapidly growing strains of *Mycobacterium.* J Biol Chem 1995; 270: 12380-9.

[57]   Nigou J, Gilleron M, Puzo G. Lipoarabinomannans: from structure to biosynthesis. Biochimie 2003; 85: 153-66.

[58]   Nigou J, Zelle-Rieser C, Gilleron M, Thurnher M, Puzo G. Mannosylated lipoarabinomannans inhibit IL-12 production by human dendritic cells: evidence for a negative signal delivered through the mannose receptor. J Immunol 2001; 166: 7477-85.

[59]   Knutson KL, Hmama Z, Herrera-Velit P, Rochford R, Reiner NE. Lipoarabinomannan of *Mycobacterium tuberculosis* promotes protein tyrosine dephosphorylation and inhibition of mitogen-activated protein kinase in human mononuclear phagocytes. Role of the Src homology 2 containing tyrosine phosphatase 1. J Biol Chem 1998; 273: 645-52.

[60]   Geijtenbeek TB, Van Vliet SJ, Koppel EA *et al.* Mycobacteria target DC-SIGN to suppress dendritic cell function. J Exp Med 2003; 197: 7-17.

[61]   Dahl KE, Shiratsuchi H, Hamilton BD, Ellner JJ, Toossi Z. Selective induction of transforming growth factor beta in human monocytes by lipoarabinomannan of *Mycobacterium tuberculosis.* Infect Immun 1996; 64: 399-405.

[62]   Maeda N, Nigou J, Herrmann JL *et al.* The cell surface receptor DC-SIGN discriminates between *Mycobacterium* species through selective recognition of the mannose caps on lipoarabinomannan. J Biol Chem 2003; 278: 5513-6.

[63]   Jones BW, Heldwein KA, Means TK, Saukkonen JJ, Fenton MJ. Differential roles of Toll-like receptors in the elicitation of proinflammatory responses by macrophages. Ann Rheum Dis 2001; 60 Suppl 3 :iii6-12.

[64]   Gilleron M, Nigou J, Nicolle D, Quesniaux V, Puzo G. The acylation state of mycobacterial lipomannans modulates innate immunity response through toll-like receptor 2. Chem Biol 2006; 13: 39-47.

[65]   Drage MG, Pecora ND, Hise AG *et al.* TLR2 and its co-receptors determine responses of macrophages and dendritic cells to lipoproteins of *Mycobacterium tuberculosis.* Cell Immunol 2009; 258: 29-37.

[66]   Moss JE, Aliprantis AO, Zychlinsky A. The regulation of apoptosis by microbial pathogens. Int Rev Cytol 1999; 187: 203-59.

[67]   Lopez M, Sly LM, Luu Y, Young D, Cooper H, Reiner NE. The 19-kDa *Mycobacterium tuberculosis* protein induces macrophage apoptosis through Toll-like receptor-2. J Immunol 2003; 170: 2409-16.

[68]   Dao DN, Kremer L, Guerardel Y *et al.* *Mycobacterium tuberculosis* lipomannan induces apoptosis and interleukin-12 production in macrophages. Infect Immun 2004; 72: 2067-74.

[69]   Doyle SE, O'Connell RM, Miranda GA *et al.* Toll-like Receptors Induce a Phagocytic Gene Program through p38. J Exp Med 2004; 199: 81-90.

[70]   Yoshida A, Inagawa H, Kohchi C, Nishizawa T, Soma G. The role of toll-like receptor 2 in survival strategies of *Mycobacterium tuberculosis* in macrophage phagosomes. Anticancer Res 2009; 29: 907-10.

[71]   Henderson RA, Watkins SC, Flynn JL. Activation of human dendritic cells following infection with *Mycobacterium tuberculosis.* J Immunol 1997; 159: 635-43.

[72]   Hertz CJ, Kiertscher SM, Godowski PJ *et al.* Microbial lipopeptides stimulate dendritic cell maturation *via* Toll-like receptor 2. J Immunol 2001; 166: 2444-50.

[73] Tsuji S, Matsumoto M, Takeuchi O *et al*. Maturation of human dendritic cells by cell wall skeleton of *Mycobacterium bovis* bacillus Calmette-Guerin: involvement of toll-like receptors. Infect Immun 2000; 68: 6883-90.

[74] Noss EH, Harding CV, Boom WH. *Mycobacterium tuberculosis* inhibits MHC class II antigen processing in murine bone marrow macrophages. Cell Immunol 2000; 201: 63-74.

[75] Noss EH, Pai RK, Sellati TJ *et al*. Toll-like receptor 2-dependent inhibition of macrophage class II MHC expression and antigen processing by 19-kDa lipoprotein of *Mycobacterium tuberculosis*. J Immunol 2001; 167: 910-8.

[76] Gehring AJ, Rojas RE, Canaday DH, Lakey DL, Harding CV, Boom WH. The *Mycobacterium tuberculosis* 19-kilodalton lipoprotein inhibits gamma interferon-regulated HLA-DR and Fc gamma R1 on human macrophages through Toll-like receptor 2. Infect Immun 2003; 71: 4487-97.

[77] Pai RK, Pennini ME, Tobian AA, Canaday DH, Boom WH, Harding CV. Prolonged toll-like receptor signaling by *Mycobacterium tuberculosis* and its 19-kilodalton lipoprotein inhibits gamma interferon-induced regulation of selected genes in macrophages. Infect Immun 2004; 72: 6603-14.

[78] Tobian AA, Potter NS, Ramachandra L *et al*. Alternate class I MHC antigen processing is inhibited by Toll-like receptor signaling pathogen-associated molecular patterns: *Mycobacterium tuberculosis* 19-kDa lipoprotein, CpG DNA, and lipopolysaccharide. J Immunol 2003; 171: 1413-22.

[79] Post FA, Manca C, Neyrolles O, Ryffel B, Young DB, Kaplan G. *Mycobacterium tuberculosis* 19-kilodalton lipoprotein inhibits Mycobacterium smegmatis-induced cytokine production by human macrophages *in vitro*. Infect Immun 2001; 69: 1433-9.

[80] Abou-Zeid C, Gares MP, Inwald J *et al*. Induction of a type 1 immune response to a recombinant antigen from *Mycobacterium tuberculosis* expressed in Mycobacterium vaccae. Infect Immun 1997; 65: 1856-62.

[81] Rao V, Dhar N, Tyagi AK. Modulation of host immune responses by overexpression of immunodominant antigens of *Mycobacterium tuberculosis* in bacille Calmette-Guerin. Scand J Immunol 2003; 58: 449-61.

[82] Yeremeev VV, Stewart GR, Neyrolles O *et al*. Deletion of the 19kDa antigen does not alter the protective efficacy of BCG. Tuber Lung Dis 2000; 80: 243-7.

[83] Rao V, Dhar N, Shakila H, Singh R, Khera A, Jain R, *et al*. Increased expression of *Mycobacterium tuberculosis* 19 kDa lipoprotein obliterates the protective efficacy of BCG by polarizing host immune responses to the Th2 subtype. Scand J Immunol 2005;61:410-7.

[84] Redecke V, Hacker H, Datta SK *et al*. Cutting edge: activation of Toll-like receptor 2 induces a Th2 immune response and promotes experimental asthma. J Immunol 2004; 172: 2739-43.

[85] Roura-Mir C, Wang L, Cheng TY *et al*. *Mycobacterium tuberculosis* regulates CD1 antigen presentation pathways through TLR-2. J Immunol 2005; 175: 1758-66.

[86] Nau GJ, Richmond JF, Schlesinger A, Jennings EG, Lander ES, Young RA. Human macrophage activation programs induced by bacterial pathogens. Proc Natl Acad Sci U S A 2002; 99: 1503-8.

[87] Schnare M, Barton GM, Holt AC, Takeda K, Akira S, Medzhitov R. Toll-like receptors control activation of adaptive immune responses. Nat Immunol 2001; 2: 947-50.

[88] Way SS, Kollmann TR, Hajjar AM, Wilson CB. Protective cell-mediated immunity to *Listeria monocytogenes* in the absence of myeloid differentiation factor 88. J Immunol 2003; 171: 533-7.

[89] Torres D, Barrier M, Bihl F *et al*. Toll-like receptor 2 is required for optimal control of *Listeria monocytogenes* infection. Infect Immun 2004; 72: 2131-9.

[90] Fremond CM, Yeremeev V, Nicolle DM, Jacobs M, Quesniaux VF, Ryffel B. Fatal *Mycobacterium tuberculosis* infection despite adaptive immune response in the absence of MyD88. J Clin Invest 2004; 114: 1790-9.

[91] Shi S, Blumenthal A, Hickey CM, Gandotra S, Levy D, Ehrt S. Expression of many immunologically important genes in *Mycobacterium tuberculosis*-infected macrophages is independent of both TLR2 and TLR4 but dependent on IFN-alphabeta receptor and STAT1. J Immunol 2005; 175: 3318-28.

[92] Kleinnijenhuis J, Joosten LA, van de Veerdonk FL *et al*. Transcriptional and inflammasome-mediated pathways for the induction of IL-1beta production by *Mycobacterium tuberculosis*. Eur J Immunol 2009; 39: 1914-22.

[93] Yadav M, Schorey JS. The beta-glucan receptor dectin-1 functions together with TLR2 to mediate macrophage activation by mycobacteria. Blood 2006; 108: 3168-75.

[94] Lee HM, Yuk JM, Shin DM, Jo EK. Dectin-1 is Inducible and Plays an Essential Role for Mycobacteria-Induced Innate Immune Responses in Airway Epithelial Cells. J Clin Immunol 2009; 29: 795-805.

[95] Bowdish DM, Sakamoto K, Kim MJ *et al*. MARCO, TLR2, and CD14 are required for macrophage cytokine responses to mycobacterial trehalose dimycolate and *Mycobacterium tuberculosis*. PLoS Pathog 2009;5:e1000474.

[96] Schlesinger LS, Bellinger-Kawahara CG, Payne NR, Horwitz MA. Phagocytosis of *Mycobacterium tuberculosis* is mediated by human monocyte complement receptors and complement component C3. J Immunol 1990; 144: 2771-80.

[97]   Schlesinger LS, Hull SR, Kaufman TM. Binding of the terminal mannosyl units of lipoarabinomannan from a virulent strain of *Mycobacterium tuberculosis* to human macrophages. J Immunol 1994; 152: 4070-9.

[98]   Kang BK, Schlesinger LS. Characterization of mannose receptor-dependent phagocytosis mediated by *Mycobacterium tuberculosis* lipoarabinomannan. Infect Immun 1998; 66: 2769-77.

[99]   Tailleux L, Schwartz O, Herrmann JL *et al.* DC-SIGN is the major *Mycobacterium tuberculosis* receptor on human dendritic cells. J Exp Med 2003; 197: 121-7.

[100]   Tanne A, Ma B, Boudou F *et al.* A murine DC-SIGN homologue contributes to early host defense against *Mycobacterium tuberculosis*. J Exp Med 2009; 206: 2205-20.

[101]   Leemans JC, Florquin S, Heikens M, Pals ST, van der Neut R, Van Der Poll T. CD44 is a macrophage binding site for *Mycobacterium tuberculosis* that mediates macrophage recruitment and protective immunity against tuberculosis. J Clin Invest 2003; 111: 681-9.

[102]   Court N, Vasseur V, Vacher R *et al.* Partial redundancy of the pattern recognition receptors, scavenger receptors, and C-type lectins for the long-term control of *Mycobacterium tuberculosis* infection. J Immunol 2010; 184: 7057-70.

[103]   Fortune SM, Solache A, Jaeger A *et al.* *Mycobacterium tuberculosis* inhibits macrophage responses to IFN-gamma through myeloid differentiation factor 88-dependent and -independent mechanisms. J Immunol 2004; 172: 6272-80.

[104]   Pathak SK, Basu S, Basu KK *et al.* Direct extracellular interaction between the early secreted antigen ESAT-6 of *Mycobacterium tuberculosis* and TLR2 inhibits TLR signaling in macrophages. Nat Immunol 2007; 8: 610-8.

[105]   Gringhuis SI, den Dunnen J, Litjens M, van Het Hof B, van Kooyk Y, Geijtenbeek TB. C-type lectin DC-SIGN modulates Toll-like receptor signaling *via* Raf-1 kinase-dependent acetylation of transcription factor NF-kappaB. Immunity 2007; 26: 605-16.

[106]   Pathak SK, Basu S, Bhattacharyya A, Pathak S, Kundu M, Basu J. *Mycobacterium tuberculosis* lipoarabinomannan-mediated IRAK-M induction negatively regulates Toll-like receptor-dependent interleukin-12 p40 production in macrophages. J Biol Chem 2005; 280: 42794-800.

[107]   Beatty WL, Rhoades ER, Ullrich HJ, Chatterjee D, Heuser JE, Russell DG. Trafficking and release of mycobacterial lipids from infected macrophages. Traffic 2000; 1: 235-47.

[108]   Nigou J, Gilleron M, Cahuzac B *et al.* The phosphatidyl-myo-inositol anchor of the lipoarabinomannans from *Mycobacterium bovis* bacillus Calmette Guerin. Heterogeneity, structure, and role in the regulation of cytokine secretion. J Biol Chem 1997; 272: 23094-103.

[109]   Zhang N, Torrelles JB, McNeil MR *et al.* The Emb proteins of mycobacteria direct arabinosylation of lipoarabinomannan and arabinogalactan *via* an N-terminal recognition region and a C-terminal synthetic region. Mol Microbiol 2003; 50: 69-76.

[110]   Krutzik SR, Modlin RL. The role of Toll-like receptors in combating mycobacteria. Semin Immunol 2004;16:35-41.

[111]   Reiling N, Ehlers S, Holscher C. MyDths and un-TOLLed truths: sensor, instructive and effector immunity to tuberculosis. Immunol Lett 2008; 116: 15-23.

[112]   Abel B, Thieblemont N, Quesniaux VJ *et al.* Toll-like receptor 4 expression is required to control chronic *Mycobacterium tuberculosis* infection in mice. J Immunol 2002; 169: 3155-62.

[113]   Branger J, Leemans JC, Florquin S, Weijer S, Speelman P, Van Der Poll T. Toll-like receptor 4 plays a protective role in pulmonary tuberculosis in mice. Int Immunol 2004; 16: 509-16.

[114]   Tjarnlund A, Guirado E, Julian E, Cardona PJ, Fernandez C. Determinant role for Toll-like receptor signaling in acute mycobacterial infection in the respiratory tract. Microbes Infect 2006; 8: 1790-800.

[115]   Reiling N, Holscher C, Fehrenbach A *et al.* Cutting edge: Toll-like receptor (TLR)2- and TLR4-mediated pathogen recognition in resistance to airborne infection with *Mycobacterium tuberculosis*. J Immunol 2002; 169: 3480-4.

[116]   Shim TS, Turner OC, Orme IM. Toll-like receptor 4 plays no role in susceptibility of mice to *Mycobacterium tuberculosis* infection. Tuberculosis (Edinb) 2003; 83: 367-71.

[117]   Kamath AB, Alt J, Debbabi H, Behar SM. Toll-like receptor 4-defective C3H/HeJ mice are not more susceptible than other C3H substrains to infection with *Mycobacterium tuberculosis*. Infect Immun 2003; 71: 4112-8.

[118]   Drennan MB, Nicolle D, Quesniaux VJ *et al.* Toll-Like Receptor 2-Deficient Mice Succumb to *Mycobacterium tuberculosis* Infection. Am J Pathol 2004; 164: 49-57.

[119]   Sugawara I, Yamada H, Li C, Mizuno S, Takeuchi O, Akira S. Mycobacterial infection in TLR2 and TLR6 knockout mice. Microbiol Immunol 2003; 47: 327-36.

[120]   Bafica A, Scanga CA, Feng CG, Leifer C, Cheever A, Sher A. TLR9 regulates Th1 responses and cooperates with TLR2 in mediating optimal resistance to *Mycobacterium tuberculosis*. J Exp Med 2005; 202: 1715-24.

[121]   Holscher C, Reiling N, Schaible UE *et al.* Containment of aerogenic *Mycobacterium tuberculosis* infection in mice does not require MyD88 adaptor function for TLR2, -4 and -9. Eur J Immunol 2008; 38: 680-94.

[122] Sugawara I, Yamada H, Mizuno S, Takeda K, Akira S. Mycobacterial infection in MyD88-deficient mice. Microbiol Immunol 2003; 47: 841-7.

[123] Feng CG, Scanga CA, Collazo-Custodio CM *et al.* Mice lacking myeloid differentiation factor 88 display profound defects in host resistance and immune responses to *Mycobacterium avium* infection not exhibited by Toll-like receptor 2 (TLR2)- and TLR4-deficient animals. J Immunol 2003; 171: 4758-64.

[124] Scanga CA, Bafica A, Feng CG, Cheever AW, Hieny S, Sher A. MyD88-deficient mice display a profound loss in resistance to *Mycobacterium tuberculosis* associated with partially impaired Th1 cytokine and nitric oxide synthase 2 expression. Infect Immun 2004; 72: 2400-4.

[125] Flynn JL, Goldstein MM, Chan J *et al.* Tumor necrosis factor-alpha is required in the protective immune response against *Mycobacterium tuberculosis* in mice. Immunity 1995; 2: 561-72.

[126] Jacobs M, Brown N, Allie N, Ryffel B. Fatal *Mycobacterium bovis* BCG infection in TNF-LT-alpha-deficient mice. Clin Immunol 2000; 94: 192-9.

[127] Jacobs M, Marino MW, Brown N *et al.* Correction of defective host response to *Mycobacterium bovis* BCG infection in TNF-deficient mice by bone marrow transplantation. Lab Invest 2000; 80: 901-14.

[128] Wieland CW, Koppel EA, den Dunnen J *et al.* Mice lacking SIGNR1 have stronger T helper 1 responses to *Mycobacterium tuberculosis.* Microbes Infect 2007; 9: 134-41.

[129] Schaefer M, Reiling N, Fessler C *et al.* Decreased pathology and prolonged survival of human DC-SIGN transgenic mice during mycobacterial infection. J Immunol 2008; 180: 6836-45.

[130] Kang TJ, Chae GT. Detection of Toll-like receptor 2 (TLR2) mutation in the lepromatous leprosy patients. FEMS Immunol Med Microbiol 2001; 31: 53-8.

[131] Kang TJ, Lee SB, Chae GT. A polymorphism in the toll-like receptor 2 is associated with IL-12 production from monocyte in lepromatous leprosy. Cytokine 2002; 20: 56-62.

[132] Kang TJ, Yeum CE, Kim BC, You EY, Chae GT. Differential production of interleukin-10 and interleukin-12 in mononuclear cells from leprosy patients with a Toll-like receptor 2 mutation. Immunology 2004; 112: 674-80.

[133] Yim JJ, Lee HW, Lee HS *et al.* The association between microsatellite polymorphisms in intron II of the human Toll-like receptor 2 gene and tuberculosis among Koreans. Genes Immun 2006; 7: 150-5.

[134] Caws M, Thwaites G, Dunstan S *et al.* The influence of host and bacterial genotype on the development of disseminated disease with *Mycobacterium tuberculosis.* PLoS Pathog 2008; 4: e1000034.

[135] Velez DR, Wejse C, Stryjewski ME, Abbate E *et al.* Variants in toll-like receptors 2 and 9 influence susceptibility to pulmonary tuberculosis in Caucasians, African-Americans, and West Africans. Hum Genet 2010; 127: 65-73

[136] Ogus AC, Yoldas B, Ozdemir T *et al.* The Arg753GLn polymorphism of the human toll-like receptor 2 gene in tuberculosis disease. Eur Respir J 2004; 23: 219-23.

[137] Hawn TR, Misch EA, Dunstan SJ *et al.* A common human TLR1 polymorphism regulates the innate immune response to lipopeptides. Eur J Immunol 2007; 37: 2280-9.

[138] Johnson CM, Lyle EA, Omueti KO *et al.* Cutting edge: A common polymorphism impairs cell surface trafficking and functional responses of TLR1 but protects against leprosy. J Immunol 2007; 178: 7520-4.

[139] Ma X, Liu Y, Gowen BB, Graviss EA, Clark AG, Musser JM. Full-exon resequencing reveals toll-like receptor variants contribute to human susceptibility to tuberculosis disease. PLoS One 2007; 2: e1318.

[140] Davila S, Hibberd ML, Hari Dass R *et al.* Genetic association and expression studies indicate a role of toll-like receptor 8 in pulmonary tuberculosis. PLoS Genet 2008; 4: e1000218.

[141] Hawn TR, Dunstan SJ, Thwaites GE *et al.* A polymorphism in Toll-interleukin 1 receptor domain containing adaptor protein is associated with susceptibility to meningeal tuberculosis. J Infect Dis 2006; 194: 1127-34.

[142] Dissanayeke SR, Levin S, Pienaar S *et al.* Polymorphic variation in TIRAP is not associated with susceptibility to childhood TB but may determine susceptibility to TBM in some ethnic groups. PLoS One 2009; 4: e6698.

[143] Khor CC, Chapman SJ, Vannberg FO *et al.* A Mal functional variant is associated with protection against invasive pneumococcal disease, bacteremia, malaria and tuberculosis. Nat Genet 2007; 39: 523-8.

[144] Nejentsev S, Thye T, Szeszko JS *et al.* Analysis of association of the TIRAP (MAL) S180L variant and tuberculosis in three populations. Nat Genet 2008; 40:2 61-2; author reply 262-3.

[145] Castiblanco J, Varela DC, Castano-Rodriguez N, Rojas-Villarraga A, Hincapie ME, Anaya JM. TIRAP (MAL) S180L polymorphism is a common protective factor against developing tuberculosis and systemic lupus erythematosus. Infect Genet Evol 2008; 8: 541-4.

[146] Hamann L, Kumpf O, Schuring RP *et al.* Low frequency of the TIRAP S180L polymorphism in Africa, and its potential role in malaria, sepsis, and leprosy. BMC Med Genet 2009; 10: 65.

[147] Ku CL, von Bernuth H, Picard C *et al.* Selective predisposition to bacterial infections in IRAK-4-deficient children: IRAK-4-dependent TLRs are otherwise redundant in protective immunity. J Exp Med 2007; 204: 2407-22.

[148] von Bernuth H, Picard C, Jin Z *et al.* Pyogenic bacterial infections in humans with MyD88 deficiency. Science 2008; 321: 691-6.

[149] Chatterjee D, Khoo KH. Mycobacterial lipoarabinomannan: an extraordinary lipoheteroglycan with profound physiological effects. Glycobiology 1998; 8: 113-20.

CHAPTER 7

Bacterial Infections and Pneumonia: What is the Role of Toll-Like Receptors?

Sylvia Knapp[*]

Center for Molecular Medicine of the Austrian Academy of Sciences & Department of Medicine 1, Division of Infectious Diseases and Tropical Medicine, Medical University Vienna, Vienna, 1090, Austria

Abstract: Bacterial pneumonia is an important disease and the most frequent cause of death due to an infection worldwide. Host defense against inhaled pathogens is essential in preventing microbes from gaining access to the lower respiratory tract where they might cause tissue damage. The innate immune system provides the first line of defense and hence is involved in the recognition of invading pathogens. In order to detect microbial motifs, innate immune cells express a panel of so-called pattern recognition receptors. The most important recognition receptors are Toll-like receptors (TLRs) of which 10 have been identified in humans. Each TLR can identify a specific set of microbial motifs, which then leads to the activation of innate immune cells and the release of proinflammatory mediators. The distinct role of selected TLRs during bacterial pneumonia has been extensively studied in animal models. While host defense against *Streptococcus pneumoniae* depends on the simultaneous involvement of TLR2, TLR4 and TLR9, the immune response during most Gram-negative pneumonias requires the presence of TLR4. Although these data disclosed important information they also revealed a high redundancy in the requirements for TLRs *in vivo*. Genetic association studies in humans in turn confirmed the redundancy since only deficiencies in common downstream signaling molecules were found associated with increased susceptibility to bacterial pneumonia. Immunotherapeutic possibilities that could target TLRs directly are therefore limited, and currently confined to TLRs' role as adjuvants and activators of adaptive immune responses in vaccine development.

Keywords: TLRs, bacterial pneumonia, *Streptococcus pneumonia*, Gram-negative pneumonias.

1. POPULATION FREQUENCIES OF BACTERIAL PNEUMONIA

Pneumonia and lower respiratory tract infections are the second leading cause of illness worldwide and a major cause of day life disability [1]. According to the global burden of disease report issued by the world health organization (WHO), the global incidence of pneumonia exceeded 400 million cases in 2004 alone [2]. Of note, these numbers do not include upper respiratory tract infections, tuberculosis or episodes of pneumonia in HIV-infected people, hence slightly underestimating the actual burden of disease. In accordance with the high incidence of pneumonia worldwide, lower respiratory tract infections are the leading cause of disability adjusted life years (DALYs), which is a combined measure of years of life lost due to death and years of 'healthy' life lost due to a disease or disability. One DALY compares to one year of healthy life lost. Using this analysis method, the WHO reported lower respiratory tract infections to account for 94 million DALYs in 2004 [2].

While the greatest numbers of pneumonia cases are reported in developing countries [2], it should not be underestimated that pneumonia is a very serious health care problem in the Western world, and as such the seventh leading cause of death in the U.S. [3]. Adding to the importance of pneumonia as the single most frequent cause of disease and death due to an infection worldwide [4], several studies indicate that bacterial pneumonia is the leading cause of systemic inflammation and sepsis [5].

From a clinical perspective, two major entities of bacterial pneumonia are differentiated, namely community-acquired (CAP) and hospital-acquired pneumonia (HAP). This distinction is important, because

*Address correspondence to Sylvia Knapp: Center for Molecular Medicine & Department of Medicine 1, Division of Infectious Diseases and Tropical Medicine, Medical University Vienna, Waehringer Guertel 18-20, Vienna, 1090, Austria; Tel: +43-1-40400-5139; E-mail: sylvia.knapp@meduniwien.ac.at

the causative pathogens and the resulting clinical presentation differ greatly between these two forms of pneumonia. While the most important pathogens in CAP are *Streptococcus pneumoniae (S. pneumoniae)*, *Haemophilus influenzae (H. influenzae)* or *Mycoplasma* [6], HAP is mainly caused by Gram-negative microbes such as *Pseudomonas aeruginosa (Pseudomonas)*, *Klebsiella pneumoniae (Klebsiella)*, or *Acinetobacter baumannii (A. baumannii)* and mostly associated with underlying pulmonary conditions or intensive care patients receiving mechanical ventilation [7, 8]. This distinction is quite obviously important when appropriate antibiotic treatment is considered.

2. PATHOPHYSIOLOGY OF BACTERIAL PNEUMONIA

Host defense against respiratory pathogens involves a multitude of cells and mediators. Mild infections are contained and prevented from gaining access to the lower respiratory tract by physical barriers, mucociliary clearance mechanisms and the release of antimicrobial peptides [9]. More severe infections or failure of local defense mechanisms will allow pathogens to gain access to the lower respiratory tract and to get into contact with a number of specialized cells that will try to eliminate these invaders. Among the most important immune cells in the alveolar compartment are alveolar macrophages, which are resident phagocytes with an exceptional potential of eliminating all kinds of particulate matter. As such, alveolar macrophages are considered important in identifying the presence of inhaled microbes and to initiate and orchestrate the inflammatory response. The release of chemokines by alveolar macrophages in turn leads to the attraction and migration of neutrophils to the site of infection [10, 11]. Recruited neutrophils phagocytose and kill ingested bacteria with reactive oxygen species, antimicrobial peptides and various enzymes that are stored in their granules. After having performed their duties, neutrophils rapidly undergo apoptosis after which they are cleared by surrounding macrophages [12].

3. THE ROLE OF TLRs IN PNEUMONIA

The most important initial step in fighting bacterial infections is for immune cells to appropriately recognize the presence of pathogens within the lungs. The identification of microbes is achieved *via* the interaction with so-called pattern-recognition receptors. Toll-like receptors (TLR) are prototypic pattern recognition receptors that efficiently sense the presence of invading pathogens. As such TLRs recognize three types of conserved motifs derived from microbes, namely lipids, proteins or nucleic acids. To this end 10 human TLRs have been described and numerous pathogen-associated ligands were discovered over the last 10 years [13].

Depending on the localization of these TLRs, cell surface expressed receptors like TLR1, TLR2, TLR4, TLR5 and TLR6 are distinguished from endosomal TLRs, which cover TLR3, TLR7, TLR8 and TLR9 [14]. All endosomal TLRs recognize nucleic acids, such as viral, bacterial - but also mammalian - RNA or DNA. TLR3 detects double stranded (ds) RNA from viruses [15] and endogenous RNA from damaged and necrotic cells [16, 17]. TLR7 and TLR8 sense the presence of ssRNA [18, 19], and TLR9 recognizes unmethylated CpG DNA motifs [20]. Ligands for cell surface TLRs are more heterogeneous. The best characterized cell-membrane TLR is TLR4, which senses the presence of lipopolysaccharide (LPS), a major cell wall component of Gram-negative bacteria [21]. TLR2 is a rather promiscuous receptor that heterodimerizes with TLR1 or TLR6 for signaling, and recognizes various bacterial ligands including lipoproteins, lipoteichoic acid, or lipoarabinomannan [22-25]. TLR5 recognizes bacterial flagellin, a component of flagellated bacteria such as *Pseudomonas* [26]. It is worth mentioning that many TLRs do not only detect microbial motifs but are also able to sense tissue damage by recognizing endogenous danger molecules [27]. As such TLR4 detects oxidized phospholipids [28, 29] and myeloid related protein 8/14 (Mrp8/14) [30], whereas HMGB1 [31] and hyaluronan [32] are sensed by TLR2 and TLR4.

Activation of TLRs by respective ligands leads to the recruitment of adaptor proteins, like MyD88 (myeloid differentiation primary response gene 88) and Mal (MyD88 adapter like, also called TIRAP) or TRIF (TIR-domain containing adapter inducing IFN-β) and TRAM (TRIF related adapter molecule), and the induction of a signaling cascade that will ultimately result in the nuclear translocation of nuclear factor κB (NFκB) and/or interferon regulatory factors (IRF) [33] (Fig. **1**). NFκB activation induces transcription of genes for pro-inflammatory cytokines such as TNF-α or IL-1 and chemokines, while interferon regulatory factors mediate a type I interferon response. All TLRs with the exception of TLR3 recruit MyD88, and only TLR3 and TLR4 associate with TRIF. While all TLRs are capable of inducing NFκB mediated responses, only TLR4 and the endosomal TLRs (*i.e.* TLR3, TLR7-9) additionally trigger a type I interferon response.

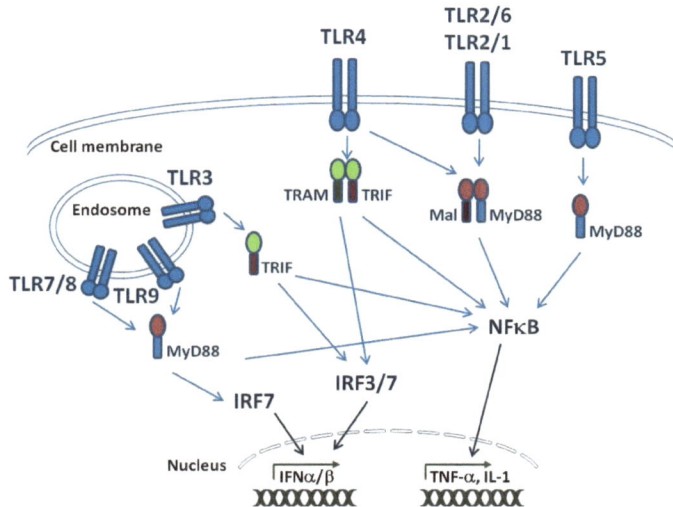

Figure 1: TLR signaling.

During bacterial infections TLR2, TLR4, TLR5 and TLR9 are considered to be crucial in the recognition of microbes and to induce the resulting host defense mechanisms against inhaled bacteria. However, no general conclusion can be drawn, as each bacterial species elicits a 'special' and often unique inflammatory response, which depends on the interplay of distinct pathogen recognition receptors.

4. EXPRESSION OF TLRs IN THE PNEUMONIC LUNG

Because the lungs are continuously exposed to the outside world and hence encounter various microbes on a regular basis, it only makes sense that TLRs are expressed on multiple cell types within the respiratory tract. The three most important resident pulmonary cell types involved in host defense against invading pathogens are alveolar macrophages, epithelial cells and dendritic cells (DCs).

Alveolar macrophages, which are sentinel phagocytes and strategically located in the alveoli, are considered important effector cells that are among the first cells to detect the presence of invading pathogens. The TLR expression pattern of alveolar macrophages has been studied by several investigators. Reports that assessed mRNA levels of various TLRs in human alveolar macrophages found TLR1, 2, 4, 7 and 8 expressed, but could not detect TLR9 mRNA [34]. A more recent study applying RT-PCR and FACS methods, however, identified TLR2, 4 and 9 expressed on human alveolar macrophages [35]. What seems to be a consistent finding in human and murine alveolar macrophages upon inflammation is the fact that TLR4 is rapidly downregulated while TLR2 expression increases [34, 36].

Respiratory epithelial cells are increasingly recognized as important cells in terms of sensing the presence of pathogens [37]. As such, airway epithelial cells are known to mediate an inflammatory response and studies by Skerett *et al.* elegantly confirmed the importance of these cells *in vivo* [38]. Making use of transgenic mice harboring a dominant negative IκBα construct under the control of the surfactant protein C promoter, the authors showed that LPS induced lung inflammation was significantly diminished in the absence of functional NFκB activation in distal respiratory epithelial cells [38]. Since NFκB activation is a classical downstream effect of TLRs, it is not unexpected that respiratory epithelial cells express a wide array of these pattern recognition receptors among which TLR2, TLR4, TLR5 and TLR9 have been identified [39, 40].

DCs are another sentinel myeloid cell type present within the pulmonary compartment. Respiratory tract DCs are considered important in their ability to present antigens to lymphocytes in draining lymph nodes, and thus activate adaptive immune responses [41]. However, recent evidence suggests that alveolar macrophages are also quite potent antigen presenting cells that have the capacity to migrate to draining lymph nodes [42]. Depending on the localization of DCs within the lung, intraepithelial DCs are differentiated from interstitial and inflammatory DCs; on a functional and phenotypic basis conventional (cDCs) and plasmacytoid (pDCs) are considered the two main DC-subsets [43]. Although the precise roles of these distinct DC subsets within the lungs during bacterial pneumonia are not entirely understood, their crucial function in host defense is illustrated by the fact that intraepithelial DCs extend their dendrites into the airspace, where they sample and screen for microbial ligands entering the lower respiratory tract [44, 45]. To fulfill their function in host defense DCs express a wide array of TLRs. Because each subset of lung DCs is hard to isolate and analyze for TLR expression, primary blood-derived (human) or spleen DCs (mouse) were investigated in most studies [46]: summarizing these data it seems that cDCs express most TLRs (*i.e.* TLR1 to TLR9), while pDCs are selectively expressing high levels of TLR7 and TLR9. These data are mostly based on mRNA levels and thus do not allow to understand protein expression and functionality.

5. FUNCTION AND ACTIVATION OF TLRs DURING PNEUMONIA

The biological function of distinct TLRs during pneumonia has been investigated in great detail over the last years with most data coming from mouse studies of bacterial pneumonia and the use of respective TLR-deficient animals [47, 48]. Depending on the causative pathogen or bacterial ligand investigated, the individual contribution of selected TLRs has been elucidated (Table **1**). Data from lung inflammation models using purified bacterial ligands clearly confirmed the importance of individual TLRs in recognizing their respective ligands *in vivo*. As such LPS-induced lung inflammation was abolished in the absence of functional TLR4 signaling [49, 50]. Mycobacterial lipoarabinomannan- and staphylococcal or pneumococcal lipoteichoic acid-induced pneumonitis was absent in TLR2-knock out animals [51-53]. Follow-up studies investigated the respective role of cell subsets within the lungs that might mediate the TLR-induced inflammatory response. Hollingsworth *et al.* made use of chimeric TLR4 mice and showed that TLR4 on cells of hematopoietic origin was required for LPS-induced lung inflammation [54]. Based on these data and earlier reports in macrophage-depleted mice, alveolar macrophages seem to be the TLR4-dependent initiators of the inflammatory response to inhaled LPS [55].

Focusing on clinically relevant pneumonia, several groups explored the functional contribution of TLRs to host defense and survival during lung infections with bacteria (Table **1**). Arguing that Gram-positive bacteria contain several TLR2 ligands, such as lipoteichoic acid and lipopeptides, we studied the role of TLR2 in host response to *S. pneumoniae*, and anticipated a reduced inflammatory response in TLR2-deficient mice upon pulmonary infection. We discovered that TLR2 contributes to chemokine release and the attraction of neutrophils to the lungs (Fig. **2**), but absence of TLR2 was surprisingly not associated with altered bacterial elimination nor differences in survival [56].

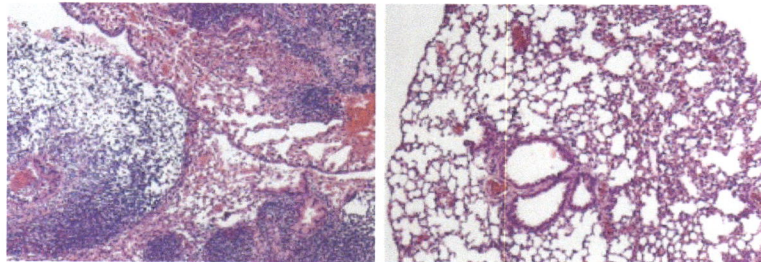

Figure 2: Lung histology (hematoxylin-eosin staining) 48h following induction of pneumococcal pneumonia in wild type (left panel) and TLR2-defieicnt (right panel) mice. Magnification x 40.

Arguing that other TLR ligands might compensate for the loss of TLR2-mediated signaling, pneumolysin, the major pore-forming toxin released by all virulent *S. pneumoniae* strains, was identified to signal *via*

TLR4 [57]. Accordingly, TLR4-deficient mice suffering from pneumococcal pneumonia showed a modest survival disadvantage over wild type animals, thus supporting this idea *in vivo* [58]. Moreover, bacterial pneumonia induced by pneumolysin-deficient *S. pneumoniae* clearly depended on the presence of TLR2 [59]. Albiger *et al.* addressed the function of TLR9 and MyD88 during murine pneumococcal pneumonia and revealed that TLR9 and MyD88 contribute to bacterial uptake and killing by macrophages and thereby impact host defense against this pathogen [60]. Together, these data from various TLR-deficient animals infected with *S. pneumoniae* clearly illustrate the high redundancy in the requirement for distinct TLRs. Hence, TLR2, TLR4 and TLR9 together mediate the effective host response to this pathogen, and the absence of one TLR can be compensated by other TLRs during Gram-positive pneumonia.

The functional requirement for TLRs during Gram-negative pneumonia was approached in a similar manner in mice. In contrast to Gram-positive bacteria, Gram-negative microbes share a very potent immunostimulatory molecule in their cell wall, namely the TLR4 agonist LPS.

Consequently, TLR4 plays the most important role in the inflammatory response to Gram-negative bacterial infections *in vivo*. An impaired inflammatory response in TLR4-deficient mice has been demonstrated after infections with *Klebsiella pneumoniae* [58], *Acinetobacter baumannii* [50], *Escherichia coli* [61] or *Pseudomonas aeruginosa* [62]. However, while the inflammatory response depended on TLR4 in all above mentioned pneumonia models, bacterial clearance was only affected in TLR4-deficient mice infected with *A. baumannii* or *Klebsiella*. Rather unexpectedly, the absence of TLR2 improved host defense during *Pseudomonas* and *A. baumannii* infection, but the precise reason for this is unclear [50, 62]. Because *Pseudomonas* is a flagellated bacterium, the role of TLR5 was also studied during pneumonia induced by this pathogen. Although the specific expression pattern of TLR5 within the lungs is not entirely resolved, the immune response of epithelial cells to flagellated *Pseudomonas* strongly depends on the presence of TLR5 [40]. *In vivo*, flagellin has been shown to mask the requirement for other TLRs such as TLR4 and TLR2 [62] and TLR5-deficient mice showed a severely impaired inflammatory response to *Pseudomonas* [63].

Furthermore, host defense against *Klebsiella* depends on the presence of MyD88 and Mal, although TRIF was also found to partially contribute *in vivo* [64, 65]. While TLR4 is one of the initiating receptors explaining the importance of MyD88 [58], TLR9 also seems to play a contributing role during *Klebsiella* infections [66]. Likewise, protective immunity against *Haemophilus influenzae* requires the involvement of TLR4 and MyD88 [67, 68], while TLR9 does not play a role [69]. Hence, while TLR4 seems to be the major TLR required in combating pneumonia induced by *A. baumannii* and *Haemophilus,* and TLR4 and TLR9 are essential against *Klebsiella* infections, TLR5 is a major recognition receptor involved in host defense against *Pseudomonas.*

Table 1: Roles of TLRs and Myd88 investigated upon infection with indicated pathogens *in vivo*.

Receptor	*Pathogen*	*Refs.*
TLR2	*S. pneumoniae*	[56, 59]
	A. baumannii	[50]
	Legionella	[70-72]
	Pseudomonas	[62, 73, 74]
TLR4	*S. pneumoniae*	[57, 58]
	Klebsiella	[58]
	A. baumannii	[50]
	Pseudomonas	[62]
	Legionella	[70, 72, 75]
	Haemophilus	[67]
TLR5	*Pseudomonas*	[62, 63]
	Legionella	[76, 77]
TLR9	*S. pneumoniae*	[60]

Table 1: cont….

	Legionella	[76]
	Klebsiella	[66].
	Haemophilus	[69]
MyD88	S. pneumoniae	[60]
	Legionella	[70, 71, 76, 78]
	Pseudomonas	[73, 79]
	Haemophilus	[68]

Legionella pneumophila is an intracellular pathogen that can give rise to serious lung infections, also known as Legionnaire's disease. The requirement for TLR-mediated host defense pathways has been investigated in murine models of disease and TLR2- and MyD88-dependent signaling seems to be required for control of bacterial replication [70-72]. Mice deficient in MyD88 succumbed to infection, whereas TLR4 did not play a role [70, 72, 75]. However, in an attempt to delineate the role of MyD88 in more detail, TLR-independent MyD88-mediated responses were shown to contribute to host defense against this pathogen [70, 78]. Different groups also studied the potential role of other TLRs like TLR5 and TLR9 and did not find a direct role [76], while others detected an impaired neutrophil migration in TLR5 deficient mice infected with *Legionella* [77] .

6. ROLE OF TLRs IN BACTERIAL PNEUMONIA IN HUMANS

The requirement and functional role of TLRs in humans suffering from bacterial pneumonia is less well understood. The high redundancy in the need for TLRs in combating bacterial pneumonia likely explains the lack of serious phenotypes in humans with single nucleotide polymorphisms (SNPs) in TLRs [80-82]. The only exception might be Legionnaire's disease, where patients with TLR5 mutation were shown to exhibit enhanced susceptibility, while TLR4 mutations seem to protect from this disease [83, 84]. However, because all TLRs converge in their signaling pathways, deficiencies in downstream signaling molecules would affect multiple TLRs at once and might therefore impact host defense and susceptibility to bacterial pneumonia. As such, SNPs of Interleukin-1 receptor associated kinase (IRAK)4, which is a signaling molecule downstream of all MyD88-dependent TLR mediated responses [85], have been identified in children suffering from recurrent pulmonary infections with *S. pneumoniae* but also *Staphylococcus aureus* [86, 87]. Although children and young adults harboring this IRAK4 SNP suffer from recurrent infections, adults live mostly without any infectious complication – a fact that is not entirely understood thus far, but indicates the possibility that alternative pathways can compensate for IRAK4 deficiency. These serious infectious complications in children with IRAK4 SNPs might not only stem from impaired TLR-signaling but most likely involve interleukin-1 receptor (IL-1R) associated responses, since IL-1R signaling also depends on MyD88-IRAK4 pathways and IL-1R has been shown to exert protective effects during pneumococcal pneumonia [88]. Likewise, nine children with functional MyD88 deficiency that were identified suffered from recurrent pyogenic infections, including pneumococcal pneumonia, *S. aureus* and *Pseudomonas* infections [89]. However, just like with IRAK4 deficiency, functional MyD88 deficiency does not result in an increased susceptibility to infectious diseases in adults.

Another genetic association study addressed the role of a SNP (S180L) in the adaptor protein Mal, which is required for MyD88-dependent signaling in response to TLR2 and TLR4 activation (Fig. **1**) [90]. This report showed reduced TLR2-induced NFκB activation in the presence of Mal S180L. While homozygous carriers had an increased risk for invasive pneumococcal diseases, heterozygosity was associated with protection from pneumococcal disease [90]. These findings are quite surprising and led the authors to speculate that homozygosity might abolish crucial signaling events, while heterozygosity possibly modulates inflammation and hence provides an optimized inflammatory response. The same report also demonstrated protection from tuberculosis and malaria in Mal S180L heterozygous individuals [90], and it will be interesting to see data from patients with Gram-negative pneumonia such as induced by *Pseudomonas* and *A. baumannii*, where TLR2 deficiency was protective in animal models [50, 62].

NFκB activation is the prime downstream target of most TLRs and multiple other receptors involved in immunity [91]. Several investigators studied the role of mutations in NFκB related genes and infections. The genetic cause for a rare immunodeficiency called anhidrotic ectodermal dysplasia with immunodeficiency (EDA-ID) was identified to be linked to a hypomorphic mutation of the NFκB essential modulator (NEMO) [80]. The infectious phenotype of these patients involves recurrent infections with *S. pneumoniae, S. aureus* and *Haemophilus influenzae*. Another group of investigators studied various mutations in NFκB associated IκB inhibitory genes, such as NFκBIA, NFκBIB, NFκBIE, NFκBIZ, and correlated data with clinical evidence of invasive pneumococcal disease. In summary, while the most common mutations of NFκBIA and NFκBIE were linked to protection from pneumococcal disease [92], several mutations in NFκBIZ were associated with disease in homozygous carriers whereas protection from pneumococcal disease was discovered in heterozygosity [93]. Collectively, these investigations clearly point towards a quite complex regulation of immune responses during pneumococcal infection and support the idea of a well-balanced and tightly modulated immune response against *S. pneumoniae*.

7. IMMUNOTHERAPEUTIC POSSIBILITIES AND FUTURE APPLICATIONS

Immunotherapeutic approaches targeting TLRs are currently widely investigated [94]. Beside the established therapy with the TLR7 agonist imiquimod for papillomas and some forms of skin tumors, few new drug targets have reached clinical practice. Regarding therapeutic approaches for bacterial pneumonia, no TLR-directed therapies are currently studied. The only novel, TLR-based therapeutic approach that is related to bacterial pneumonia, is the use of TLR agonists as potent adjuvants in vaccine development. As such TLR9 agonists are currently under investigation for pneumococcal vaccines [95]. In addition, several TLR antagonists are currently studied for the treatment of sepsis, such as Eritoran, a lipid A analogue that inhibits TLR4 activation [96]. Considering the fact that bacterial pneumonia is the single most frequent source of sepsis [97], these novel therapies might indirectly affect pneumonia therapy as they address complications of severe bacterial pneumonia.

REFERENCES

[1]   Mizgerd JP. Lung infection--a public health priority. PLoS Med 2006; 3: e76.
[2]   Global Burden of Disease 2004. http://wwwwhoint/healthinfo/global_burden_disease/2004_report_update/ en/indexhtml. 2008; accessed July 4, 2010.
[3]   Deaths: Leading Causes for 2002. National Vital Statistics Report 2005; 53: 1-90.
[4]   Morens DM, Folkers GK, Fauci AS. The challenge of emerging and re-emerging infectious diseases. Nature 2004; 430: 242-49.
[5]   Wheeler AP and Bernard GR. Treating patients with severe sepsis. N Engl J Med 1999; 340: 207-14..
[6]   Finch RG. Epidemiological features and chemotherapy of community-acquired respiratory tract infections. J Antimicrob Chemother 1990; 26: E53-61.
[7]   Chastre J and Fagon J-Y. Ventilator-associated Pneumonia. Am J Respir Crit Care Med 2002; 165: 867-903.
[8]   Park DR. The microbiology of ventilator-associated pneumonia. Respir Care 2005; 50: 742-63; discussion 63-5.
[9]   Knowles MR and Boucher RC. Mucus clearance as a primary innate defense mechanism for mammalian airways. The Journal of Clinical Investigation 2002; 109: 571-77.
[10]   Maus UA, Koay MA, Delbeck T, *et al*. Role of resident alveolar macrophages in leukocyte traffic into the alveolar air space of intact mice. Am J Physiol Lung Cell Mol Physiol 2002; 282: L1245-52..
[11]   Standiford TJ, Kunkel SL, Greenberger MJ, Laichalk LL and Strieter RM. Expression and regulation of chemokines in bacterial pneumonia. J Leukoc Biol 1996; 59: 24-8.
[12]   Cox G, Crossley J and Xing Z. Macrophage engulfment of apoptotic neutrophils contributes to the resolution of acute pulmonary inflammation *in vivo*. Am J Respir Cell Mol Biol 1995; 12: 232-7..
[13]   Akira S, Uematsu S and Takeuchi O. Pathogen Recognition and Innate Immunity. Cell 2006; 124: 783-801.
[14]   Barton GM and Kagan JC. A cell biological view of Toll-like receptor function: regulation through compartmentalization. Nat Rev Immunol 2009; 9: 535-42.
[15]   Alexopoulou L, Holt AC, Medzhitov R and Flavell RA. Recognition of double-stranded RNA and activation of NF-kappaB by Toll- like receptor 3. Nature 2001; 413: 732-8..

[16]　Cavassani KA, Ishii M, Wen H, *et al.* TLR3 is an endogenous sensor of tissue necrosis during acute inflammatory events. J Exp Med 2008; 205: 2609-21.

[17]　Lai Y, Di Nardo A, Nakatsuji T, *et al.* Commensal bacteria regulate Toll-like receptor 3-dependent inflammation after skin injury. Nat Med 2009; 15: 1377-82.

[18]　Diebold SS, Kaisho T, Hemmi H, Akira S and Reis e Sousa C. Innate Antiviral Responses by Means of TLR7-Mediated Recognition of Single-Stranded RNA. Science 2004; 303: 1529-31.

[19]　Heil F, Hemmi H, Hochrein H, *et al.* Species-Specific Recognition of Single-Stranded RNA *via* Toll-like Receptor 7 and 8. Science 2004; 303: 1526-29.

[20]　Hemmi H, Takeuchi O, Kawai T, *et al.* A Toll-like receptor recognizes bacterial DNA. Nature 2000; 408: 740-5..

[21]　Hoshino K, Takeuchi O, Kawai T, *et al.* Cutting edge: Toll-like receptor 4 (TLR4)-deficient mice are hyporesponsive to lipopolysaccharide: evidence for TLR4 as the Lps gene product. J Immunol 1999; 162: 3749-52..

[22]　Takeuchi O, Hoshino K, Kawai T, *et al.* Differential roles of TLR2 and TLR4 in recognition of gram-negative and gram-positive bacterial cell wall components. Immunity 1999; 11: 443-51..

[23]　Takeuchi O, Hoshino K and Akira S. Cutting edge: TLR2-deficient and MyD88-deficient mice are highly susceptible to *Staphylococcus aureus* infection. J Immunol 2000; 165: 5392-6..

[24]　Schroder NW, Morath S, Alexander C, *et al.* Lipoteichoic acid (LTA) of *Streptococcus pneumoniae* and *Staphylococcus aureus* activates immune cells *via* Toll-like receptor (TLR)-2, lipopolysaccharide-binding protein (LBP), and CD14, whereas TLR-4 and MD-2 are not involved. J Biol Chem 2003; 278: 15587-94..

[25]　Means TK, Lien E, Yoshimura A, *et al.* The CD14 ligands lipoarabinomannan and lipopolysaccharide differ in their requirement for Toll-like receptors. J Immunol 1999; 163: 6748-55..

[26]　Hayashi F, Smith KD, Ozinsky A, *et al.* The innate immune response to bacterial flagellin is mediated by Toll- like receptor 5. Nature 2001; 410: 1099-103..

[27]　Knapp S. Update on the role of Toll-like receptors during bacterial infections and sepsis. WMW Wiener Medizinische Wochenschrift 2010; 160: 107-11.

[28]　Miller YI, Viriyakosol S, Binder CJ, *et al.* Minimally Modified LDL Binds to CD14, Induces Macrophage Spreading *via* TLR4/MD-2, and Inhibits Phagocytosis of Apoptotic Cells. J Biol Chem 2003; 278: 1561-68.

[29]　Imai Y, Kuba K, Neely GG, *et al.* Identification of oxidative stress and Toll-like receptor 4 signaling as a key pathway of acute lung injury. Cell 2008; 133: 235-49.

[30]　Vogl T, Tenbrock K, Ludwig S, *et al.* Mrp8 and Mrp14 are endogenous activators of Toll-like receptor 4, promoting lethal, endotoxin-induced shock. Nat Med 2007; 13: 1042-9.

[31]　Park JS, Svetkauskaite D, He Q, *et al.* Involvement of Toll-like Receptors 2 and 4 in Cellular Activation by High Mobility Group Box 1 Protein. J Biol Chem 2004; 279: 7370-77.

[32]　Jiang D, Liang J, Fan J, *et al.* Regulation of lung injury and repair by Toll-like receptors and hyaluronan. Nat Med 2005; 11: 1173-79.

[33]　Kawai T and Akira S. TLR signaling. Semin Immunol 2007; 19: 24-32.

[34]　Maris NA, Dessing MC, de Vos AF, *et al.* Toll-like receptor mRNA levels in alveolar macrophages after inhalation of endotoxin. Eur Respir J 2006; 28: 622-26.

[35]　Juarez E, Nunez C, Sada E, *et al.* Differential expression of Toll-like receptors on human alveolar macrophages and autologous peripheral monocytes. Respir Res 2010; 11: 2.

[36]　Oshikawa K and Sugiyama Y. Gene expression of Toll-like receptors and associated molecules induced by inflammatory stimuli in the primary alveolar macrophage. Biochem Biophys Res Commun 2003; 305: 649-55.

[37]　Hippenstiel S, Opitz B, Schmeck B and Suttorp N. Lung epithelium as a sentinel and effector system in pneumonia - molecular mechanisms of pathogen recognition and signal transduction. Respiratory Research 2006; 7: 97.

[38]　Skerrett SJ, Liggitt HD, Hajjar AM, *et al.* Respiratory epithelial cells regulate lung inflammation in response to inhaled endotoxin. Am J Physiol Lung Cell Mol Physiol 2004; 287: L143-52.

[39]　Greene CM, Carroll TP, Smith SGJ, *et al.* TLR-Induced Inflammation in Cystic Fibrosis and Non-Cystic Fibrosis Airway Epithelial Cells. J Immunol 2005; 174: 1638-46.

[40]　Zhang Z, Louboutin J-P, Weiner DJ, Goldberg JB and Wilson JM. Human Airway Epithelial Cells Sense *Pseudomonas aeruginosa* Infection *via* Recognition of Flagellin by Toll-Like Receptor 5. Infect Immun 2005; 73: 7151-60.

[41]　von Garnier C, Filgueira L, Wikstrom M, *et al.* Anatomical Location Determines the Distribution and Function of Dendritic Cells and Other APCs in the Respiratory Tract. J Immunol 2005; 175: 1609-18.

[42]　Kirby AC, Coles MC and Kaye PM. Alveolar Macrophages Transport Pathogens to Lung Draining Lymph Nodes. J Immunol 2009; 183: 1983-89.

[43]   Lambrecht BN and Hammad H. Biology of Lung Dendritic Cells at the Origin of Asthma. Immunity 2009; 31: 412-24.

[44]   Jahnsen FL, Strickland DH, Thomas JA, *et al.* Accelerated Antigen Sampling and Transport by Airway Mucosal Dendritic Cells following Inhalation of a Bacterial Stimulus. J Immunol 2006; 177: 5861-67.

[45]   GeurtsvanKessel CH, Willart MAM, van Rijt LS, *et al.* Clearance of influenza virus from the lung depends on migratory langerin+CD11b but not plasmacytoid dendritic cells. J Exp Med 2008; 205: 1621-34.

[46]   Reis e Sousa C. Toll-like receptors and dendritic cells: for whom the bug tolls. Semin Immunol 2004; 16: 27-34.

[47]   Mizgerd JP. Acute Lower Respiratory Tract Infection. N Engl J Med 2008; 358: 716-27.

[48]   Opitz B, van Laak V, Eitel J and Suttorp N. Innate Immune Recognition in Infectious and Noninfectious Diseases of the Lung. Am J Respir Crit Care 2010; 181: 1294-309.

[49]   Hollingsworth JW, II, Cook DN, Brass DM, *et al.* The Role of Toll-like Receptor 4 in Environmental Airway Injury in Mice. Am J Respir Crit Care 2004; 170: 126-32.

[50]   Knapp S, Wieland CW, Florquin S, *et al.* Differential Roles of CD14 and Toll-like Receptors 4and 2 in Murine Acinetobacter Pneumonia. Am J Respir Crit Care Med 2006; 173: 122-9.

[51]   Wieland CW, Knapp S, Florquin S, *et al.* Non-mannose-capped Lipoarabinomannan Induces Lung Inflammation *via* Toll-like Receptor 2. Am J Respir Crit Care Med 2004; .

[52]   Dessing MC, Schouten M, Draing C, *et al.* Role played by Toll-like receptors 2 and 4 in lipoteichoic acid-induced lung inflammation and coagulation. J Infect Dis 2008; 197: 245-52.

[53]   Knapp S, von Aulock S, Leendertse M, *et al.* Lipoteichoic acid-induced lung inflammation depends on TLR2 and the concerted action of TLR4 and the platelet-activating factor receptor. J Immunol 2008; 180: 3478-84.

[54]   Hollingsworth JW, Chen BJ, Brass DM, *et al.* The Critical Role of Hematopoietic Cells in Lipopolysaccharide-induced Airway Inflammation. Am J Respir Crit Care 2005; 171: 806-13.

[55]   Koay MA, Gao X, Washington MK, *et al.* Macrophages Are Necessary for Maximal Nuclear Factor-kappa B Activation in Response to Endotoxin. Am J Respir Cell Mol Biol 2002; 26: 572-78.

[56]   Knapp S, Wieland CW, van 't Veer C, *et al.* Toll-Like Receptor 2 Plays a Role in the Early Inflammatory Response to Murine Pneumococcal Pneumonia but Does Not Contribute to Antibacterial Defense. J Immunol 2004; 172: 3132-38.

[57]   Malley R, Henneke P, Morse SC, *et al.* Recognition of pneumolysin by Toll-like receptor 4 confers resistance to pneumococcal infection. Proc Natl Acad Sci U S A 2003; 100: 1966-71..

[58]   Branger J, Knapp S, Weijer S, *et al.* Role of Toll-like receptor 4 in gram-positive and gram-negative pneumonia in mice. Infect Immun 2004; 72: 788-94.

[59]   Dessing MC, Florquin S, Paton JC and van der Poll T. Toll-like receptor 2 contributes to antibacterial defence against pneumolysin-deficient pneumococci. Cellular Microbiology 2008; 10: 237-46.

[60]   Albiger B, Dahlberg S, Sandgren A, *et al.* Toll-like receptor 9 acts at an early stage in host defence against pneumococcal infection. Cell Microbiol 2007; 9: 633-44.

[61]   Lee JS, Frevert CW, Matute-Bello G, *et al.* TLR-4 pathway mediates the inflammatory response but not bacterial elimination in *E. coli* pneumonia. Am J Physiol Lung Cell Mol Physiol 2005; 289: L731-38.

[62]   Skerrett SJ, Wilson CB, Liggitt HD and Hajjar AM. Redundant Toll-like receptor signaling in the pulmonary host response to *Pseudomonas aeruginosa. Am* J Physiol Lung Cell Mol Physiol 2007; 292: L312-22.

[63]   Morris AE, Liggitt HD, Hawn TR and Skerrett SJ. Role of Toll-like receptor 5 in the innate immune response to acute *P. aeruginosa* pneumonia. Am J Physiol Lung Cell Mol Physiol 2009; 297: L1112-19.

[64]   Cai S, Batra S, Shen L, Wakamatsu N and Jeyaseelan S. Both TRIF- and MyD88-Dependent Signaling Contribute to Host Defense against Pulmonary *Klebsiella* Infection. J Immunol 2009; 183: 6629-38.

[65]   Jeyaseelan S, Young SK, Yamamoto M, *et al.* Toll/IL-1R Domain-Containing Adaptor Protein (TIRAP) Is a Critical Mediator of Antibacterial Defense in the Lung against *Klebsiella pneumoniae* but Not *Pseudomonas aeruginosa.* J Immunol 2006; 177: 538-47.

[66]   Deng JC, Moore TA, Newstead MW, *et al.* CpG Oligodeoxynucleotides Stimulate Protective Innate Immunity against Pulmonary *Klebsiella* Infection. J Immunol 2004; 173: 5148-55.

[67]   Wang X, Moser C, Louboutin J-P, *et al.* Toll-Like Receptor 4 Mediates Innate Immune Responses to *Haemophilus influenzae* Infection in Mouse Lung. J Immunol 2002; 168: 810-15.

[68]   Wieland CW, Florquin S, Maris NA, *et al.* The MyD88-Dependent, but Not the MyD88-Independent, Pathway of TLR4 Signaling Is Important in Clearing Nontypeable *Haemophilus influenzae* from the Mouse Lung. J Immunol 2005; 175: 6042-49.

[69]   Wieland CW, Florquin S and van der Poll T. Toll-like receptor 9 is not important for host defense against *Haemophilus influenzae.* Immunobiology 2009; In Press: .

[70] Archer KA and Roy CR. MyD88-Dependent Responses Involving Toll-Like Receptor 2 Are Important for Protection and Clearance of *Legionella pneumophila* in a Mouse Model of Legionnaires' Disease. Infect Immun 2006; 74: 3325-33.

[71] Hawn Thomas R, Smith Kelly D, Aderem A and Skerrett Shawn J. Myeloid Differentiation Primary Response Gene (88) and Toll Like Receptor 2 Deficient Mice Are Susceptible to Infection with Aerosolized *Legionella pneumophila*. The Journal of Infectious Diseases 2006; 193: 1693-702.

[72] Fuse ET, Tateda K, Kikuchi Y, *et al.* Role of Toll-like receptor 2 in recognition of *Legionella pneumophila* in a murine pneumonia model. J Med Microbiol 2007; 56: 305-12.

[73] Power MR, Peng Y, Maydanski E, Marshall JS and Lin T-J. *The Development of Early Host Response to Pseudomonas aeruginosa* Lung Infection Is Critically Dependent on Myeloid Differentiation Factor 88 in Mice. J Biol Chem 2004; 279: 49315-22.

[74] Lorenz E, Chemotti DC, Vandal K and Tessier PA. Toll-Like Receptor 2 Represses Nonpilus Adhesin-Induced Signaling in Acute Infections with the *Pseudomonas aeruginosa* pilA Mutant. Infect Immun 2004; 72: 4561-69.

[75] Lettinga K, Florquin S, Speelman P, *et al.* Toll Like Receptor 4 Is Not Involved in Host Defense against Pulmonary *Legionella pneumophila* Infection in a Mouse Model. The Journal of Infectious Diseases 2002; 186: 570-73.

[76] Archer KA, Alexopoulou L, Flavell RA and Roy CR. Multiple MyD88-dependent responses contribute to pulmonary clearance of *Legionella pneumophila*. Cellular Microbiology 2009; 11: 21-36.

[77] Hawn TR, Berrington WR, Smith IA, *et al.* Altered Inflammatory Responses in TLR5-Deficient Mice Infected with *Legionella pneumophila*. J Immunol 2007; 179: 6981-87.

[78] Sporri R, Joller N, Albers U, Hilbi H and Oxenius A. MyD88-Dependent IFN-{gamma} Production by NK Cells Is Key for Control of Legionella pneumophila Infection. J Immunol 2006; 176: 6162-71.

[79] Skerrett SJ, Liggitt HD, Hajjar AM and Wilson CB. Cutting Edge: Myeloid Differentiation Factor 88 Is Essential for Pulmonary Host Defense against *Pseudomonas aeruginosa* but Not Staphylococcus aureus. J Immunol 2004; 172: 3377-81.

[80] Ku CL, Yang K, Bustamante J, *et al.* Inherited disorders of human Toll-like receptor signaling: immunological implications. Immunol Rev 2005; 203: 10-20.

[81] Texereau J, Chiche JD, Taylor W, *et al.* The Importance of Toll-Like Receptor 2 Polymorphisms in Severe Infections. Clin Infect Dis 2005; 41: S408-S15.

[82] Schwartz David A and Cook Donald N. Polymorphisms of the Toll Like Receptors and Human Disease. Clin Infect Dis 2005; 41: S403-S07.

[83] Hawn TR, Verbon A, Lettinga KD, *et al.* A Common Dominant TLR5 Stop Codon Polymorphism Abolishes Flagellin Signaling and Is Associated with Susceptibility to Legionnaires' Disease. J Exp Med 2003; 198: 1563-72.

[84] Hawn TR, Verbon A, Janer M, *et al.* Toll-like receptor 4 polymorphisms are associated with resistance to Legionnaires' disease. PNAS 2005; 102: 2487-89.

[85] Kim TW, Staschke K, Bulek K, *et al.* A critical role for IRAK4 kinase activity in Toll-like receptor-mediated innate immunity. J Exp Med 2007; 204: 1025-36.

[86] Picard C, Puel A, Bonnet M, *et al.* Pyogenic bacterial infections in humans with IRAK-4 deficiency. Science 2003; 299: 2076-9.

[87] Ku C-L, von Bernuth H, Picard C, *et al.* Selective predisposition to bacterial infections in IRAK-4 deficient children: IRAK-4 dependent TLRs are otherwise redundant in protective immunity. J Exp Med 2007; 204: 2407-22.

[88] Rijneveld AW, Florquin S, Branger J, *et al.* TNF-alpha compensates for the impaired host defense of IL-1 type I receptor-deficient mice during pneumococcal pneumonia. J Immunol 2001; 167: 5240-6..

[89] von Bernuth H, Picard C, Jin Z, *et al.* Pyogenic Bacterial Infections in Humans with MyD88 Deficiency. Science 2008; 321: 691-96.

[90] Khor CC, Chapman SJ, Vannberg FO, *et al.* A Mal functional variant is associated with protection against invasive pneumococcal disease, bacteremia, malaria and tuberculosis. Nat Genet 2007; 39: 523-28.

[91] Kawai T and Akira S. Signaling to NF-[kappa]B by Toll-like receptors. Trends in Molecular Medicine 2007; 13: 460-69.

[92] Chapman SJ, Khor CC, Vannberg FO, *et al.* I{kappa}B Genetic Polymorphisms and Invasive Pneumococcal Disease. Am J Respir Crit Care 2007; 176: 181-87.

[93] Chapman SJ, Khor CC, Vannberg FO, *et al.* NFKBIZ polymorphisms and susceptibility to pneumococcal disease in European and African populations. Genes Immun 2010; 11: 319-25.

[94] Hennessy EJ, Parker AE and O'Neill LAJ. Targeting Toll-like receptors: emerging therapeutics? Nat Rev Drug Discov 2010; 9: 293-307.

[95]   Sogaard Ole S, Lohse N, Harboe Zitta B, *et al.* Improving the Immunogenicity of Pneumococcal Conjugate Vaccine in HIV Infected Adults with a Toll Like Receptor 9 Agonist Adjuvant: A Randomized, Controlled Trial. Clin Infect Dis 2010; 51: 42-50.

[96]   Tidswell M, Tillis W, Larosa SP, *et al.* Phase 2 trial of eritoran tetrasodium (E5564), a toll-like receptor 4 antagonist, in patients with severe sepsis. Crit Care Med 2010; 38: 72-83.

[97]   Bernard GR, Wheeler AP, Russell JA, *et al.* The effects of ibuprofen on the physiology and survival of patients with sepsis. The Ibuprofen in Sepsis Study Group. N Engl J Med 1997; 336: 912-8.

CHAPTER 8

TLRs and Viral Infection in the Lung

Stephanie Traub and Sebastian L. Johnston[*]

Department of Respiratory Medicine, National Heart & Lung Institute, Imperial College London W2 1PG, London UK

Abstract: In response to viral infection and array of innate an adaptive immune cells, in conjunction with the airway epithelium, orchestrate and inflammatory response to eliminate the invading virus. Pattern recognition receptors and Toll-like receptors (TLRs) in particular have an important role in these events. Here we describe the expression and function of TLRs by infiltrating and resident cells within the airways and describe their roles in responding to infection of the upper and lower respiratory tract with respiratory syncytial virus, rhinoviruses, adenoviruses and influenza virus. We discuss factors affecting host susceptibility to infection and resolution of pulmonary viral infection and describe how TLRs and their signaling pathways represent promising targets for prophylactic and therapeutic interventions in this context.

Keywords: TLRs, respiratory syncytial virus, rhinoviruses, adenoviruses and influenza virus, therapeutics.

1. INTRODUCTION

Breathing exposes the respiratory tract to pathogens and foreign particles. Therefore, the respiratory system includes many mechanisms for defence against entering bacteria and viruses. Most respiratory virus infections in early childhood are upper respiratory tract infections and are caused by infections with seasonal viruses. It is believed that around one third of respiratory tract infections affect the lower respiratory tract however there are viruses that infect the upper respiratory tract that are also important [1-4].

Pulmonary host defence consists of several defence mechanisms including natural barriers. Mucus production by mucus membranes and mucociliary clearance play a crucial role in removal and elimination of pathogens from the lung. Equally important are the non-specific innate immune cells and specific adaptive immune cells in recognising and clearing viral pathogens from the lung. Innate immune cells such as neutrophils, alveolar macrophages and dendritic cells and their products are the first line of defence against pathogens that succeed in overcoming the physical barriers. Epithelial cells are now recognised as central players in controlling subsequent specific immune responses together with antigen-presenting cells, in which T and B cells are activated and recruited to produce a variety of antigen-specific antibodies [5]. Other cells, such as natural killer (NK), natural killer T (NKT) and γδ T cells are recruited and expand in the lung to support immune responses. Activated mast cells, eosinophils and basophils infiltrate into the airway, especially in allergen-related disease and are regarded as potent inflammatory cells.

The essential role of immune system, both the innate and adaptive, is recognising foreign non-self molecules in particular pathogens. It does this *via* specific receptors, called pattern recognition receptors (PRRs) that can initiate innate and specific adaptive immune responses. This chapter focuses on recent findings regarding the recognition of viral pathogens by members of the PRR family of Toll-like receptors (TLRs) and their role in the induction of mucosal immune responses.

2. PATTERN RECOGNITION BY TLRs

Pattern recognition receptors recognise non-self molecules, which are mostly conserved structures of pathogens, and are known as pathogen-associated molecular pattern (PAMPs). PRRs include members of

*Address correspondence to Sebastian L. Johnston:** Department of Respiratory Medicine, National Heart & Lung Institute, Imperial College London W2 1PG, London UK Tel: +44 20 7594 3764 Fax: +44 20 7262 8913; Email: s.johnston@imperial.ac.uk

Catherine M. Greene (Ed)

the Toll-like receptor (TLR) family, the NOD-like receptor (NLR) family, RIG-I-like receptor (RLR) family and cytosolic DNA sensors [6-11]. The TLR family consists so far of 13 mammalian TLRs (TLR1-TLR13) of which 10 can be found in humans and 13 have been identified in mice. They can be divided regarding their localisation; either they are located on the cell surface, like TLR1, 2, 4-6 and 10 or in the endosomal compartment like TLR3, 7-9 [9]. TLRs recognise bacterial tri- or diacylated lipopetides (TLR2 in cooperation with TLR1 or TLR6, respectively) as well as lipoteichoic acids, glycolipids and yeast molecules [12-15]. The endosomal TLRs TLR3 and TLR7/TLR8 detect single (ssRNA) and double stranded RNA (dsRNA), respectively, with TLR9 recognising viral and bacterial CpG DNA motifs [16-18]. Lipopolysaccharide is the ligand for TLR4, but this TLR may also be activated by viral proteins [19-22]. TLR5 recognises bacterial flagellin [23].

3. TLR EXPRESSION IN THE LUNG

Lung defence mechanisms have to be effective at recognising pathogens. In recent years it has become increasingly clear that members of the TLR family and other members of the PRR family play an important role in the recognition of pathogens. Several studies have shown that different lung cell types like epithelial cells, alveolar macrophages and endothelial cells express different TLRs. Similarly immune cells that infiltrate the lung such as eosinophils, neutrophils, dendritic cells (DC) subsets, T cells, B cells and mast cells bear different combinations of TLRs and contribute to viral recognition.

3.1. Epithelial Cells

Epithelial cells are not just regarded as an epithelial barrier, but as active participants in the process of inducing and regulating inflammation. Epithelial cells have been shown to express TLRs. Airway epithelial cells express TLR1-TLR11 [24-33]. Functional expression in bronchial epithelial cells has been shown for TLR1-6 and TLR9 by stimulation with the corresponding TLR-specific ligands [26]. Protein expression of TLR2 [31, 34, 35], TLR3 [36], TLR4 [31, 37], TLR5 [31, 33, 35] and TLR9 [38] has been demonstrated in pulmonary epithelial cells. TLR4 is present on both the cell surface and intracellularly [37], whilst TLR2 is principally localized on the surface [39, 40].

Stimulation of epithelial cells with influenza A virus has demonstrated a role for TLR3 in the expression of proinflammatory cytokines [41, 42]. The TLR3 agonists dsRNA or polyI:C can induce cytokine release and activation of downstream molecules in a TLR3 dependent manner in airway epithelial cells [43-45]. Human rhinovirus increases the expression of TLR3 mRNA and protein in human bronchial epithelial cells [28] and it has been shown in siRNA studies targeting TRIF that human rhinovirus signals *via* TLR3 [46]. Taken together it is increasingly clear that epithelial cells play an important role in recognition of viruses and other pathogens and participate in modulating immune responses in the lung by release of cytokines and chemokines [47, 48].

3.2. Alveolar Macrophages

Resting alveolar macrophages are believed to play a major role in lung defence by monitoring pathogenic organisms entering the lung. They are equipped to do this because of their phagocytic, antigen processing and immunomodulatory functions. Alveolar macrophages express functional TLR2-5 and TLR9 [49, 50], but TLR expression seems to be lower than in other cell types [49], however inhalation of LPS by human volunteers has been shown to enhance the expression of TLR1, 2, 7, 8 and CD14 (a co-receptor for TLR4 and MD-2) [51]. Whilst TLR2 and TLR4 ligands can increase expression of TLR2, TLR4 and TLR9, other molecules such as surfactant protein A and LPS have been shown to down regulate TLR2 and TLR4 expression [51, 52].

3.3. Endothelial Cells

The pulmonary endothelium forms a semiselective barrier that regulates the exchange of fluids, macromolecules and cells between the vascular compartment and tissue spaces. During inflammation the endothelial barrier becomes more permissive to allow leukocyte trafficking from the blood to the interstitium through intercellular gaps [53]. The role of TLRs in lung endothelial cells is not yet quite clear. Most of the studies regarding TLR expression have used non-pulmonary endothelial cells [54-57]. Rat and mouse pulmonary endothelial cells have been shown to express TLR2, TLR4 [58, 59] and TLR9 [60]. TLR9 is functional in lung endothelial cells and its activation can result in cytokine release [60]. Further studies should reveal the role of TLRs in endothelial cells and their possible role in defence against viral infection in the lung.

3.4. Eosinophils

Eosinophils have an important role in asthma etiology however they also regulate clearance of some viruses from the lung. Human peripheral blood eosinophils express TLR1, TLR2, TLR4-7, TLR9 and TLR10. Ligands for TLR2, TLR5 and TLR7 can induce upregulation of cell surface molecules and cytokine release [61]. The TLR7 ligand R848 induces superoxide release and promotes cell survival in eosinophils [62]. Interestingly eosinophils have been shown to contribute to clearance of RSV from the lung [63, 64]. Several authors suggest a link of TLR-mediated activation of eosinophils by viral and bacterial infections with exacerbation of allergic asthma. TLR-activated eosinophils could induce proinflammatory cytokines for the recruitment and infiltration of neutrophils and further eosinophils, and the TLR-induced upregulation of adhesion molecules on the surface of eosinophils could trigger their attachment and subsequent degranulation. Thus eosinophils may contribute to the exacerbation of allergic inflammation in the presence of infections [32, 55, 56, 61, 62, 65]. Further studies are necessary to clarify the role of TLRs on eosinophils in recognition of viral infections and their role in exacerbation of allergic diseases.

3.5. Neutrophils

Neutrophils play a prominent role in inflammatory responses and clearance of viruses from the lung. Neutrophils express all TLRs except TLR3 and activation of TLRs on neutrophils can induce cytokine release, superoxide generation and increase phagocytosis [61, 66, 67]. TLR8 in particular has been implicated in neutrophilic responses under conditions of oxidative stress, which occurs during viral infections. Additionally, TLR8 plays a role in priming human neutrophils for leukotriene induction [68, 69] leading to the hypothesis that TLR8 may be an anti-viral receptor for recognizing ssRNA, which is present during various phases of viral replication [70]. In neutrophils TLR7 is essential for influenza virus recognition and inflammatory cytokine production [71, 72]. Moreover TLR-dependent promotion of neutrophil migration [73], neutrophil apoptosis and phagocytic clearance by neutrophils as well as the ability of these cells to release multiple cytokines have been proposed to be other important mechanisms for the resolution of virus induced airway inflammation [74].

3.6. Dendritic Cells

Dendritic cells (DCs) have a central role in the initiation of immune responses and in linking innate and adaptive immunity. DCs are efficient antigen-presenting cells, producers of IFNs, other cytokines and chemokines and can induce T cell proliferation after their migration to the regional lymph node. DCs express a variety of TLRs and exposure to TLR ligands is thought to be expecially important for dendritic cell maturation and priming [75]. Most of our knowledge about DCs has been gained by characterization of DCs from compartments other than the lung. Two types of DC subtypes have been described; plasmacytoid DC (pDC) with high expression of TLR7/8 and TLR9 [76, 77] and myeloid or conventional DC (mDC or cDC) that express TLR2-4, TLR7 and TLR9 [78, 79]. Lung-specific DC subsets and their features have also been studied [80-84]. Three subtypes of DCs have been described in the lung: myeloid DC type 1 (mDC1) and mDC2, that express TLR1-4, TLR6 and TLR8, and pDC that can express TLR7 and TLR9. TLR3 ligands can induce cytokine release from mDC1, but not mDC2, whereas pDC showed cytokine release after stimulation with ligands for TLR7 and TLR9. Additionally, mDC1 have been shown to induce strong T cell proliferation, with mDC2 inducing an intermediate effect, whilst pDC hardly induce any T cell proliferation [85]. pDCs can limit RSV replication, pulmonary inflammation and airway hyperresponsiveness induced by RSV [86] and are found in increased numbers after RSV infection in the lung [87]. TLR-dependent viral recognition by DCs induces proinflammatorty cytokine and chemokine production as well as expression of type I IFN which is essential for induction of transcription of genes which play a role in host resistance to viral infections. Additionally, key components of the innate and adaptive immunity are activated by DC activation. These events include maturation of antigen presenting cells and production of cytokines involved in activation of T, B and NK-cells [76, 88]. Also direct physical contact between DCs and NK cells, monocytes, T helper cells, cytotoxic T cells, regulatory T cells and B cells are important in tailoring immune responses against viruses and other pathogens [89].

3.7. T Cells

DCs carry out surveillance of the mucosal surface of the respiratory tract by sampling antigens and presenting them to naive T cells in the draining lymph nodes [90]. This primary response of T cells to inhaled antigens is important for the generation of effector and memory T cells during infection. One type of effector T cells, the virus-specific CD8+ effector T cells leave the regional lymph nodes and travel to the sites of viral replication in somatic tissues [91]. Stimulation of CD4+ T cells results in their differentiation into Th1, Th2, Th9, Th17 or Th22 cells [92]. Other T cells with immunoregulatory properties exist, such as CD4⁻CD8⁻ T cells and T regulatory (Treg) cells [93]. Different T cell subtypes can express different TLRs and these different TLR expression pattern can occur depending on their functional status. Mouse CD8+ T cells express TLR1 to TLR13 [94]. Functionality of TLRs on T cells has been demonstrated in studies where costimulation with a TLR2 ligand induced enhanced proliferation, survival and effector function in antigen-activated CD8 T cells and reduced the need for costimulatory signals from DCs [95]. Human CD8+ T cells express TLR2-4, TLR7 and TLR9 [96]; CD4+ T cells express at least TLR3, TLR6, TLR7 and TLR9 [97]. Enhanced survival of mouse CD4+ cells has been observed after stimulation with the TLR3 ligand polyI:C and the TLR9 ligand CpG, but ligands for TLR2 and TLR4 had no effect on proliferation and survival [98]. Nor are TLR2 or TLR4 ligands likely to affect naive human CD4+ T cells as they do not express significant levels of TLR2 and TLR4 [99]. Regulatory T cells such as CD4+CD25+ Treg cells express TLR2, TLR4, TLR5, TLR7/8 and TLR9 [100-102] and there is evidence that these cells are regulated by TLR ligands. For example ligands for TLR2, TLR5 and TLR8 modulate the proliferation and suppressive function of CD4+CD25+ Treg cells [103, 104], TLR7 signaling can enhance the suppressor function of CD4+CD25+ Treg cells, while TLR8 activation reverses the immunosuppressive function of CD4+CD25+ Treg cells [17, 105, 106]. Similar responses have been reported for TLR9 [107]. Additionally, costimulation of CD3 and TLR9 induces proliferation in CD4+CD25+ Treg cells [108]. It has become increasingly clear that many different T cell subsets express TLRs. Therefore, TLR expression on T cells and TLR dependent activation of APCs that provides costimulatory signals to T cells are likely to be two important mechanisms in generating effective immune responses against viral infections.

3.8. B Cells

T helper cells potentiate immune responses by activation of B cells. The T helper cell - B cell interaction is important because naive B cells require a signal *via* the B cell receptor complex and an additional costimulatory signal (CD40 ligation) to produce specific antibodies against bacteria, viruses and tumour cells. However, several other mechanisms of B cell activation implicating TLRs have been suggested [109, 110]. For example T cell independent type II (TI-2) antigens are known to be recognised by B cell subsets such as marginal zone B cells. TLRs expressed by these cells provide B cell costimulatory signals [111]. Moreover, others have shown evidence that T-cell dependent responses to virus particles induce a shift of immunoglobulin isotypes when TLR7 and TLR9 ligands are coupled to virus-like particles [112]. B cells express TLRs, but like T cells TLR expression and responsiveness differs strongly in different B cell subsets, and also between mouse and human B cells. For example, human B cells are unresponsive to TLR4 ligands, whereas mouse B cells secret cytokines and proliferate after stimulation with the TLR4 ligand LPS [77, 113, 114]. In contrast, TLR7 and TLR9 are expressed by all B cell subsets and can be activated by their cognate ligands [77, 114-118]. In human B cells TLR7 expression depends on type I IFN priming that up-regulates the *de novo* synthesis of TLR7 mRNA and sensitizes B cells for TLR7 ligands [114]. TLR3 seems to be only expressed in marginal zone B cells in the spleen [117, 119]. In another B cell subtype, the B-1 B cells, TLR8 mRNA expression has been reported [117]. Additionally, downstream molecules of TLR signaling have been shown to be important for changes in immunoglobulin isotype pattern changes after stimulation of B cells with influenza virus [120]. Studies with influenza virus in MyD88 or TLR7-deficient mice showed impaired anti-influenza immunoglobulin responses [120-123]. Thus B cells and B cell subsets appear to have an important role in defence against viral infections and TLRs play a role in fine-tuning antibody-mediated defences and B cell activation [124].

3.9. Mast Cells

Mast cells are resident in several tissues, but their numbers increase at sites of allergic inflammation. Mast cells are located at mucosal surfaces where exposure to invading viruses occurs, but their ability to respond to viral infections is less clear. Human mast cells express TLR1, TLR2, TLR4-7 and TLR 9. Stimulation with RSV, influenza virus or polyI:C induces cytokine production by mast cells [125]. However, only one study has shown a possible contribution of mast cells to innate immune responses against viral infections *via* the production of type I IFNs [125]. In the absence of antigen mast cells can be activated by IgE and TLR ligands (*e.g.* LPS or PGN) and costimulation with both molecules can lead to increased cytokine production [126]. Mast cells play a role in virus-induced asthma exacerbations [127], suggesting a possible link of amplification mechanisms *via* TLR ligands. However, the contribution of TLRs in mast cells is less understood.

Tissue-, compartment- and cell-specific TLR expression patterns seems to be a necessary requirement to allow the immune system to react to local exposure to infectious viruses. Also effector functions and especially IFN production by resident and infiltrating cells after recognition of TLR ligands, such as occurs in epithelial and dendritic cells are important mechanisms for viral clearance.

4. VIRAL INFECTIONS AND INNATE IMMUNE RESPONSES OF THE LUNG

4.1. Respiratory Viruses

Viral respiratory tract infections are common infectious illnesses. Since the introduction of sensitive molecular diagnostic techniques virus detection rates in large population studies are much higher than previously recorded using standard methodologies [4, 128, 129]. The most consistently found viruses in upper or lower respiratory tract infections are human rhinoviruses (RV), influenza viruses, respiratory syncytial virus (RSV), parainfluenza viruses, coronaviruses, adenoviruses, enteroviruses and human metapneumovirus [4, 130-132]. Effective identification and elimination of respiratory viruses by the host is therefore important as well as restricting the immune response to a minimal and not a systemic infection.

4.2. Innate Immune Response to Viral Infections

In the past several years, the essential role for TLRs in the recognition and fight against viral infections and the initiation of an effective immune response has become increasingly clear. TLRs participate in viral sensing of human viruses. TLR2 is involved in recognition of measles virus [133] and herpes simplex virus [134]; TLR3 recognises dsRNA from RNA viruses like reoviruses, picornaviruses, RSV and influenza A [16, 135, 136]; TLR4 was found to participate in the inflammatory cytokine response to the fusion (F) protein of RSV [137]; TLR7 and TLR8 sense ssRNA such as influenza A virus [71, 138] and vesicular stomatitis virus [139]; TLR9 was shown to induce inflammatory responses to dsDNA viruses like adenoviruses [140] and herpes simplex virus [139]. In this next section we will focus on the role of TLRs in innate immune responses for the most important respiratory viruses in the lung.

4.2.1. Respiratory Syncytical Virus

Respiratory syncytical virus (RSV) is a negative-sense ssRNA virus of the paramyxoviridae family. RSV is a major lung respiratory pathogen usually causing mild illnesses. However, in immune compromised patients, infants and the elderly severe respiratory diseases can occur with significant morbidity and mortality [141]. RSV triggers an inflammatory response by the host and large amounts of proinflammatory cytokines and chemokines are released by airway epithelial cells, macrophages and DCs [142, 143]. TLR4 was the first TLR found to play a role in RSV infection *via* its recognition of the F protein [137, 144]. These results have been controversially discussed [145, 146]. Interestingly, TLR4 polymorphisms have been linked epidemiologically with increased severity of RSV disease in children [147, 148]. Other groups have shown a role for TLR3 mediated cytokine and chemokine induction [48, 149] and up-regulation of TLR3 [36] in RSV-infected epithelial cells. TLR7-/- mice infected with RSV showed increased mucus production as well as altered cytokine production [150, 151] while a study in MyD88-/- mice, which is an adaptor protein for all TLRs except TLR3, described accumulation of eosinophils, augmented mucus production and decreased cDC recruitment to the lung during RSV infection [152]. Others have reported activation of NFκB and upregulation of TLR3 and TLR7 in the lung after infection of RSV [153]. A study in infants with RSV-associated bronchiolitis showed a difference in gene expression of TLR7 and TLR8 and mRNAs of other viral sensors [154].

4.2.2. Influenza Viruses

Influenza A and B viruses are negative-sense ssRNA viruses of the orthomyxoviridae family. Influenza epidemics occur every winter and infected patients are often co-infected with bacteria. Influenza virus A can be recognized by TLR3 and TLR7. Murine pDCs secrete IFN-α after stimulation with influenza *via* TLR7 or other non-pulmonary viruses [138, 139]. Studies in influenza-infected mice showed TLR3 upregulation. Influenza infected TLR3-/- mice displayed reduced cytokine levels as well as lower CD8 lymphocyte numbers in the airway [155]. Others demonstrated an essential role for TLR7 in the recognition of influenza and inflammatory cytokine production by murine neutrophils [71].

4.2.3. Rhinoviruses

Rhinoviruses (RV) have single-stranded positive sense RNA genomes and belong to the picornaviridae family. RVs often cause mild respiratory infections known as the common cold. However, in infants, rhinovirus infection can cause more serious lower respiratory infection. RVs also play an important role in precipitating exacerbations of asthma [156-158]. RV can increase the expression of TLR3 mRNA and protein on human bronchial epithelial cells and induce TLR3-dependent cytokine and chemokine release in human bronchial epithelial cells [28, 159]. Others have found similar results, indicating a role of TLR3 in RV recognition, whilst additional viral sensors like MDA5, but not RIG-I, also play a role in RV recognition [46]. In an animal model of cigarette smoke, cigarette smoke extract was capable of increasing RV-induced TLR3 expression and RV-induced cytokine release in alveolar epithelial cells [160]. A coinfection model of influenza virus and RV showed that influenza infection increases airway epithelial cell ICAM-1 and TLR3 expression leading to enhanced binding of RV and increased RV-induced chemokine release [161]. Others have also reported RV-induced upregulation of ICAM-1, TLR3 and cytokine expression [162] and TSLP production [163] in airway epithelial cells.

4.2.4. Adenoviruses

Adenoviruses are non-enveloped dsDNA viruses causing both upper and lower respiratory tract infections. Most infections are mild and need no treatment. However, in immunocompromised patients, the young and occasionally in healthy adults severe symptoms can occur. Adenovirus activates innate immune responses *via* its dsDNA through TLR-dependent and independent pathways [140, 164, 165]. For pDCs it has been reported that recognition of adenoviruses is mediated by TLR9 [166], for cDC and macrophages adenovirus sensing is independent of TLR9 [165] but results in both cases in TLR9-dependent proinflammatory cytokine responses [167]. Furthermore, adenovirus-infected MyD88-/- mice had lower amounts of inflammatory cytokines in their plasma [168]. A later study showed after an *in vivo* infection with adenovirus that type I IFN activated NK cells accumulated in the liver indicating a possible role of TLR-dependent signaling in adenovirus recognition [169]. Only one study has investigated the role of TLR pathways in adenoviral infection of a human alveolar epithelial cell line where it was demonstrated that MyD88 and TRIF knock-down cell lines induced less IL-6 and IFNβ than normal cells [170].

Recent research on innate and adaptive immunity has identified molecules and molecular pathways involved in the host's immune response to respiratory viruses. Members of the TLR family are important pathogen recognition receptors for viral genomes and proteins, mainly TLR3, TLR4, TLR7/8 and TLR9, which play important roles in triggering antiviral immune responses including type I IFN production and apoptosis. The different and redundant roles of certain TLRs in viral recognition and the specific reaction of the innate immune system may reflect the necessity to react to specific characteristics of viruses. Also different gene expression patterns induced by TLRs as well as the tissue and cell-type dependent expression of TLRs are likely to have a large influence on the outcome of viral infection.

5. VIRAL LUNG DISEASE: POPULATION FREQUENCIES AND HOST SUSCEPTIBILITY

The resistance to infections involves an interplay between environmental and genetic factors. Increasing evidence suggests that human genetic factors play a role in immunodeficiency and susceptibility to infectious diseases [171, 172]. Recent advances in sequencing and mapping of the human genome have established genome-wide maps of single nucleotide polymorphisms [173]. Polymorphisms and genes have been identified which have been clearly linked to increased susceptibility to infections. Ethnic differences in the distribution of these polymorphisms exist. Polymorphisms in the genes encoding TLRs and their signaling proteins have been described which are associated with altered susceptibility to viral infections. In this next section we will focus on the role of TLR polymorphisms for respiratory viral infections in human studies.

TLR4 missense mutations in infants have been associated with the development of severe RSV infection [147, 148, 174]. A TLR4 SNP and the level of CD14 (an adaptor protein of TLR signaling) are associated with the development of RSV bronchiolitis in the Japanese population, indicating that different genetic factors in ethnic groups contribute to the development of viral infections [175]. In a study in China patients have been screened for SNPs in TLRs associated with viral infection, including TLR2-4 and TLR7-9. This study revealed TLR polymorphisms correlating to ethnic populations and suggest that the observed divergence of virus susceptibility in ethnic population could be associated with ethnic specific polymorphisms in TLRs [176].

For non-respiratory viruses other polymorphisms have been shown to have a role. For example SNPS in TLR3 or UNC-93B, an intracellular protein downstream induced by TLR3 signaling, are associated with herpes simplex virus 1 encephalitis [177-179]. Significantly lower expression of IFNα and both of its receptor subunits was found in patients with hepatitis C virus infection with a variant allele of TLR7 [180] but not TLR3 [181]. A number of other studies have addressed this [182, 183]. Although their effect is not known regarding respiratory viruses NEMO (NFκB essential modifier) mutations have been shown to lead to deficient NK cell cytotoxicity [184] and are associated with a higher incidence of herpesvirus infections [185] whilst mutations in STAT1 (Signal Transducers and Activators of Transcription protein 1) lead to impaired STAT1-dependent response of type I IFN and result in susceptibility to viral disease [186].

In individuals with IRAK-4 deficiency (a protein kinase involved in TLR signaling) it has been reported that patients may control viral infections by using redundant TLRs and/or TLR-independent production of IFNs [187]. The IRAK-4 defect abolishes type I and III IFN *via* TLR7-9, but patients have a functional TLR3.

These examples show evidence for higher susceptibility to viral infections in patients with polymorphisms in TLRs and genes that participate in TLR signaling. However, the diversity of the immune system and other TLR-independent pathways may protect the body against viral infections and replace missing or defective paths of the immune system.

6. IMMUNOTHERAPEUTIC POSSIBILITIES

TLRs and their signaling pathways represent promising targets for prophylactic and therapeutic interventions including infectious diseases, inflammatory diseases, allergies, autoimmune diseases and cancer. In some cases artificial TLR activation could be of therapeutic value in promoting antiviral immunity, however in suppressing excessive inflammation, TLR antagonists could be of interest in a number of clinical contexts. TLR agonists have also been used to stimulate the immune system as adjuvants in vaccine development. Therefore, TLR agonists are used as small molecule immune potentiators (SMIPs) in adjuvants to stimulate specific and desired immune responses [188]. For example, synthetic dsRNA had been added to an adjuvant to improve its potency for flu vaccines [189]. CpG oligonucleotides have been used as TLR9-dependent immune potentiators [190] and have been shown to be potent mucosal adjuvants in mice by selective recruitment of DCs and NK cells which allow a better clearance of respiratory pathogens [191]. Preclinical studies have shown that CpG oligonucleotides when co-administrated with allergens and vaccines induce strong immune responses by activating CD4 Th1 cells and CD8 T cells [192, 193]. Others have found utilizing ligands for TLR2/6, TLR3 and TLR9 in combination with a HIV envelope vaccine resulted in a better T cell response [194].

Antagonists of TLRs could also be used to block overwhelming immune responses. For example intracellular RNA sensors such as TLR3, TLR7 or TLR8 could be the optimal target for vaccination against

RNA viruses; peptide epitopes extended with an agonist of TLRs could lead to induction of protective immunity against viruses. Recently, studies have shown that changes in modifications of CpG-oligonucleotides led to antagonism of TLR7 and TLR9 [195] and these may be suitable candidates for diseases where inappropriate and uncontrolled TLR activation is implicated. Although unrelated to viral infection, soluble forms of TLR2 have been found in human breast milk, plasma and monocyte supernatants which lead to interaction between sTLR2 and CD14 in response to bacterial lipopeptide and therefore a neutralisation of bacterial products [196]. In line with this, an alternatively spliced TLR4 protein, which occurs in the mouse and is found as a soluble TLR has been shown to reduce LPS-mediated cytokine production in mouse macrophages [197]. These are examples for promising candidates for the development of new approaches for the treatment of infectious diseases by using specific inhibitors of TLRs. A selection of TLR-based drugs have been identified and are currently being evaluated in preclinical studies and clinical trials. Imiquimod, a synthetic agonist which activates TLR7 has already been approved for its actions in preventing papilloma-induced genital warts [198] and imiquimod is effective as treatment of inflammatory dermatologic disease and skin cancers [199, 200].

TLR-based vaccines for malaria, anthrax, influenza and hepatitis B virus have been evaluated in clinical trials [201-203]. Several companies have different TLR-based molecules in preclinical development such as a TLR7 agonist IPH-32XX for use in cancers, autoimmune diseases and infectious diseases [204]. Ampligen (polyI:polyC12U) which is a synthetically produced TLR3 agonist has been tested against chronic fatigue syndrome [205]. Cliniquest have identified an endogenous human protein CQ-07001 shown to be an agonist of TLR3 that is currently undergoing preclinical development. VAX-102 a TLR5 agonist from VaxInnate Corporation is in phase I trials for influenza infection [206]. Both preclinical and clinical data support a role of TLR-based agonist and antagonists and the possibility to control different diseases.

7. RECENT ADVANCES

It is recognized that several TLRs play important roles as pattern recognition receptors in virus-induced diseases. Especially TLR3, TLR7/8 and TLR9 are engaged in sensing of viruses and viral motifs. However, recently other cytoplasmic proteins have been identified as player in the recognition of viral nucleic acids. These include three families: the RIG-I-like receptors (RLRs), DNA-binding factors and nucleotide-binding domain-leucine-rich repeat-containing molecules (NLRs).

RIG-I, MDA5 and LGP2 belong to the RLR family of helicases [207]. Activation of these RNA helicases leads to the induction of type I IFN and antiviral and inflammatory responses against infection [208]. RIG-I recognises a large number of viruses including RSV, influenza A virus, vesicular stomatitis virus, ebola virus and dengue virus [209, 210]. Picornavirus RNA, sendai virus and polyI:C are recognised by MDA5 [46, 211]. Studies in LGP2-/- mice suggest that LGP2 is a positive regulator of RLRs and is essential for type I IFN production [212, 213].

Recent studies identified a cytoplasmic DNA receptor called DNA-dependent activator of IFN-regulatory factors (DAI/ZVP-1) which binds B-form DNA and trigger signaling to type I IFN production. Stimulation of mouse fibroblasts with B-DNA, vaccinia virus or polyI:C led to DAI dependent IFNβ mRNA expression [7]. Further studies would have to identify the role of DAI in the recognition of viral infections.

The inflammasome is a multiprotein complex [10] and recent work has highlighted a role of the NLR pathway in the recognition of DNA or RNA in virus infection. The NLRP3 inflammasome was found to be activated and led to secretion of IL-1β in adenovirus and vaccinia virus infection [214, 215]. Also for influenza A triggering of the inflammasome through NLRP3 has been reported [216-219].

In this context viral immune evasion strategies have been identified that target PRRs and their downstream signaling molecules [220]. For example, paramyxovirus V proteins bind to MDA-5 [221, 222] and influenza virus NS1 binds to RIG-I [223] preventing RNA detection and IFN induction. Viral evasion mechanisms have also been identified for the downstream molecules of TLR3 and TLR7. NS3/4A from hepatitis C virus, for example, cleaves TRIF, a TLR3 adaptor molecule [224] and inhibitory proteins of

RSV and measles virus have been shown to inhibit TLR7 and TLR9-induced type I IFN induction [225]. These findings suggest that both TLRs and cytosolic RNA/DNA sensors play an important role in the detection of viral infections at different stages.

8. CONCLUSION

TLRs participate in recognising and clearing viruses from the lung however factors that lead to their aberrant expression, such as inactivating SNPs, or interfere with their signaling activity (*e.g.* viral immune evasion strategies) can have deleterious effects for the host. A more in-depth understanding the expression, function and idiosyncratic properties of TLRs is required for the development of TLR-directed therapeutic strategies for the treatment of pulmonary viral infections.

REFERENCES

[1] Valero N, Larreal Y, Arocha F, *et al.* [Viral etiology of acute respiratory infections]. Invest Clin 2009; 50: 359-68.

[2] Jansen RR, Schinkel J, Dek I, *et al.* Quantitation of respiratory viruses in relation to clinical course in children with acute respiratory tract infections. Pediatr Infect Dis J 2010; 29: 82-4.

[3] Tregoning JS, Schwarze J. Respiratory viral infections in infants: causes, clinical symptoms, virology, and immunology. Clin Microbiol Rev 2010; 23: 74-98.

[4] Lieberman D, Shimoni A, Keren-Naus A, Steinberg R, Shemer-Avni Y. Identification of respiratory viruses in adults: nasopharyngeal versus oropharyngeal sampling. J Clin Microbiol 2009; 47: 3439-43.

[5] Suzuki T, Chow CW, Downey GP. Role of innate immune cells and their products in lung immunopathology. Int J Biochem Cell Biol 2008; 40: 1348-61.

[6] Fritz JH, Ferrero RL, Philpott DJ, Girardin SE. Nod-like proteins in immunity, inflammation and disease. Nat Immunol 2006; 7: 1250-7.

[7] Takaoka A, Wang Z, Choi MK, *et al.* DAI (DLM-1/ZBP1) is a cytosolic DNA sensor and an activator of innate immune response. Nature 2007; 448: 501-5.

[8] Yoneyama M, Fujita T. Structural mechanism of RNA recognition by the RIG-I-like receptors. Immunity 2008; 29: 178-81.

[9] Beutler BA. TLRs and innate immunity. Blood 2009; 113: 1399-407.

[10] Martinon F, Mayor A, Tschopp J. The inflammasomes: guardians of the body. Annu Rev Immunol 2009; 27: 229-65.

[11] Opitz B, Eitel J, Meixenberger K, Suttorp N. Role of Toll-like receptors, NOD-like receptors and RIG-I-like receptors in endothelial cells and systemic infections. Thromb Haemost 2009; 102: 1103-9.

[12] Aliprantis AO, Yang RB, Mark MR, *et al.* Cell activation and apoptosis by bacterial lipoproteins through toll-like receptor-2. Science 1999; 285: 736-9.

[13] Morath S, Stadelmaier A, Geyer A, Schmidt RR, Hartung T. Synthetic lipoteichoic acid from *Staphylococcus aureus* is a potent stimulus of cytokine release. J Exp Med 2002; 195: 1635-40.

[14] Takeuchi O, Kawai T, Muhlradt PF, *et al.* Discrimination of bacterial lipoproteins by Toll-like receptor 6. Int Immunol 2001; 13: 933-40.

[15] Takeuchi O, Sato S, Horiuchi T, *et al.* Cutting edge: role of Toll-like receptor 1 in mediating immune response to microbial lipoproteins. J Immunol 2002; 169: 10-4.

[16] Alexopoulou L, Holt AC, Medzhitov R, Flavell RA. Recognition of double-stranded RNA and activation of NF-kappaB by Toll-like receptor 3. Nature 2001; 413: 732-8.

[17] Heil F, Hemmi H, Hochrein H, *et al.* Species-specific recognition of single-stranded RNA *via* toll-like receptor 7 and 8. Science 2004; 303: 1526-9.

[18] Hemmi H, Takeuchi O, Kawai T, *et al.* A Toll-like receptor recognizes bacterial DNA. Nature 2000; 408: 740-5.

[19] Poltorak A, He X, Smirnova I, *et al.* Defective LPS signaling in C3H/HeJ and C57BL/10ScCr mice: mutations in Tlr4 gene. Science 1998; 282: 2085-8.

[20] Lagos D, Vart RJ, Gratrix F, *et al.* Toll-like receptor 4 mediates innate immunity to Kaposi sarcoma herpesvirus. Cell Host Microbe 2008; 4: 470-83.

[21] Hutchens MA, Luker KE, Sonstein J, Nunez G, Curtis JL, Luker GD. Protective effect of Toll-like receptor 4 in pulmonary vaccinia infection. PLoS Pathog 2008; 4: e1000153.

[22] Schabbauer G, Luyendyk J, Crozat K, *et al.* TLR4/CD14-mediated PI3K activation is an essential component of interferon-dependent VSV resistance in macrophages. Mol Immunol 2008; 45: 2790-6.

[23] Hayashi F, Smith KD, Ozinsky A, *et al.* The innate immune response to bacterial flagellin is mediated by Toll-like receptor 5. Nature 2001; 410: 1099-103.

[24] Homma T, Kato A, Hashimoto N, *et al.* Corticosteroid and cytokines synergistically enhance toll-like receptor 2 expression in respiratory epithelial cells. Am J Respir Cell Mol Biol 2004; 31: 463-9.

[25] Sha Q, Truong-Tran AQ, Plitt JR, Beck LA, Schleimer RP. Activation of airway epithelial cells by toll-like receptor agonists. Am J Respir Cell Mol Biol 2004; 31: 358-64.

[26] Mayer AK, Muehmer M, Mages J, *et al.* Differential recognition of TLR-dependent microbial ligands in human bronchial epithelial cells. J Immunol 2007; 178: 3134-42.

[27] Cai Z, Shi Z, Sanchez A, *et al.* Transcriptional regulation of Tlr11 gene expression in epithelial cells. J Biol Chem 2009; 284: 33088-96.

[28] Hewson CA, Jardine A, Edwards MR, Laza-Stanca V, Johnston SL. Toll-like receptor 3 is induced by and mediates antiviral activity against rhinovirus infection of human bronchial epithelial cells. J Virol 2005; 79: 12273-9.

[29] Schmeck B, Huber S, Moog K, *et al.* Pneumococci induced TLR- and Rac1-dependent NF-kappaB-recruitment to the IL-8 promoter in lung epithelial cells. Am J Physiol Lung Cell Mol Physiol 2006; 290: L730-L7.

[30] Armstrong L, Medford AR, Uppington KM, *et al.* Expression of functional toll-like receptor-2 and -4 on alveolar epithelial cells. Am J Respir Cell Mol Biol 2004; 31: 241-5.

[31] Muir A, Soong G, Sokol S, *et al.* Toll-like receptors in normal and cystic fibrosis airway epithelial cells. Am J Respir Cell Mol Biol 2004; 30: 777-83.

[32] Greene CM, Carroll TP, Smith SG, *et al.* TLR-induced inflammation in cystic fibrosis and non-cystic fibrosis airway epithelial cells. J Immunol 2005; 174: 1638-46.

[33] Zhang Z, Louboutin JP, Weiner DJ, Goldberg JB, Wilson JM. Human airway epithelial cells sense *Pseudomonas aeruginosa* infection *via* recognition of flagellin by Toll-like receptor 5. Infect Immun 2005; 73: 7151-60.

[34] Droemann D, Goldmann T, Branscheid D, *et al.* Toll-like receptor 2 is expressed by alveolar epithelial cells type II and macrophages in the human lung. Histochem Cell Biol 2003; 119: 103-8.

[35] Adamo R, Sokol S, Soong G, Gomez MI, Prince A. *Pseudomonas aeruginosa* flagella activate airway epithelial cells through asialoGM1 and toll-like receptor 2 as well as toll-like receptor 5. Am J Respir Cell Mol Biol 2004; 30: 627-34.

[36] Groskreutz DJ, Monick MM, Powers LS, Yarovinsky TO, Look DC, Hunninghake GW. Respiratory syncytial virus induces TLR3 protein and protein kinase R, leading to increased double-stranded RNA responsiveness in airway epithelial cells. J Immunol 2006; 176: 1733-40.

[37] Guillot L, Medjane S, Le-Barillec K, *et al.* Response of human pulmonary epithelial cells to lipopolysaccharide involves Toll-like receptor 4 (TLR4)-dependent signaling pathways: evidence for an intracellular compartmentalization of TLR4. J Biol Chem 2004; 279: 2712-8.

[38] Droemann D, Albrecht D, Gerdes J, *et al.* Human lung cancer cells express functionally active Toll-like receptor 9. Respir Res 2005; 6: 1.

[39] Hertz CJ, Wu Q, Porter EM, *et al.* Activation of Toll-like receptor 2 on human tracheobronchial epithelial cells induces the antimicrobial peptide human beta defensin-2. J Immunol 2003; 171: 6820-6.

[40] Soong G, Reddy B, Sokol S, Adamo R, Prince A. TLR2 is mobilized into an apical lipid raft receptor complex to signal infection in airway epithelial cells. J Clin Invest 2004; 113: 1482-9.

[41] Le Goffic R, Pothlichet J, Vitour D, *et al.* Cutting Edge: Influenza A virus activates TLR3-dependent inflammatory and RIG-I-dependent antiviral responses in human lung epithelial cells. J Immunol 2007; 178: 3368-72.

[42] Guillot L, Le Goffic R, Bloch S, *et al.* Involvement of toll-like receptor 3 in the immune response of lung epithelial cells to double-stranded RNA and influenza A virus. J Biol Chem 2005; 280: 5571-80.

[43] Gern JE, French DA, Grindle KA, *et al.* Double-stranded RNA induces the synthesis of specific chemokines by bronchial epithelial cells. Am J Respir Cell Mol Biol 2003; 28: 731-7.

[44] Matsukura S, Kokubu F, Kurokawa M, *et al.* Synthetic double-stranded RNA induces multiple genes related to inflammation through Toll-like receptor 3 depending on NF-kappaB and/or IRF-3 in airway epithelial cells. Clin Exp Allergy 2006; 36: 1049-62.

[45] Koff JL, Shao MX, Ueki IF, Nadel JA. Multiple TLRs activate EGFR *via* a signaling cascade to produce innate immune responses in airway epithelium. Am J Physiol Lung Cell Mol Physiol 2008; 294: L1068-75.

[46] Wang Q, Nagarkar DR, Bowman ER, *et al.* Role of double-stranded RNA pattern recognition receptors in rhinovirus-induced airway epithelial cell responses. J Immunol 2009; 183: 6989-97.

[47] Oshansky CM, Barber JP, Crabtree J, Tripp RA. Respiratory syncytial virus F and G proteins induce interleukin 1alpha, CC, and CXC chemokine responses by normal human bronchoepithelial cells. J Infect Dis 2010; 201: 1201-7.

[48]   Rudd BD, Burstein E, Duckett CS, Li X, Lukacs NW. Differential role for TLR3 in respiratory syncytial virus-induced chemokine expression. J Virol 2005; 79: 3350-7.

[49]   Juarez E, Nunez C, Sada E, Ellner JJ, Schwander SK, Torres M. Differential expression of Toll-like receptors on human alveolar macrophages and autologous peripheral monocytes. Respir Res 2010; 11: 2.

[50]   Fenhalls G, Squires GR, Stevens-Muller L, *et al.* Associations between toll-like receptors and interleukin-4 in the lungs of patients with tuberculosis. Am J Respir Cell Mol Biol 2003; 29: 28-38.

[51]   Maris NA, Dessing MC, de Vos AF, *et al.* Toll-like receptor mRNA levels in alveolar macrophages after inhalation of endotoxin. Eur Respir J 2006; 28: 622-6.

[52]   Henning LN, Azad AK, Parsa KV, Crowther JE, Tridandapani S, Schlesinger LS. Pulmonary surfactant protein A regulates TLR expression and activity in human macrophages. J Immunol 2008; 180: 7847-58.

[53]   Moore TM, Chetham PM, Kelly JJ, Stevens T. Signal transduction and regulation of lung endothelial cell permeability. Interaction between calcium and cAMP. Am J Physiol 1998; 275: L203-22.

[54]   Pegu A, Qin S, Fallert Junecko BA, Nisato RE, Pepper MS, Reinhart TA. Human lymphatic endothelial cells express multiple functional TLRs. J Immunol 2008; 180: 3399-405.

[55]   Fischer S, Nishio M, Peters SC, *et al.* Signaling mechanism of extracellular RNA in endothelial cells. FASEB J 2009; 23: 2100-9.

[56]   Loos T, Dekeyzer L, Struyf S, *et al.* TLR ligands and cytokines induce CXCR3 ligands in endothelial cells: enhanced CXCL9 in autoimmune arthritis. Lab Invest 2006; 86: 902-16.

[57]   Lundberg AM, Drexler SK, Monaco C, *et al.* Key differences in TLR3/poly I:C signaling and cytokine induction by human primary cells: a phenomenon absent from murine cell systems. Blood 2007; 110: 3245-52.

[58]   Andonegui G, Bonder CS, Green F, *et al.* Endothelium-derived Toll-like receptor-4 is the key molecule in LPS-induced neutrophil sequestration into lungs. J Clin Invest 2003; 111: 1011-20.

[59]   Li Y, Xiang M, Yuan Y, *et al.* Hemorrhagic shock augments lung endothelial cell activation: role of temporal alterations of TLR4 and TLR2. Am J Physiol Regul Integr Comp Physiol 2009; 297: R1670-80.

[60]   Li J, Ma Z, Tang ZL, Stevens T, Pitt B, Li S. CpG DNA-mediated immune response in pulmonary endothelial cells. Am J Physiol Lung Cell Mol Physiol 2004; 287: L552-8.

[61]   Wong CK, Cheung PF, Ip WK, Lam CW. Intracellular signaling mechanisms regulating toll-like receptor-mediated activation of eosinophils. Am J Respir Cell Mol Biol 2007; 37: 85-96.

[62]   Nagase H, Okugawa S, Ota Y, *et al.* Expression and function of Toll-like receptors in eosinophils: activation by Toll-like receptor 7 ligand. J Immunol 2003; 171: 3977-82.

[63]   Phipps S, Lam CE, Mahalingam S, *et al.* Eosinophils contribute to innate antiviral immunity and promote clearance of respiratory syncytial virus. Blood 2007; 110: 1578-86.

[64]   Rosenberg HF, Domachowske JB. Eosinophils, eosinophil ribonucleases, and their role in host defense against respiratory virus pathogens. J Leukoc Biol 2001; 70: 691-8.

[65]   Mansson A, Cardell LO. Role of atopic status in Toll-like receptor (TLR)7- and TLR9-mediated activation of human eosinophils. J Leukoc Biol 2009; 85: 719-27.

[66]   Hayashi F, Means TK, Luster AD. Toll-like receptors stimulate human neutrophil function. Blood 2003; 102: 2660-9.

[67]   O'Mahony DS, Pham U, Iyer R, Hawn TR, Liles WC. Differential constitutive and cytokine-modulated expression of human Toll-like receptors in primary neutrophils, monocytes, and macrophages. Int J Med Sci 2008; 5: 1-8.

[68]   Yanagisawa S, Koarai A, Sugiura H, *et al.* Oxidative stress augments toll-like receptor 8 mediated neutrophilic responses in healthy subjects. Respir Res 2009; 10: 50.

[69]   Janke M, Poth J, Wimmenauer V, *et al.*Selective and direct activation of human neutrophils but not eosinophils by Toll-like receptor 8. J Allergy Clin Immunol 2009; 123: 1026-33.

[70]   Hattermann K, Picard S, Borgeat M, Leclerc P, Pouliot M, Borgeat P. The Toll-like receptor 7/8-ligand resiquimod (R-848) primes human neutrophils for leukotriene B4, prostaglandin E2 and platelet-activating factor biosynthesis. FASEB J 2007; 21: 1575-85.

[71]   Wang JP, Bowen GN, Padden C, *et al.* Toll-like receptor-mediated activation of neutrophils by influenza A virus. Blood 2008; 112: 2028-34.

[72]   Wang JP, Liu P, Latz E, Golenbock DT, Finberg RW, Libraty DH. Flavivirus activation of plasmacytoid dendritic cells delineates key elements of TLR7 signaling beyond endosomal recognition. J Immunol 2006; 177: 7114-21.

[73]   Lefebvre JS, Marleau S, Milot V, *et al.* Toll-like receptor ligands induce polymorphonuclear leukocyte migration: key roles for leukotriene B4 and platelet-activating factor. FASEB J 2010; 24: 637-47.

[74]   Fox S, Leitch AE, Duffin R, Haslett C, Rossi AG. Neutrophil apoptosis: relevance to the innate immune response and inflammatory disease. J Innate Immun 2010; 2: 216-27.

[75] Barton GM. Viral recognition by Toll-like receptors. Semin Immunol 2007; 19: 33-40.

[76] Gilliet M, Cao W, Liu YJ. Plasmacytoid dendritic cells: sensing nucleic acids in viral infection and autoimmune diseases. Nat Rev Immunol 2008; 8: 594-606.

[77] Hornung V, Rothenfusser S, Britsch S, *et al.* Quantitative expression of toll-like receptor 1-10 mRNA in cellular subsets of human peripheral blood mononuclear cells and sensitivity to CpG oligodeoxynucleotides. J Immunol 2002; 168: 4531-7.

[78] Matsumoto M, Funami K, Tanabe M, *et al.* Subcellular localization of Toll-like receptor 3 in human dendritic cells. J Immunol 2003; 171: 3154-62.

[79] Kokkinopoulos I, Jordan WJ, Ritter MA. Toll-like receptor mRNA expression patterns in human dendritic cells and monocytes. Mol Immunol 2005; 42: 957-68.

[80] Cochand L, Isler P, Songeon F, Nicod LP. Human lung dendritic cells have an immature phenotype with efficient mannose receptors. Am J Respir Cell Mol Biol 1999; 21: 547-54.

[81] Sertl K, Takemura T, Tschachler E, Ferrans VJ, Kaliner MA, Shevach EM. Dendritic cells with antigen-presenting capability reside in airway epithelium, lung parenchyma, and visceral pleura. J Exp Med 1986; 163: 436-51.

[82] Leonard CT, Soccal PM, Singer L, *et al.*Dendritic cells and macrophages in lung allografts: A role in chronic rejection? Am J Respir Crit Care Med 2000; 161: 1349-54.

[83] Todate A, Chida K, Suda T, *et al.* Increased numbers of dendritic cells in the bronchiolar tissues of diffuse panbronchiolitis. Am J Respir Crit Care Med 2000; 162: 148-53.

[84] Demedts IK, Brusselle GG, Vermaelen KY, *et al.* Identification and characterization of human pulmonary dendritic cells. Am J Respir Cell Mol Biol 2005; 32: 177-84.

[85] Demedts IK, Bracke KR, Maes T *et al.* Different roles for human lung dendritic cell subsets in pulmonary immune defense mechanisms. Am J Respir Cell Mol Biol 2006; 35: 387-93.

[86] Wang H, Peters N, Schwarze J. Plasmacytoid dendritic cells limit viral replication, pulmonary inflammation, and airway hyperresponsiveness in respiratory syncytial virus infection. J Immunol 2006; 177: 6263-70.

[87] Smit JJ, Rudd BD, Lukacs NW. Plasmacytoid dendritic cells inhibit pulmonary immunopathology and promote clearance of respiratory syncytial virus. J Exp Med 2006; 203: 1153-9.

[88] Perry AK, Chen G, Zheng D, Tang H, Cheng G. The host type I interferon response to viral and bacterial infections. Cell Res 2005; 15: 407-22.

[89] Fitzgerald-Bocarsly P, Feng D. The role of type I interferon production by dendritic cells in host defense. Biochimie 2007; 89: 843-55.

[90] Plantinga M, Hammad H, Lambrecht BN. Origin and functional specializations of DC subsets in the lung. Eur J Immunol 2010; 40: 2112-8.

[91] Welsh RM, Che JW, Brehm MA, Selin LK. Heterologous immunity between viruses. Immunol Rev 2010; 235: 244-66.

[92] Wan YY. Multi-tasking of helper T cells. Immunology 2010; 130: 166-71.

[93] Palomares O, Yaman G, Azkur AK, Akkoc T, Akdis M, Akdis CA. Role of Treg in immune regulation of allergic diseases. Eur J Immunol 2010; 40: 1232-40.

[94] Salem ML, Diaz-Montero CM, El-Naggar SA, Chen Y, Moussa O, Cole DJ. The TLR3 agonist poly(I:C) targets CD8+ T cells and augments their antigen-specific responses upon their adoptive transfer into naive recipient mice. Vaccine 2009; 27: 549-57.

[95] Mercier BC, Cottalorda A, Coupet CA, Marvel J, Bonnefoy-Berard N. TLR2 engagement on CD8 T cells enables generation of functional memory cells in response to a suboptimal TCR signal. J Immunol 2009; 182: 1860-7.

[96] Hammond T, Lee S, Watson MW, *et al.* Toll-like receptor (TLR) expression on CD4+ and CD8+ T-cells in patients chronically infected with hepatitis C virus. Cell Immunol 2010; 264: 150-5.

[97] Sutmuller RP, den Brok MH, Kramer M, *et al.* Toll-like receptor 2 controls expansion and function of regulatory T cells. J Clin Invest 2006; 116: 485-94.

[98] Gelman AE, Zhang J, Choi Y, Turka LA. Toll-like receptor ligands directly promote activated CD4+ T cell survival. J Immunol 2004; 172: 6065-73.

[99] Babu S, Blauvelt CP, Kumaraswami V, Nutman TB. Cutting edge: diminished T cell TLR expression and function modulates the immune response in human filarial infection. J Immunol 2006; 176: 3885-9.

[100] Caramalho I, Lopes-Carvalho T, Ostler D, Zelenay S, Haury M, Demengeot J. Regulatory T cells selectively express toll-like receptors and are activated by lipopolysaccharide. J Exp Med 2003; 197: 403-11.

[101] Liu G, Zhang L, Zhao Y. Modulation of immune responses through direct activation of Toll-like receptors to T cells. Clin Exp Immunol 2010; 160: 168-75.

[102] MacLeod H, Wetzler LM. T cell activation by TLRs: a role for TLRs in the adaptive immune response. Sci STKE 2007; 2007: pe48.

[103] Liu G, Zhao Y. Toll-like receptors and immune regulation: their direct and indirect modulation on regulatory CD4+ CD25+ T cells. Immunology 2007; 122: 149-56.

[104] Rahman AH, Taylor DK, Turka LA. The contribution of direct TLR signaling to T cell responses. Immunol Res 2009; 45: 25-36.

[105] Forward NA, Furlong SJ, Yang Y, Lin TJ, Hoskin DW. Signaling through TLR7 enhances the immunosuppressive activity of murine CD4+CD25+ T regulatory cells. J Leukoc Biol 2009; 87: 117-25.

[106] Peng G, Guo Z, Kiniwa Y, *et al.* Toll-like receptor 8-mediated reversal of CD4+ regulatory T cell function. Science 2005; 309: 1380-4.

[107] Wang HY, Lee DA, Peng G *et al.* Tumor-specific human CD4+ regulatory T cells and their ligands: implications for immunotherapy. Immunity 2004; 20: 107-18.

[108] Chiffoleau E, Heslan JM, Heslan M, Louvet C, Condamine T, Cuturi MC. TLR9 ligand enhances proliferation of rat CD4+ T cell and modulates suppressive activity mediated by CD4+ CD25+ T cell. Int Immunol 2007; 19: 193-201.

[109] Ruprecht CR, Lanzavecchia A. Toll-like receptor stimulation as a third signal required for activation of human naive B cells. Eur J Immunol 2006; 36: 810-6.

[110] Avalos AM, Busconi L, Marshak-Rothstein A. Regulation of autoreactive B cell responses to endogenous TLR ligands. Autoimmunity 2010; 43: 76-83.

[111] Vos Q, Lees A, Wu ZQ, Snapper CM, Mond JJ. B-cell activation by T-cell-independent type 2 antigens as an integral part of the humoral immune response to pathogenic microorganisms. Immunol Rev 2000; 176: 154-70.

[112] Jegerlehner A, Maurer P, Bessa J, Hinton HJ, Kopf M, Bachmann MF. TLR9 signaling in B cells determines class switch recombination to IgG2a. J Immunol 2007; 178: 2415-20.

[113] Mandler R, Finkelman FD, Levine AD, Snapper CM. IL-4 induction of IgE class switching by lipopolysaccharide-activated murine B cells occurs predominantly through sequential switching. J Immunol 1993; 150: 407-18.

[114] Bekeredjian-Ding IB, Wagner M, Hornung V, Giese T, Schnurr M, Endres S, Hartmann G. Plasmacytoid dendritic cells control TLR7 sensitivity of naive B cells *via* type I IFN. J Immunol 2005; 174: 4043-50.

[115] Bernasconi NL, Onai N, Lanzavecchia A. A role for Toll-like receptors in acquired immunity: up-regulation of TLR9 by BCR triggering in naive B cells and constitutive expression in memory B cells. Blood 2003; 101: 4500-4.

[116] Bourke E, Bosisio D, Golay J, Polentarutti N, Mantovani A. The toll-like receptor repertoire of human B lymphocytes: inducible and selective expression of TLR9 and TLR10 in normal and transformed cells. Blood 2003; 102: 956-63.

[117] Gururajan M, Jacob J, Pulendran B. Toll-like receptor expression and responsiveness of distinct murine splenic and mucosal B-cell subsets. PLoS One 2007; 2: e863.

[118] Barr TA, Brown S, Ryan G, Zhao J, Gray D. TLR-mediated stimulation of APC: Distinct cytokine responses of B cells and dendritic cells. Eur J Immunol 2007; 37: 3040-53.

[119] Genestier L, Taillardet M, Mondiere P, Gheit H, Bella C, Defrance T. TLR agonists selectively promote terminal plasma cell differentiation of B cell subsets specialized in thymus-independent responses. J Immunol 2007;178(12):7779-86.

[120] Heer AK, Shamshiev A, Donda A, *et al.* TLR signaling fine-tunes anti-influenza B cell responses without regulating effector T cell responses. J Immunol 2007; 178: 2182-91.

[121] Graham MB, Braciale TJ. Resistance to and recovery from lethal influenza virus infection in B lymphocyte-deficient mice. J Exp Med 1997; 186: 2063-8.

[122] Kopf M, Brombacher F, Bachmann MF. Role of IgM antibodies versus B cells in influenza virus-specific immunity. Eur J Immunol 2002; 32: 2229-36.

[123] Coro ES, Chang WL, Baumgarth N. Type I IFN receptor signals directly stimulate local B cells early following influenza virus infection. J Immunol 2006; 176: 4343-51.

[124] Bekeredjian-Ding I, Jego G. Toll-like receptors--sentries in the B-cell response. Immunology 2009; 128: 311-23.

[125] Kulka M, Alexopoulou L, Flavell RA, Metcalfe DD. Activation of mast cells by double-stranded RNA: evidence for activation through Toll-like receptor 3. J Allergy Clin Immunol 2004; 114: 174-82.

[126] Qiao H, Andrade MV, Lisboa FA, Morgan K, Beaven MA. FcepsilonR1 and toll-like receptors mediate synergistic signals to markedly augment production of inflammatory cytokines in murine mast cells. Blood 2006; 107: 610-8.

[127] Takenaka H, Ushio H, Niyonsaba F, *et al.* Synergistic augmentation of inflammatory cytokine productions from murine mast cells by monomeric IgE and toll-like receptor ligands. Biochem Biophys Res Commun 2010; 391: 471-6.

[128] Kehl SC, Kumar S. Utilization of nucleic acid amplification assays for the detection of respiratory viruses. Clin Lab Med 2009; 29: 661-71.

[129] Elnifro EM, Ashshi AM, Cooper RJ, Klapper PE. Multiplex PCR: optimization and application in diagnostic virology. Clin Microbiol Rev 2000; 13: 559-70.

[130] He J, Bose ME, Beck ET, *et al.* Rapid multiplex reverse transcription-PCR typing of influenza A and B virus, and subtyping of influenza A virus into H1, 2, 3, 5, 7, 9, N1 (human), N1 (animal), N2, and N7, including typing of novel swine origin influenza A (H1N1) virus, during the 2009 outbreak in Milwaukee, Wisconsin. J Clin Microbiol 2009; 47: 2772-8.

[131] Heikkinen T, Jarvinen A. The common cold. Lancet 2003; 361: 51-9.

[132] Manoha C, Espinosa S, Aho SL, Huet F, Pothier P. Epidemiological and clinical features of hMPV, RSV and RVs infections in young children. J Clin Virol 2007; 38: 221-6.

[133] Bieback K, Lien E, Klagge IM, *et al.* Hemagglutinin protein of wild-type measles virus activates toll-like receptor 2 signaling. J Virol 2002; 76: 8729-36.

[134] Kurt-Jones EA, Chan M, Zhou S, *et al.* Herpes simplex virus 1 interaction with Toll-like receptor 2 contributes to lethal encephalitis. Proc Natl Acad Sci U S A 2004; 101: 1315-20.

[135] Lau YF, Tang LH, Ooi EE, Subbarao K. Activation of the innate immune system provides broad-spectrum protection against influenza A viruses with pandemic potential in mice. Virology 2010; 406: 80-7.

[136] Torres D, Dieudonne A, Ryffel B, *et al.* Double-stranded RNA exacerbates pulmonary allergic reaction through TLR3: implication of airway epithelium and dendritic cells. J Immunol 2010;185(1):451-9.

[137] Kurt-Jones EA, Popova L, Kwinn L, *et al.* Pattern recognition receptors TLR4 and CD14 mediate response to respiratory syncytial virus. Nat Immunol 2000; 1: 398-401.

[138] Diebold SS, Kaisho T, Hemmi H, Akira S, Reis e Sousa C. Innate antiviral responses by means of TLR7-mediated recognition of single-stranded RNA. Science 2004; 303: 1529-31.

[139] Lund J, Sato A, Akira S, Medzhitov R, Iwasaki A. Toll-like receptor 9-mediated recognition of Herpes simplex virus-2 by plasmacytoid dendritic cells. J Exp Med 2003; 198: 513-20.

[140] Appledorn DM, Patial S, McBride A, *et al.* Adenovirus vector-induced innate inflammatory mediators, MAPK signaling, as well as adaptive immune responses are dependent upon both TLR2 and TLR9 *in vivo.* J Immunol 2008; 181: 2134-44.

[141] Hall CB. Respiratory syncytial virus and parainfluenza virus. N Engl J Med 2001; 344: 1917-28.

[142] Miller AL, Bowlin TL, Lukacs NW. Respiratory syncytial virus-induced chemokine production: linking viral replication to chemokine production *in vitro* and *in vivo.* J Infect Dis 2004; 189: 1419-30.

[143] Olszewska-Pazdrak B, Casola A, Saito T, *et al.* Cell-specific expression of RANTES, MCP-1, and MIP-1alpha by lower airway epithelial cells and eosinophils infected with respiratory syncytial virus. J Virol 1998; 72: 4756-64.

[144] Shingai M, Azuma M, Ebihara T, *et al.* Soluble G protein of respiratory syncytial virus inhibits Toll-like receptor 3/4-mediated IFN-beta induction. Int Immunol 2008; 20: 1169-80.

[145] Ehl S, Bischoff R, Ostler T, *et al.* The role of Toll-like receptor 4 versus interleukin-12 in immunity to respiratory syncytial virus. Eur J Immunol 2004; 34: 1146-53.

[146] Faisca P, Tran Anh DB, Thomas A, Desmecht D. Suppression of pattern-recognition receptor TLR4 sensing does not alter lung responses to pneumovirus infection. Microbes Infect 2006; 8: 621-7.

[147] Tal G, Mandelberg A, Dalal I, *et al.* Association between common Toll-like receptor 4 mutations and severe respiratory syncytial virus disease. J Infect Dis 2004; 189: 2057-63.

[148] Tulic MK, Hurrelbrink RJ, Prele CM, *et al.* TLR4 polymorphisms mediate impaired responses to respiratory syncytial virus and lipopolysaccharide. J Immunol 2007; 179: 132-40.

[149] Liu P, Jamaluddin M, Li K, Garofalo RP, Casola A, Brasier AR. Retinoic acid-inducible gene I mediates early antiviral response and Toll-like receptor 3 expression in respiratory syncytial virus-infected airway epithelial cells. J Virol 2007; 81: 1401-11.

[150] Lindell D, Morris S, Mukherjee S, Lukacs N. TLR-7 Mediated Responses to Respiratory Syncytial Virus (RSV). Journal of Immunolgy 2009; 182: 133-45.

[151] Lukacs NW, Smit JJ, Mukherjee S, Morris SB, Nunez G, Lindell DM. Respiratory virus-induced TLR7 activation controls IL-17-associated increased mucus *via* IL-23 regulation. J Immunol 2010; 185: 2231-9.

[152] Rudd BD, Schaller MA, Smit JJ, *et al.* MyD88-mediated instructive signals in dendritic cells regulate pulmonary immune responses during respiratory virus infection. J Immunol 2007; 178: 5820-7.

[153] Huang S, Wei W, Yun Y. Upregulation of TLR7 and TLR3 gene expression in the lung of respiratory syncytial virus infected mice. Wei Sheng Wu Xue Bao 2009; 49: 239-45.

[154] Scagnolari C, Midulla F, Pierangeli A, *et al.* Gene expression of nucleic acid-sensing pattern recognition receptors in children hospitalized for respiratory syncytial virus-associated acute bronchiolitis. Clin Vaccine Immunol 2009; 16: 816-23.

[155] Le Goffic R, Balloy V, Lagranderie M, *et al.* Detrimental contribution of the Toll-like receptor (TLR)3 to influenza A virus-induced acute pneumonia. PLoS Pathog 2006; 2: e53.

[156] Lemanske RF, Jr., Jackson DJ, Gangnon RE, *et al.* Rhinovirus illnesses during infancy predict subsequent childhood wheezing. J Allergy Clin Immunol 2005; 116: 571-7.

[157] Message SD, Laza-Stanca V, Mallia P, *et al.* Rhinovirus-induced lower respiratory illness is increased in asthma and related to virus load and Th1/2 cytokine and IL-10 production. Proc Natl Acad Sci U S A 2008; 105: 13562-7.

[158] Johnston SL, Pattemore PK, Sanderson G, *et al.* Community study of role of viral infections in exacerbations of asthma in 9-11 year old children. BMJ 1995; 310: 1225-9.

[159] Chen Y, Hamati E, Lee PK, *et al.* Rhinovirus induces airway epithelial gene expression through double-stranded RNA and IFN-dependent pathways. Am J Respir Cell Mol Biol 2006; 34: 192-203.

[160] Wang JH, Kim H, Jang YJ. Cigarette smoke extract enhances rhinovirus-induced toll-like receptor 3 expression and interleukin-8 secretion in A549 cells. Am J Rhinol Allergy 2009; 23: e5-9.

[161] Sajjan US, Jia Y, Newcomb DC, *et al.* *H. influenzae* potentiates airway epithelial cell responses to rhinovirus by increasing ICAM-1 and TLR3 expression. FASEB J 2006; 20: 2121-3.

[162] Jang YJ, Wang JH, Kim JS, Kwon HJ, Yeo NK, Lee BJ. Levocetirizine inhibits rhinovirus-induced ICAM-1 and cytokine expression and viral replication in airway epithelial cells. Antiviral Res 2009; 81: 226-33.

[163] Kato A, Favoreto S, Jr., Avila PC, Schleimer RP. TLR3- and Th2 cytokine-dependent production of thymic stromal lymphopoietin in human airway epithelial cells. J Immunol 2007; 179: 1080-7.

[164] Nociari M, Ocheretina O, Schoggins JW, Falck-Pedersen E. Sensing infection by adenovirus: Toll-like receptor-independent viral DNA recognition signals activation of the interferon regulatory factor 3 master regulator. J Virol 2007; 81: 4145-57.

[165] Zhu J, Huang X, Yang Y. Innate immune response to adenoviral vectors is mediated by both Toll-like receptor-dependent and -independent pathways. J Virol 2007; 81: 3170-80.

[166] Iacobelli-Martinez M, Nemerow GR. Preferential activation of Toll-like receptor nine by CD46-utilizing adenoviruses. J Virol 2007; 81: 1305-12.

[167] Basner-Tschakarjan E, Gaffal E, O'Keeffe M, *et al.* Adenovirus efficiently transduces plasmacytoid dendritic cells resulting in TLR9-dependent maturation and IFN-alpha production. J Gene Med 2006; 8: 1300-6.

[168] Hartman ZC, Kiang A, Everett RS, *et al.* Adenovirus infection triggers a rapid, MyD88-regulated transcriptome response critical to acute-phase and adaptive immune responses *in vivo*. J Virol 2007; 81: 1796-812.

[169] Zhu J, Huang X, Yang Y. A critical role for type I IFN-dependent NK cell activation in innate immune elimination of adenoviral vectors *in vivo*. Mol Ther 2008; 16: 1300-7.

[170] Hartman ZC, Black EP, Amalfitano A. Adenoviral infection induces a multi-faceted innate cellular immune response that is mediated by the toll-like receptor pathway in A549 cells. Virology 2007; 358: 357-72.

[171] Kwiatkowski D. Science, medicine, and the future: susceptibility to infection. BMJ 2000; 321: 1061-5.

[172] Casanova JL, Abel L. The human model: a genetic dissection of immunity to infection in natural conditions. Nat Rev Immunol 2004; 4: 55-66.

[173] Sachidanandam R, Weissman D, Schmidt SC, *et al.* A map of human genome sequence variation containing 1.42 million single nucleotide polymorphisms. Nature 2001; 409: 928-33.

[174] Puthothu B, Forster J, Heinzmann A, Krueger M. TLR-4 and CD14 polymorphisms in respiratory syncytial virus associated disease. Dis Markers 2006; 22: 303-8.

[175] Inoue Y, Shimojo N, Suzuki Y, *et al.* CD14 -550 C/T, which is related to the serum level of soluble CD14, is associated with the development of respiratory syncytial virus bronchiolitis in the Japanese population. J Infect Dis 2007; 195: 1618-24.

[176] Cheng PL, Eng HL, Chou MH, You HL, Lin TM. Genetic polymorphisms of viral infection-associated Toll-like receptors in Chinese population. Transl Res 2007; 150: 311-8.

[177] Zhang SY, Jouanguy E, Ugolini S, *et al.* TLR3 deficiency in patients with herpes simplex encephalitis. Science 2007; 317: 1522-7.

[178] Koehn J, Huesken D, Jaritz M, *et al.* Assessing the function of human UNC-93B in Toll-like receptor signaling and major histocompatibility complex II response. Hum Immunol 2007; 68: 871-8.

[179] Casrouge A, Zhang SY, Eidenschenk C, *et al.* Herpes simplex virus encephalitis in human UNC-93B deficiency. Science 2006; 314: 308-12.

[180]   Askar E, Ramadori G, Mihm S. Toll-like receptor 7 rs179008/Gln11Leu gene variants in chronic hepatitis C virus infection. J Med Virol 2010; 82: 1859-68.

[181]   Askar E, Bregadze R, Mertens J, *et al.* TLR3 gene polymorphisms and liver disease manifestations in chronic hepatitis C. J Med Virol 2009; 8: 1204-11.

[182]   Schott E, Witt H, Neumann K, *et al.* Association of TLR7 single nucleotide polymorphisms with chronic HCV-infection and response to interferon-a-based therapy. J Viral Hepat 2008; 15: 71-8.

[183]   Schott E, Witt H, Neumann K, *et al.* A Toll-like receptor 7 single nucleotide polymorphism protects from advanced inflammation and fibrosis in male patients with chronic HCV-infection. J Hepatol 2007; 47: 203-11.

[184]   Orange JS, Brodeur SR, Jain A, *et al.* Deficient natural killer cell cytotoxicity in patients with IKK-gamma/NEMO mutations. J Clin Invest 2002; 109: 1501-9.

[185]   Orange JS, Jain A, Ballas ZK, Schneider LC, Geha RS, Bonilla FA. The presentation and natural history of immunodeficiency caused by nuclear factor kappaB essential modulator mutation. J Allergy Clin Immunol 2004; 113: 725-33.

[186]   Dupuis S, Jouanguy E, Al-Hajjar S, *et al.* Impaired response to interferon-alpha/beta and lethal viral disease in human STAT1 deficiency. Nat Genet 2003; 33: 388-91.

[187]   Yang K, Puel A, Zhang S, *et al.* Human TLR-7-, -8-, and -9-mediated induction of IFN-alpha/beta and -lambda Is IRAK-4 dependent and redundant for protective immunity to viruses. Immunity 2005; 23: 465-78.

[188]   O'Hagan DT, De Gregorio E. The path to a successful vaccine adjuvant--'the long and winding road'. Drug Discov Today 2009; 14: 541-51.

[189]   Woodhour AF, Friedman A, Tytell AA, Hilleman MR. Hyperpotentiation by synthetic double-stranded RNA of antibody responses to influenza virus vaccine in adjuvant 65. Proc Soc Exp Biol Med 1969; 131: 809-17.

[190]   Mosca F, Tritto E, Muzzi A, *et al.* Molecular and cellular signatures of human vaccine adjuvants. Proc Natl Acad Sci U S A 2008; 105: 10501-6.

[191]   Pesce I, Monaci E, Muzzi A, *et al.* Intranasal administration of CpG induces a rapid and transient cytokine response followed by dendritic and natural killer cell activation and recruitment in the mouse lung. J Innate Immun 2010; 2: 144-59.

[192]   Broide DH. Immunostimulatory sequences of DNA and conjugates in the treatment of allergic rhinitis. Curr Allergy Asthma Rep 2005; 5: 182-5.

[193]   Vollmer J. TLR9 in health and disease. Int Rev Immunol 2006; 25: 155-810.

[194]   Zhu Q, Egelston C, Gagnon S, *et al.* Using 3 TLR ligands as a combination adjuvant induces qualitative changes in T cell responses needed for antiviral protection in mice. J Clin Invest 2010; 120: 607-16.

[195]   Wang D, Bhagat L, Yu D, *et al.* Oligodeoxyribonucleotide-based antagonists for Toll-like receptors 7 and 9. J Med Chem 2009; 52: 551-8.

[196]   LeBouder E, Rey-Nores JE, Rushmere NK, *et al.* Soluble forms of Toll-like receptor (TLR)2 capable of modulating TLR2 signaling are present in human plasma and breast milk. J Immunol 2003; 171: 6680-9.

[197]   Iwami KI, Matsuguchi T, Masuda A, Kikuchi T, Musikacharoen T, Yoshikai Y. Cutting edge: naturally occurring soluble form of mouse Toll-like receptor 4 inhibits lipopolysaccharide signaling. J Immunol 2000; 165: 6682-6.

[198]   Chang YC, Madkan V, Cook-Norris R, Sra K, Tyring S. Current and potential uses of imiquimod. South Med J 2005; 98: 914-20.

[199]   Maschke J, Brauns TC, Goos M. [Imiquimod for the topical treatment of focal epithelial hyperplasia (Heck disease) in a child]. J Dtsch Dermatol Ges 2004;2 : 848-50.

[200]   Kemeny L, Nagy N. [New perspective in immunotherapy: local imiquimod treatment.]. Orv Hetil 2010; 151: 774-83.

[201]   Higgins D, Marshall JD, Traquina P, Van Nest G, Livingston BD. Immunostimulatory DNA as a vaccine adjuvant. Expert Rev Vaccines 2007; 6: 747-59.

[202]   Kanzler H, Barrat FJ, Hessel EM, Coffman RL. Therapeutic targeting of innate immunity with Toll-like receptor agonists and antagonists. Nat Med 2007; 13: 552-9.

[203]   Meyer T, Stockfleth E. Clinical investigations of Toll-like receptor agonists. Expert Opin Investig Drugs 2008; 17: 1051-65.

[204]   Panter G, Kuznik A, Jerala R. Therapeutic applications of nucleic acids as ligands for Toll-like receptors. Curr Opin Mol Ther 2009; 11: 133-45.

[205]   Jasani B, Navabi H, Adams M. Ampligen: a potential toll-like 3 receptor adjuvant for immunotherapy of cancer. Vaccine 2009; 27: 3401-4.

[206]   Huleatt JW, Nakaar V, Desai P, *et al.* Potent immunogenicity and efficacy of a universal influenza vaccine candidate comprising a recombinant fusion protein linking influenza M2e to the TLR5 ligand flagellin. Vaccine 2008; 26: 201-14.

[207] Yoneyama M, Fujita T. RNA recognition and signal transduction by RIG-I-like receptors. Immunol Rev 2009; 227: 54-65.

[208] Xu LG, Wang YY, Han KJ, Li LY, Zhai Z, Shu HB. VISA is an adapter protein required for virus-triggered IFN-beta signaling. Mol Cell 2005; 19: 727-40.

[209] Kato H, Takeuchi O, Sato S, *et al.* Differential roles of MDA5 and RIG-I helicases in the recognition of RNA viruses. Nature 2006; 441: 101-5.

[210] Loo YM, Fornek J, Crochet N, *et al.* Distinct RIG-I and MDA5 signaling by RNA viruses in innate immunity. J Virol 2008; 82: 335-45.

[211] Gitlin L, Benoit L, Song C, *et al.* Melanoma differentiation-associated gene 5 (MDA5) is involved in the innate immune response to Paramyxoviridae infection *in vivo*. PLoS Pathog 2010; 6: e1000734.

[212] Satoh T, Kato H, Kumagai Y, *et al.* LGP2 is a positive regulator of RIG-I- and MDA5-mediated antiviral responses. Proc Natl Acad Sci U S A 2010; 107: 1512-7.

[213] Venkataraman T, Valdes M, Elsby R, *et al.* Loss of DExD/H box RNA helicase LGP2 manifests disparate antiviral responses. J Immunol 2007; 178: 6444-55.

[214] Muruve DA, Petrilli V, Zaiss AK, *et al.* The inflammasome recognizes cytosolic microbial and host DNA and triggers an innate immune response. Nature 2008; 452: 103-7.

[215] Delaloye J, Roger T, Steiner-Tardivel QG, *et al.* Innate immune sensing of modified vaccinia virus Ankara (MVA) is mediated by TLR2-TLR6, MDA-5 and the NALP3 inflammasome. PLoS Pathog 2009; 5: e1000480.

[216] Ichinohe T, Lee HK, Ogura Y, Flavell R, Iwasaki A. Inflammasome recognition of influenza virus is essential for adaptive immune responses. J Exp Med 2009; 206: 79-87.

[217] Thomas PG, Dash P, Aldridge JR, Jr., *et al.* The intracellular sensor NLRP3 mediates key innate and healing responses to influenza A virus *via* the regulation of caspase-1. Immunity 2009; 30: 566-75.

[218] Allen IC, Scull MA, Moore CB, *et al.* The NLRP3 inflammasome mediates *in vivo* innate immunity to influenza A virus through recognition of viral RNA. Immunity 2009; 30: 556-65.

[219] Ichinohe T, Pang IK, Iwasaki A. Influenza virus activates inflammasomes *via* its intracellular M2 ion channel. Nat Immunol 2010; 11: 404-10.

[220] Schroder M, Bowie AG. An arms race: innate antiviral responses and counteracting viral strategies. Biochem Soc Trans 2007; 35: 1512-4.

[221] Andrejeva J, Childs KS, Young DF, *et al.* The V proteins of paramyxoviruses bind the IFN-inducible RNA helicase, mda-5, and inhibit its activation of the IFN-beta promoter. Proc Natl Acad Sci U S A 2004; 101: 17264-9.

[222] Childs K, Stock N, Ross C, Andrejeva J, *et al.* MDA-5, but not RIG-I, is a common target for paramyxovirus V proteins. Virology 2007; 359: 190-200.

[223] Pichlmair A, Schulz O, Tan CP, *et al.* RIG-I-mediated antiviral responses to single-stranded RNA bearing 5'-phosphates. Science 2006; 314: 997-1001.

[224] Li K, Foy E, Ferreon JC, *et al.* Immune evasion by hepatitis C virus NS3/4A protease-mediated cleavage of the Toll-like receptor 3 adaptor protein TRIF. Proc Natl Acad Sci U S A 2005; 102: 2992-7.

[225] Schlender J, Hornung V, Finke S, *et al.* Inhibition of toll-like receptor 7- and 9-mediated alpha/beta interferon production in human plasmacytoid dendritic cells by respiratory syncytial virus and measles virus. J Virol 2005; 79: 5507-15.

CHAPTER 9

Toll-Like Receptor Recognition of Fungal Pathogens in the Lung

Sanjay H. Chotirmall, Catherine A. Coughlan and Emer P. Reeves[*]

Respiratory Research Division, Royal College of Surgeons in Ireland, Education and Research Centre, Beaumont Hospital, Dublin 9, Ireland

Abstract: The incidence of pulmonary complications involving fungal infections has increased over the last decade and is a common cause of morbidity and mortality. *Candida* species are one of the yeast most frequently identified in clinical samples, whilst *Aspergillus* is the most commonly found filamentous fungus. The major risk factor for fungal infection is host immunosuppression includes individuals undergoing solid organ transplant and those with HIV infection. This chapter aims to provide an overview of the epidemiology and clinical features of fungal lung infection, the expression, function and activation of relevant TLRs within the airways and a discussion of currently used and new antifungal agents and strategies.

Keywords: *Candida* spp., *Aspergillus* spp., TLRs, lung.

1. INTRODUCTION

Over the last two decades the incidence of invasive fungal infections has dramatically increased. This is related to the increased numbers and the longer survival of immune-compromised patients involved in high-dose chemotherapeutic treatments and immunosuppressive regimes in autoimmune diseases. The rate of sepsis due to fungal organisms in the United States, increased by 207% from 1979 to 2000 [1]. Examples of susceptible individuals include solid-organ or hematopoietic stem cell transplant recipients and those with acquired immunodeficiency syndrome. In addition to these high risk patient groups, increased cases of pulmonary fungal and yeast infections have been reported in individuals with chronic obstructive pulmonary disease (COPD) and cystic fibrosis (CF). A number of epidemiological studies indicate that filamentous fungi and yeast, including a number of *Aspergillus* and *Candida* species (spp.) as well as *Scedosporium apiospermum* [2] and *Exophiala dermatitidis* are commonly found in the CF and COPD lung, whilst *Penicillium emersonii* and *Acrophialophora fusisporae* are encountered almost entirely in the context of CF (Table **1**). The ability to detect and identify common and emerging fungal pathogens in sputum of patient groups is of major importance, particularly in relation to hypersensitivity to *Aspergillus*, episodes of fungaemia (post-transplant period) and colonization in chronic bronchitis. Moreover, studies of candidemia have reported an increase in the incidence of non-*albicans Candida* spp. combined with azole resistance [3, 4]. These latter observations have been observed in pediatric lung transplant patients and are of particular concern as the use of azole-based prophylaxis regimes is extensive [5]. Complicating the design of novel antifungal drugs are subtleties relating to the fact that both human and fungal cells are eukaryotic and possess similar mechanisms of DNA, RNA and protein synthesis which greatly limits the number of potential antifungal drug targets. Thus as fungal infections become more resistant to current drugs, understanding epidemiological changes and the immune response to fungi is critical for the development of novel therapeutic strategies.

The host immune response adjusts according to the fungal species encountered and also to the fungal morphotype (*e.g.* the three fungal forms of *A. fumigatus* are resting conidia, swollen conidia and hyphae). A characteristic feature dictating the immune response is the fungal cell wall which is composed of chitin, mannans and glucans. The cell wall provides both structural and physical protection for the fungus, rendering it resistant to certain host defences. For example, differential surface expression of mannans and

*Address correspondence to Emer P. Reeves: Lecturer, Department of Medicine, Royal College of Surgeons in Ireland, Education and Research Centre, Beaumont Hospital, Dublin 9, Ireland; Tel: 353-1-8093877; E-mail: emerreeves@rcsi.ie

glucans influences recognition of *C. albicans* by the complement system [6]. In turn, other innate immune defences, including β-glucan receptors, mannose receptors, and toll-like receptors (TLRs), have developed to identify and react to components of fungal cell walls. The relative role of individual receptors, such as TLR2, TLR4, and TLR9, in MyD88 activation varies depending upon the infecting fungus and the site of infection. This chapter will cover the following topics (i) the epidemiology and clinical features of fungal lung infection; (ii) an overview of the expression, function and activation of relevant TLRs in the fungal-infected lung; and (iii) currently used or soon to be available antifungal agents.

Table 1: Filamentous Fungi in Individuals with Cystic Fibrosis. Adapted from Blyth *et al.*, (2010)

Filamentous Fungi	Patients (N=69)
Aspergillus spp.	48 (69.6%)
A. fumigatus	46
A. flavus	7
Other *Aspergillus* spp.	6
Scedosporium spp.	12 (17.4%)
S. aurantiacum	4
S. prolificans	4
P. boydii / S. apiospermum complex	4
Penicillium spp.	14 (20.3%)
Paecilomyces spp.	6 (8.7%)
Other hyaline hyphomycetes	6 (8.7%)
Cladosporium spp.	4 (5.8%)
Other fungi including *Alternaria*, and *Curvularia*, spp.	20.1%

2. EPIDEMIOLOGY AND MANAGEMENT OPTIONS

2.1. *Candida* Species

Candida is a budding yeast that has the ability to convert to hyphal form both in tissues and culture. Indeed, a fast method for the identification of *Candida albicans* is to suspend the organism in serum and observe germ tube formation [7]. *Candida* forms part of the normal flora of the mucus membranes in the gastrointestinal, upper respiratory and female genital tract but can also cause opportunistic infections [8]. Fungal infections account for nearly 8% of all nosocomial infections and *Candida* is responsible in 80% of all cases [9]. In the past two decades the incidence of candidemia (also known as fungemia or invasive candidiasis) has increased throughout the world [10, 11]. The National Taiwan University Hospital reported that 21.6 patients per 10,000 discharges had nosocomial candidemia [12]. Common risk factors associated with *Candida* infection include COPD, smoking, tuberculosis, diabetes mellitus, HIV infection and prolonged use of antibiotics [13]. *Candida* spp. are frequently observed in tracheobronchial secretions of intubated patients with the proportion shown to increase with the duration of mechanical ventilation to 20%, 31% and 35% after 5, 15 and 30 days, respectively [14]. A significant increase in median hospital stay (59.9 *vs.* 38.6 days, P = 0.006) and hospital mortality (34.2% *vs.* 21.0%, P = 0.003) was observed in patients with *Candida* colonization of the respiratory tract [15]. For example, the incidence of *Candida* pneumonia varies from 0.23 to 8.0% [16-18] and poses a significant risk factor for death (P<0.0001) [19]. Moreover, a meta-analysis to elucidate efficacy of inhaled corticosteroids in the treatment of severe or very severe (stage III or IV) COPD revealed an increased risk for pneumonia and oral candidiasis [20].

The most important member of the species is *C. albicans* which is associated with mucocutaneous manifestations including vulvovaginitis and oral candidiasis, but can also give rise to more severe infections such as peritonitis or invasive candidiasis. Within Peking University People's Hospital, Beijing, a retrospective analysis (3743 patients) performed in 2010 of invasive fungal infections in surgical intensive care units, revealed that *C. albicans* was the most pathogenic fungal strain and one of the main sites of infection was the lung [21]. In *Candida* pneumonia, most reports implicate *C. albicans* and in CF, *C.*

albicans causes 95% of all *Candida* infections with the remaining 5% caused by *C. glabrata, C. parapsilosis, C. krusei* and *C. dubliniensis*. *Candida* colonization in CF has been associated with a reduction in lung function [22]. A recent prospective observational study of 89 patients with CF (3,916 sputum samples over 11 years) reported that colonization with *C. albicans* significantly predicted hospital-treated exacerbation (P = 0.004) and signified a greater rate of FEV_1 decline [23]. Within this study the main factors predicting colonization by *C. albicans* in CF were pancreatic insufficiency, osteopenia and co-colonisation with *Pseudomonas*. This latter observation is supported by an animal model study illustrating a correlation between *C. albicans* colonization and an increase in prevalence of *P. aeruginosa* pneumonia [24]. Conclusions of a second prospective study of CF patients (n=56) over a 30 month period confirmed long-term persistence of *Candida* in the respiratory tract of CF patients and that transmission between siblings was a possible means of acquisition [25].

For pulmonary *Candida* infection, treatment includes fluconazole (400 mg/day) or amphotericin B (0.5-0.7 mg/kg). In addition the use of voriconazole, a triazole that depletes ergosterol in fungal cell membranes [26] and caspofungin, an echinochandin that inhibits the production of $(1,3)$-β-D glucan [27, 28], are good choices for *Candida* infection, particularly for the azole-resistant strains such as *C. glabrata* and *C. krusei*. Indeed it has been shown that second-generation triazoles and the echinocandins are more effective against *C. glabrata* and *C. krusei* [29-31] (voriconazole and posaconazole have an MIC-90 value of 0.015-0.03 µg/ml for *C. glabrata* [30]).

2.2. *Aspergillus* Species

The *Aspergillus* genus is a group of filamentous fungi which are highly dispersed within the environment and are the most commonly isolated invasive fungi [32]. Conidia/spores (Fig. **1**) of this mould are inhaled regularly and the severity of *Aspergillus* infection is dependent on the condition of the immune system of the individual. A descriptive study of a CF population revealed that almost one third of patients attending Beaumont Hospital, Ireland had *Aspergillus* in their sputum on at least one occasion with a trend toward declining lung function in those with *Aspergillus*-positive sputum [33]. Diseases caused by *Aspergillus* can be divided into three categories: (1) invasive aspergillosis (IA) in immunocompromised patients; (2) allergic responses to inhaled conidia in individuals with a hyperactive immune response, referred to as allergic bronchopulmonary aspergillosis (ABPA) and (3) chronic aspergillosis in generally immunocompetent persons, involving the formation of a fungal ball or aspergilloma.

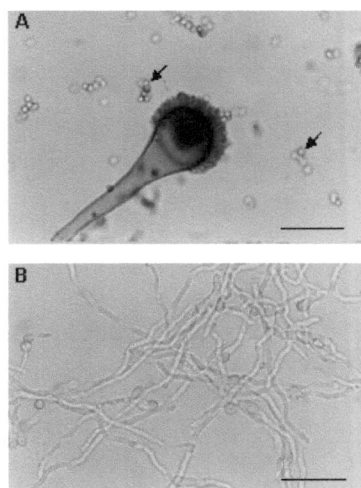

Figure 1: The sporing structure of A. fumigatus. (**A**) This microscopic image of A. fumigatus shows the long stalk (conidiophore) that supports the swollen head (vesicle) from which the spore generating cells (phialides) produce long chains of spores (conidia). Released conidia are indicated by the arrows. (**B**) Hyphae growing from *A. fumigatus* conidia. Bars: 10µM.

Pulmonary IA was first described in 1953 [34]. The incidence of IA has significantly increased in immunocompromised patients, including neutropenic patients, transplant recipients and in individuals post aggressive immunosuppressive therapy [35-37]. For high-risk patients, such as allogeneic bone marrow transplant recipients, persons with hematologic cancer, and those with signs of neutropenia or malnutrition, a positive culture result is associated with invasive disease [38]. Recently there have been an increasing number of reports that describe pulmonary IA in patients without traditional risk factors including patients with COPD. The global mortality rate of pulmonary IA in COPD patients is high, ranging from 72% to 95% [39, 40]. It is not clear why COPD patients develop pulmonary IA but underlying lung disease, surfactant protein deficiency or abnormalities [41, 42] and systemic corticosteroid treatment have been proposed as possible risk factors [40, 43], the latter by affecting phagocyte function [44].

Diagnosis requires microbiological or histopathologic demonstration of the organism in tissues but detection can also be performed using a galactomannan enzyme immunoassay, quantitative PCR of bronchoalveolar lavage samples of high risk patients [45] or early diagnosis by computed tomography scan patterns [46] (Fig. **2**). Retrospective analysis of sputum microbiology from adult CF patients (1985 to 2005) using the Royal Brompton Hospital CF database revealed that colonisation with *Aspergillus* spp. has increased significantly in the 16-25 year age group (P<0.001) [47]. Moreover the epidemiology of *A. fumigatus* is changing and in 1988 *A. fumigatus* colonization accounted for 82% of cases of invasive aspergillosis compared to 66% in 1999. In turn, the incidence of *A. terreus* colonization increased from 2% of isolates in 1996 to 15% in 2001 [48]. The incidence of fungal infections in organ transplant patients ranges from 2% to 50% depending on the type of surgery [49], however the transplanted lung is most susceptible to colonization as the respiratory tract is the primary point of entry for airborne conidia. In 2010, a prospective, multicentre study was performed to assess the incidence and epidemiology of invasive mould infections reported to the Nationwide Austrian *Aspergillus* Registry. In total 186 cases were recorded with lung transplant recipients reported to be the second highest risk for infection, with *Aspergillus* spp. (67%) being the dominant pathogens [50].

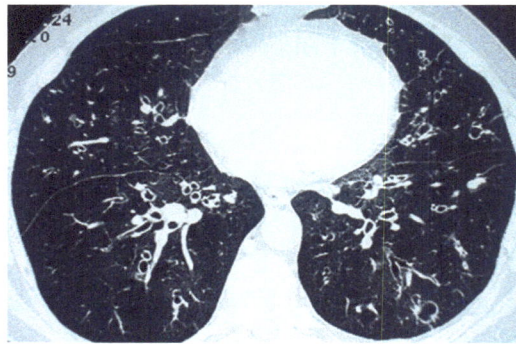

Figure 2: Computed tomography (CT) scan of the chest in a patient with cystic fibrosis colonized with *A. fumigatus* illustrating bronchiectasis and emphysematous changes.

ABPA occurs in approximately 0.9-10.9% of CF patients and is a disease mediated by an allergic response to *A. fumigatus* [51]. ABPA can progress to a chronic condition and lead to lung fibrosis and bronchiectasis if not treated with corticosteroids. An immunological response to a variety of *Aspergillus* antigens has been observed in ABPA patients resulting in elevated immunoglobulin E (IgE) levels and heightened eosinophilia and T helper 2 (Th2) responses [52]. The Th2 immune response to *A. fumigatus* associated with ABPA results in an increase of the Th2 cytokines IL-4, IL-5 and IL-13. Moreover, the response to *A. fumigatus* antigens has been imitated in CFTR deficient mice that displayed severe lung inflammation in a Th2 biased manner [53]. More recent studies have also shown that genetic events can in part determine the outcome of ABPA and whilst HLA-RR molecules (DR2, DR5 and possibly DR4 or DR7) contribute to ABPA susceptibility, in contrast HLA-DQ2 contributes to resistance [54]. In addition, polymorphisms in the promoter region of IL-10 [55] or in the IL-4 receptor alpha-chain [56] contribute a genetic risk factor for development of ABPA.

Chronic pulmonary aspergillosis (CPA) in non-immunocompromised individuals progressively destroys lung tissue resulting in the formation and expansion of cavities [57, 58]. The developed voids may contain a fungal ball (aspergilloma) and in spite of treatment, the morbidity and mortality of CPA remains high [59]. Previous or existing pulmonary conditions are often evident in CPA patients. Tuberculosis, non-tuberculous mycobacterial infection and ABPA remain the predominant risk factors for development of CPA, with COPD, prior pneumothorax or treated lung cancer also relatively common [60]. Voriconazole and posaconazole are broad spectrum antifungal drugs recommended for use as the initial therapy for patients with pulmonary IA. Both azoles are very potent against many *Aspergillus* spp., including *A. terreus* and *A. fumigatus* which are resistant to amphotericin B and itraconazole, respectively [61-64]. The echinocandins have fungistactic activities against *Aspergilllus* spp., causing damage to the fungal hyphae, however fungal recovery has been observed post drug withdrawal [65, 66].

2.3. Emerging Fungi

While historically *Candida* and *Aspergillus* spp. have caused the vast majority of opportunistic fungal infections in immunocompromised patients, other less frequently encountered filamentous fungi have emerged as important causes of respiratory fungal infections. *Cryptococcus* and *Scedosporium* spp. are examples of emerging fungi causing increased morbidity and mortality in immunocompromised patients. *Cryptococcus* infection occurs in both immunocompetent and immunosuppressed individuals, with *C. neoformans* being the most common cause acquired by inhalation. Pulmonary cryptococcosis may be asymptomatic or present non-specifically with cough, fever or pleural symptoms. *Scedosporium apiospermum* is the asexual phase of the ubiquitous saprophytic mould *Pseudoallescheria boydii* and is found worldwide in soil and associated with decaying vegetation [67]. *Scedosporium* infection can present in virtually every organ but especially in paranasal sinuses and the lungs with associated allergic bronchopulmonary mycosis [68]. Risk factors for the association of *Scedosporium* in cases of CF include bacterial co-colonization (in particular *P. aeruginosa*), use of antibiotics [69] and post-transplantation [70, 71]. *Scedosporium* spp. are resistant to traditional antifungal therapies including amphotericin B; however, voriconazole appears to be effective [72].

3. RECOGNITION OF *ASPERGILLUS* BY TOLL-LIKE RECEPTORS AND OTHER PATTERN RECOGNITION RECEPTORS IN THE LUNG

Humoral factors including complement, anatomical barriers and phagocytic cells are three key components of the human innate immune system which play important roles in the clearance of *Aspergillus* spp. [73]. Several members of the *Aspergillus* genus have been identified that colonise the airways, including *A. fumigatus*, *A. niger* and *A. terreus*. Inhaled *Aspergillus* conidia are often removed from lung epithelial surfaces *via* mucociliary action however a compromised mucociliary escalator provides an opportunistic environment for conidia germination and consequent *Aspergillus* colonisation and infection. Positioned on fungal surfaces, pathogen associated molecular patterns (PAMPs) are recognised by pattern recognition receptors (PRRs) and consequently mediate recognition of fungal invaders by the immune system [74]. Chitin, mannoproteins and β-1, 3-glutacans are the major *Aspergillus* conidia cell wall PAMPs. A linear β-glucan backbone is found within this structure to which branches of chitins, mannoproteins and further β-glucans are covalently linked (Fig. 3) [75]. Exposure of β-glucan polymers on the fungal cell surface occurs due to cell wall expansion and remodeling during conidia swelling [76]. In *Aspergillus*-induced disease, β-glucan recognition activates host defence pathways in response to fungal invasion [76].

PRRs such as TLRs and C-type lectin receptors (CLRs) are expressed by a variety of cell types including alveolar macrophages (AMs), endothelial cells, mucosal epithelial cells, lymphocytes, neutrophils and immature dendritic cells. CLRs comprise a large family of receptors that share at least one carbohydrate recognition domain originally identified in mannose binding lectin (MBL). CLRs are evolutionary conserved and have been shown to be involved in the modulation of the innate immune response and fungal recognition. Together members of the CLR and TLR families play a role in *A. fumigatus* recognition [77, 78].

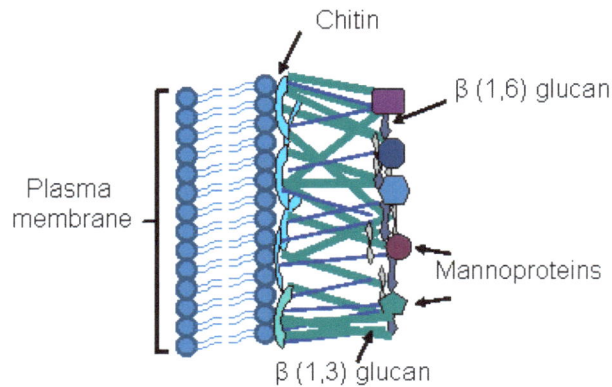

Figure 3: Fungal cell wall structure. Present is a linear β-glucan backbone with branching chitin, mannoproteins and β (1, 6) and β (1, 3) glucans. Chitin is a long-chain polymer of N-acetyl glucosamine present in the fungal cell wall and cross linking occurs between the components of the cell wall including glucans and chitin. The extremely dynamic fungal cell wall often changes in filamentous fungi during cell growth, hyphal branching and germination.

TLR2 and TLR4 in particular have major roles in recognising *A. fumigatus*. In a study performed using peritoneal macrophages *Aspergillus* conidia and hyphae were found to be differentially recognised by the immune system; TLR2 was involved in the recognition of both forms (conidia and hyphae) whereas TLR4 solely recognised the conidial form [79]. TLR2 stimulates release of IL-10 in response to *Aspergillus* hyphae, and internalization of TLR2 following ingestion of *Aspergillus* conidia can modulate the host response by downregulating cell surface TLR2 expression [80].

The chief role for TLR4 in the context of *Aspergillus* infection is recognition of the conidial phenotype however, jointly with CD14, it can mediate the recognition and response to *Aspergillus* hyphae. For example, *Aspergillus* can stimulate monocytic cells to release TNF-α, IL-1α and IL-1β in a TLR4 dependent manner [81]. CD14 is essential in this context as shown by the inhibitory effect of both TLR4 and CD14 neutralising antibodies on TNF-α release by human monocytes following stimulation with serum-optimised *A. fumigatus* hyphae [82]. By suppressing TLR4, β-glucans on *A. fumigatus* can modulate the immune response to *Aspergillus* [80]. Interestingly, increased susceptibility to invasive aspergillosis occurs in hematopoietic cell transplant recipients with inactivating TLR4 polymorphisms [83]. Additional evidence for roles for TLR2 and 4 in macrophage recognition of *Aspergillus* comes from studies in doubly deficient mice where neutrophil recruitment was found to be significantly decreased [84].

TLR9 is also implicated in the recognition of *A. fumigatus*. TLR9's natural ligand, unmethylated CpG-containing DNA, has been identified in *A. fumigatus* and recent work has highlighted its participation in cytokine production [85, 86]. TLR9 deficient mice display higher levels of hyphal damage and conidia activity compared to wild type mice [87]. Anti-allergy properties are a well known feature of TLR9, and a non-functional TLR9 SNP (allele C on T-1237C) is known to be associated with susceptibility to ABPA [88]. Anti-fungal agents including caspofungin, amphotericin B and fluconazole all upregulate expression of several TLRs in response to *A. fumigatus* and such drugs, particularly caspofungin, confer peak upregulation of TLR9 [89].

Other PRRs engaged in interactions with *A. fumigatus* include the CLR, dectin-1 [90]. Dectin-1 present on phagocytic cells is a type II transmembrane receptor that can recognise β-1,3-glutacans, a major *A. fumigatus* cell wall component also present on swollen or germinating conidia [91-93] (Fig. **4**). In *A. fumigatus* exposed macrophages, dectin-1 co-operates with TLR2 in the induction of pro-inflammatory mediators [90]. Nor does TLR2 recognise β-glucans alone, instead it co-operates with dectin-1 to mediate recognition however the underlying mechanisms for this interaction remain unclear [96]. The combined TLR2/dectin-1 recognition of *Aspergillus* hyphae induces production of reactive oxygen intermediates and the secretion of cytokines, and remains essential for phagocytosis of conidia [90]. Platelets also execute damage to *Aspergillus* hyphae by directly damaging the fungal cell wall and inducing neutrophil aggravated fungicidal effects [97].

3.1. Evasion of Innate Immune Responses by *Aspergillus* spp.

Phagocytic cells function as the first line of defence however with ever-mounting virulence of *Aspergillus*, the fungus can evade host defences by utilising various virulence factors and secondary metabolites in order to initiate human disease. In this context, dectin-1 plays a critical role in *A. fumigatus* lung immunity. Dectin-1 deficient mice experience an uncontrolled *A. fumigatus* growth within the lung and express reduced levels of cytokines and chemokines essential for recruitment of neutrophils into the lung [98].

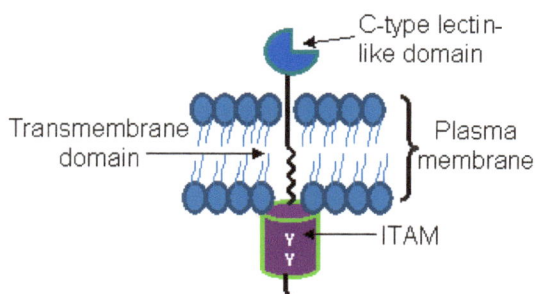

Figure 4: The C-type lectin receptor, Dectin-1. Dectin-1, a type II transmembrane protein contains an extracellular COOH terminus with one C-type lectin-like domain. The immunoreceptor tyrosine-based activation motif (ITAM) is present in the intracellular NH$_2$ terminus. ITAM is present on several pro-inflammatory receptors including T cell receptors, Fc receptors and NK receptors [94, 95]. Tyrosine phoshorylation of the ITAM-like motif is required for effective dectin-1 signaling [96].

Downregulation of complement activation may also occur in the presence of fungal pathogens such as *Aspergillus*. This occurs through binding of complement regulators to the fungal surface enabling immune evasion by the fungi [99]. For example, *Aspergillus* conidia bind host complement factors, factor H, factor H like protein-1 (FHLP-1), factor H related protein-1 (FHRP-1) and plasminogen [100]. The complement receptor 3 (CR-3) also plays a role in anti-fungal immunity in the specific binding of β-1,3-glutacans and cleavage of CR-3 on conidial surfaces [99]. Pentraxin-3 (PTX3) a secreted PRR can also bind to *Aspergillus* conidia and PTX3 deficient mice display impaired macrophage and dendritic cell fungal recognition, inappropriate generation of Th2 response and a higher susceptibility to pulmonary IA [101].

3.2. *Aspergillus*-Induced T Cell Responses and Cytokine Expression

Numerous cytokines and chemokines are induced by signaling through PRRs to regulate the host response and the development of distinct T-cell responses may arise depending on the type of aspergillosis evoked. For instance, ABPA is predominantly a Th2 response. The upregulation of pro-inflammatory and Th1 cytokines such as IL-1, IL-6, IL-18 and TNF-α, IL-12 coupled with IL-4 and IL-10 downregulation has been associated with improved prognosis for *Aspergillus* infection [102-105]. On dendritic cells (DCs) the priming of an antifungal Th1 response occurs through TLR induced MyD88 signaling [106]. Th17 cells function as negative regulators of the *Aspergillus*-induced Th1 response [107] and their anti-fungal properties are regulated by TLRs both positively and negatively *via* contrasting pathways [107].

TNF-α is a central cytokine in the defence against *A. fumigatus* and is secreted principally by AMs but crucially also by pulmonary epithelial cells. Prior work has revealed that following intrapulmonary administration of *A. fumigatus* conidia in pulmonary IA, TNF-α was detected and that neutralisation of this cytokine resulted in a decreased neutrophil recruitment to the site of infection and an increase in fungal load [103, 108]. Neutrophil recruitment to infection sites therefore requires the production of neutrophil chemokines and activators such as interleukin-8 (IL-8) and TNF-α [109].

Stimulation of neutrophils with *A. fumigatus* antigens induces TLR2 and TLR4 dependent production of IL-8 [78]. In chronic inflammatory diseases such as CF and COPD elevated levels of IL-8 are found in sputum [110]. IL-8-induced neutrophil chemotaxis and excessive neutrophil elastase (NE) release in these disease contexts can result in bronchial epithelial damage [111]. An impaired release of MIP-2, an alternate chemoattractant for neutrophil influx has also been identified in a TLR2/4 double deficient mouse model resulting in impaired neutrophil recruitment in response to *Aspergillus* infection [84]. Release of MIP-2 and TNF-α by AMs additionally occurs as a consequence of germinating *Aspergillus* conidia. These factors further induce airway neutrophil recruitment and potential epithelial damage in the context of chronic lung disease [76].

Release of the Th2 cytokines IL-4 and IL-10 also occur following *Aspergillus* hyphae exposure [112]. Neutralisation of IL-4 in mice enhances resistance to *Aspergillus* as it has been shown to down-regulate the oxidative burst and phagocytic damage to *Aspergillus* hyphae [102]. Elevated levels of IL-10 which diminish monocyte anti-hyphal activity and the oxidative burst are observed in neutropenic patients afflicted with *Aspergillus* infection [113].

4. THE ROLE OF TLRs IN THE DEFENCE AGAINST *CANDIDA* SPECIES WITHIN THE LUNG

A delicate balance exists between colonization and infection caused by *Candida* spp. in humans. What influences this equilibrium at a distinct time point depends on the functional state of the immune system and its ability to respond to the species. In reality, a continuum likely exists: commensal in the setting of immunocompetence, colonization following minor compromise and pathogenic during states of florid immunodeficiency. Many superficial structural components (mannans and mannoproteins) of the *Candida* spp. induce significant immune responses owing to their immunogenic potential and additionally determine virulence [114-116]. Mannan-deficient strains of *Candida* spp. confer diminished virulence. Innate and adaptive immunity unite in response to infection by *Candida* spp. and both play interdependent roles during the natural progression of such infections [114, 115, 117-119].

The chief PAMPs detected by the immune system lie in the *Candida* cell wall which encases β-(1,3)-glucan polysaccharide fibrils covalently linked to chitin (a β-(1,4)-linked polymer of *N*-acetyl glucosamine) and β-(1,6)-glucan. Arrayed on the *Candida* cell surface are *N*-linked [120] or *O*-linked mannosylated proteins called mannans [121]. As for *Aspergillus*, CLRs and TLRs are two major determinants of the immune response to invading *Candida* spp. A host of immune cell types (monocytes, macrophages, neutrophils and epithelial cells) can all defend against *Candida* spp. however their membrane CLR/TLR expression pattern varies. Consequently, their responses to the same *Candida* spp. may differ significantly. Both CLRs and TLRs recognize the major polysaccharide cell wall components, *N*- and *O*-linked mannans, β-mannosides, β-(1,6)-glucan and phospholipomannan. The mannan structures are detected by the mannose receptor (MR), the dendritic cell-specific ICAM3-grabbing nonintegrin (DC-SIGN), dectin-2, galectin-3 and TLR4 whereas CR3, dectin-1 and TLR2 detect the β-glucans.

PRRs in addition to receptors for opsonins such as the Fc and complement receptors are employed by cells of the immune system to phagocytose pathogens [122]. Following microbe internalization an inflammatory response results predominantly elicited by TLRs which are deployed to phagosomes. Consequently, TLR signaling and phagocytosis are not mutually exclusive events and in fact are functionally linked: TLR signaling influences phagocytosis whilst phagocytic receptors manipulate TLR signaling. This occurs *via* crosstalk between both receptor subtypes [96, 123-126]. Although mannose-binding lectin (MBL) can bind to *C. albicans* [127] and has the ability to opsonize fungal yeasts by activating the complement system [128], MBL-deficient mice do not show decreased survival to infection with *C. albicans* [129]. However dectins-1 and -2, galectin-3, DC-SIGN and MR do play important roles in the innate immune response to *C. albicans*.

Dectin-1 recognizes β-(1,3)-glucans, mediates ligand uptake and phagocytosis, and triggers cytokine production [130]. Alone it is sufficient in inducing responses to fungi however synergistic proinflammatory responses occur in cooperation with TLRs. For example in collaboration with TLR2, dectin-1 triggers proinflammatory responses by *C. albicans* or zymosan [96, 131]. These co-operative proinflammatory responses are synergized in the presence of farnesol, a quorum-sensing molecule produced by *C. albicans* that inhibits its filamentation [132]. Dectin-2 is mainly expressed on myeloid cells and maturing monocytes. It recognizes high-mannose structures [133] and interacts with the FcγR to induce TNF in response to filamentous *C. albicans* [134]. On macrophages the galectin-3 receptor mediates the recognition of β-mannosides expressed on *C. albicans*. This PAMP-PRR interaction is also enhanced by TLR2 [135]. DC-SIGN, expressed on mature DCs, recognizes high-mannose structures in *C. albicans* and mediates phagocytosis of fungal particles [136]. Finally, MR recognizes chitin, fructose, and mannose and has been implicated in the recognition of several fungi, including *C. neoformans*, *C. albicans*, and *Pneumocystis* spp. Branched *N*-bound mannans in *C. albicans* are recognised by MR and mice defective in MR display partial impairment in their host defense against *Candida* infections [137].

Following the initial observation by Lemaitre that *Drosophila melanogaster* deficient in the Toll receptor succumb readily to infection with *A. fumigatus* due to defective synthesis of the drosomycin defensin [138], the role for TLRs in antifungal defense has been extensively studied and recently a human homolog of drosomycin called drosomycin-like defensin has been described. This peptide is expressed mainly in the skin and has activity against a variety of filamentous fungi [139], however its potential as an antifungal or anti-*C. albicans* therapeutic has not yet been exploited. Early studies on TLRs revealed that TLR2 and TLR6 co-operate in recognition of the fungal structure zymosan derived from *Saccharomyces cerevisiae* [140]. With respect to *C. albicans,* blocking of TLR2 has been shown to lead to decreased monocyte production of TNF and IL-1β after stimulation with *C. albicans* [141]. Furthermore TLR2$^{-/-}$ mice have decreased TNF and MIP-2 production and reduced neutrophil recruitment after challenge with *Candida* [142]. TLR1 and TLR6, two receptors capable of forming heterodimers with TLR2, may also have a minor role in *C. albicans* recognition [143]. Further evidence for an anti-fungal role for TLR2 comes from studies showing that TLR2-deficient macrophages have an increased ability to contain *C. albicans* [144], and that TLR2 signaling can promote Th2-type or T-reg-type responses in response to *C. albicans* [145, 146] (Fig. **5**). TLR4 participates in antifungal host defense by recognizing *O*-linked mannan structures and mediating proinflammatory responses. TLR9 has the potential to recognize fungal DNA and blocking TLR9 either pharmacologically in human monocytes or genetically in TLR9-deficient mouse macrophages leads to a reduced production of cytokines, mainly IL-10, in response to stimulation with *C. albicans* [147]. However the contribution of TLR9 to fungal recognition can be extended to include its role in interactions between anti-fungal agents and polymorphonuclear cells in response to fungal infection.

This is an active area of ongoing work [89]. Such interaction may involve TLR1, TLR2, TLR4 and TLR9, in response to infection with *Aspergillus* and/or *Candida* spp. Caspofungin has thus far shown the broadest capacity to allow fungi to stimulate TLR upregulation with a particular functional relevance for TLR9 in this context [89]. In addition to interacting with anti-fungal agents, phagocytic cells play critical roles in the immune response to *C. albicans* and the TLRs additionally influence the regulation of neutrophil survival. For instance, TLR2 participates in the response to pathogenic yeasts and confers an increase to the functional lifespan of the neutrophil.

In TLR2$^{-/-}$ mice, reduced leucocyte chemotaxis to the site of infection coupled with diminished chemokine release facilitates widespread pathogen dissemination to immune organs such as the spleen and lymph nodes. Increased frequency of apoptotic neutrophils in the inflammatory exudates and falls in nitric oxide production and phagocytic/myeloperoxidase activity are also observed in these mice. TLR2 signals are therefore vital to both neutrophil activation and survival following *Candida albicans* infection [148].

Recognition of *C. albicans* by the innate immune system can also occur through MR and DC-SIGN recognizing branched *N*-linked mannans, and TLR4 recognizing linear *O*-linked mannans. CR3 responds to β-(1,6)-glucan and dectin-1 whilst galectin-3 in combination with TLR2 each recognize β-glucan/phospholipomannan and β-mannosides, respectively. It is likely that these recognition receptors can operate in combination and that stimulation *via* multiple PAMP–PRR combinations might increase both the sensitivity and the specificity of the immune recognition process. Notwithstanding these elegant recognition systems, *C. albicans* frequently colonizes and subsequently infects immunocompromised individuals.

Although TLRs are well described to recognize specific molecular signatures present on *Candida* spp. they additionally influence adaptive immune responses that follow this initial recognition. This synchronized action of both innate and adaptive responses to the organism is crucial in mediating protective effects against the species [149]. For instance, a diminished number of IFN-γ producing CD4 T lymphocytes are observed following *in-vitro* challenge of splenocytes obtained from MyD88$^{-/-}$ mice following infection with a low virulence *Candida* spp. illustrating that TLR pathways are essential in the generation of an adequate Th1 response [150]. Although Th1 cells provide protection against *C. albicans via* a pro-inflammatory pathway this must be delicately balanced. In this context both Th2 and regulatory T (Treg) cells which can be controlled by TLR2 are employed [146, 149, 151, 152]. Treg cells maintain peripheral tolerance and keep excessive pro-inflammatory responses that lead to tissue injury in check by curbing CD4+ and CD8+ T lymphocytes and preventing hyporesponsiveness to invading *Candida* spp. [146, 149, 153-155] (Fig. **5**).

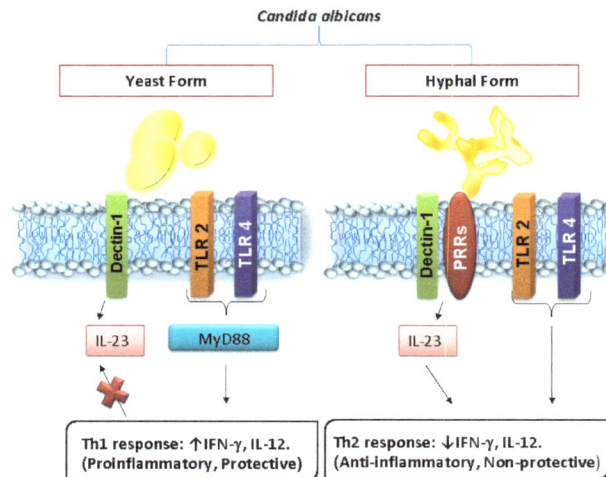

Figure 5: Differential immunological response to yeast and hyphal forms of *Candida albicans*. The yeast form of the organism stimulates TLR2 *via* a MyD88 dependent pathway which causes release of IL-12/IFN-γ and a protective Th1-based pro-inflammatory response. TLR4 also contributes to this interaction. In a MyD88-independent pathway, dectin-1 triggers IL-23 production (Th17 response) which is consequently inhibited by the over-riding Th1 predominance to the overall response. Over time, secretion of IL-10 (a Th2 cytokine) and Treg cells balance this response avoiding it becoming damaging to the host. The hyphal form of the organism stimulates TLR2 (involving TLR4) however for unknown reasons promotes a contrasting non-protective Th2 response. This may be attributed to interactions between the TLRs with other PRRs (such as dectin-1) that, preferentially identifies the yeast form of the organism. Consequently, the hyphal form favors activation of Dectin-2 also promoting a Th17 response which is not inhibited so contributes to the Th2 environment.

TLRs on DCs release immunomodulating cytokines (IL-4, IL-10 and IL-12) and upregulate co-stimulatory molecules, both indispensable steps during pathogen specific adaptive responses [156]. Following *Candida* phagocytosis by DCs, distinct responses to the yeast and hyphal forms are observed: yeasts prime Th1 cells and release IL-12 whilst hyphae prime Th2 cells and induce IL-4 release [157] (Fig. **5**). Treg supression from TLR-activated DCs *in vivo* is designed to limit excessive cell responses however release from this suppression is possible and permits the activation of *Candida* specific T-cells. For such a release to occur, TLR-MyD88 activation on DCs is required followed by IL-6 release culminating in a predominant Th1 response. Additionally, interactions between naïve CD4 T cells and TLR-MyD88 activated DCs are required for an adequate *in vivo* memory response to infection: Th1 cells induced with a lack of MyD88 and Treg have been shown experimentally to fail in memory acquisition [156, 158-160]. Paradoxically, immune evasion by *Candida* spp. can also surprisingly occur through TLRs. This evasion has been demonstrated by a TLR2-based suppressive effect that results in a compromised immunity against *Candida* *albicans*. This in turn is modulated by a release of IL-10 and induction of Treg cells [145, 161]. These mechanisms do however remain controversial because they contrast the observation that IL-10 release by DCs is MyD88-dependent. Furthermore, the activation of Treg cells by IL-10 producing DCs is necessary for ongoing anti-*Candida* memory and consequently the inadequate Th1 response of TLR2$^{-/-}$ mice may be explained by a lack of IL-10 production by DCs [106, 154]. Finally Th17 cells have recently been illustrated to have an anti-*Candida* role in immunity and TLRs may contribute to this Th17 response to *Candida* infection. Future studies are required to fully understand these complex interactions between arms of the innate and adaptive immune systems [107, 162].

5. CONCLUSIONS AND PERSPECTIVES

A better understanding of the complex signaling networks that underpin and protect the host against fungal pathogens remains a major challenge in this field and will undoubtedly drive the development of future therapeutics [163]. Our ultimate challenge remains translating our current understanding of fungal interaction with CLRs/TLRs to develop realistic treatments targeting the at-risk populations. Prevention and/or treatment of fungal infection remains complex with rapid emergence of resistant strains with potent virulence. One approach may be to focus on the interactions between the innate and adaptive immune systems described above. Acquired responses to *Aspergillus* and *Candida* depends on several factors - differential surface fungal ligand exposure, fungal form (yeast or hyphal) and the subsequent interaction with PRRs mainly dectins and TLRs. Each of these may be targeted, however a unifying method may lie in the development of a vaccine against fungal species. Such development is already underway and must take into account the interdependent roles of CLRs/TLRs in the respective immune response. TLRs strongly induce an inflammatory response but CLRs have the ability to modulate such a response through enhancing or inhibiting cytokine production. It is only with a thorough understanding of these natural host defence systems that we can select targets to induce the strong adjuvant effect required of a vaccine to allow effective adaptive immune response and protection against *Candida* [164] and *Aspergillus* spp [165].

Modulation of CLR expression and activity also represent important therapeutic strategies that remain, as yet, underexplored. A newly identified CLR, Mincle, has been shown to participate in macrophage recognition of *C. albicans*. Although it remains to be shown which PAMP expressed by *C. albicans* directly activates Mincle, the role of this receptor in fungal innate immunity has been clearly demonstrated. Inhibition studies have shown decreased TNF production by macrophages following stimulation by *Candida* yeast cells and Mincle knockout mice display hypersusceptibility to *Candida* infection [166]. It will be interesting to determine the expression and function of Mincle by immune and epithelial cells in individuals prone to infections with *Candida* spp.

Although we present extensive data illustrating a specific role for TLRs in the recognition and response to *Aspergillus* and *Candida* spp. in the human host, little is known precisely about the specificity of the individual fungal ligands and whether such described ligands act alone or in unison with other proteins. While accepted that such signaling is a complex process, encompassing interactions between the TLRs and other PRRs, the participation of accessory proteins such as CD14 and MD2 cannot be underestimated. Targeting accessory proteins may bear fruit in the development of future therapeutic strategies. An alternate approach may lie in evaluating the phagocytic process directed at fungi. Following initial recognition of surface located fungal ligands by phagocytes, there ensues a cascade of events. Post-phagocytosis, intracellular TLRs positioned at the endosomal membrane may trigger further host responses to ligands not necessarily exposed at the fungal surface. This second wave of host responses remain a valuable avenue for further research and in turn may dictate our progress of future immune based treatments used in *Aspergillus*/*Candida* specific disease [167-170].

REFERENCES

[1]   Martin GS, Mannino DM, Eaton S, Moss M. The epidemiology of sepsis in the United States from 1979 through 2000. N Engl J Med 2003; 348: 1546-54.

[2]   Nagano Y, Millar BC, Goldsmith CE, Elborn JS, Rendall J, Moore JE. Emergence of *Scedosporium apiospermum* in patients with cystic fibrosis. Arch Dis Child 2007; 92: 607.

[3]   Cuenca-Estrella M, Rodriguez D, Almirante B *et al. In vitro* susceptibilities of bloodstream isolates of *Candida* species to six antifungal agents: results from a population-based active surveillance programme, Barcelona, Spain, 2002-2003. J Antimicrob Chemother 2005; 55: 194-9.

[4]   Pfaller MA, Diekema DJ, Jones RN *et al.* International surveillance of bloodstream infections due to *Candida* species: frequency of occurrence and *in vitro* susceptibilities to fluconazole, ravuconazole, and voriconazole of isolates collected from 1997 through 1999 in the SENTRY antimicrobial surveillance program. J Clin Microbiol 2001; 39: 3254-9.

[5]   Dummer JS, Lazariashvilli N, Barnes J, Ninan M, Milstone AP. A survey of anti-fungal management in lung transplantation. J Heart Lung Transplant 2004; 23: 1376-81.

[6]   Boxx GM, Kozel TR, Nishiya CT, Zhang MX. Influence of mannan and glucan on complement activation and C3 binding by *Candida albicans*. Infect Immun 2010; 78: 1250-9.

[7]   Kavanagh. Medical Mycology. Cellular and Molecular Techniques: John Wiley & Sons, Ltd 2007.

[8]   Naglik JR, Challacombe SJ, Hube B. *Candida albicans* secreted aspartyl proteinases in virulence and pathogenesis. Microbiol Mol Biol Rev 2003; 67: 400-28.

[9]   Rose HD, Sheth NK. Pulmonary candidiasis. A clinical and pathological correlation. Arch Intern Med 1978; 138: 964-5.

[10]   Hsueh PR, Teng LJ, Yang PC, Ho SW, Luh KT. Emergence of nosocomial candidemia at a teaching hospital in Taiwan from 1981 to 2000: increased susceptibility of *Candida* species to fluconazole. Microb Drug Resist 2002; 8: 311-9.

[11]   Tortorano AM, Kibbler C, Peman J, Bernhardt H, Klingspor L, Grillot R. Candidaemia in Europe: epidemiology and resistance. Int J Antimicrob Agents 2006; 27: 359-66.

[12]   Ruan SY, Lee LN, Jerng JS, Yu CJ, Hsueh PR. *Candida glabrata* fungaemia in intensive care units. Clin Microbiol Infect 2008; 14: 136-40.

[13]   Jha BJ, Dey S, Tamang MD, Joshy ME, Shivananda PG, Brahmadatan KN. Characterization of Candida species isolated from cases of lower respiratory tract infection. Kathmandu Univ Med J (KUMJ) 2006; 4: 290-4.

[14]   Azoulay E, Timsit JF, Tafflet M *et al. Candida* colonization of the respiratory tract and subsequent *Pseudomonas* ventilator-associated pneumonia. Chest 2006; 129: 110-7.

[15]   Delisle MS, Williamson DR, Perreault MM, Albert M, Jiang X, Heyland DK. The clinical significance of *Candida* colonization of respiratory tract secretions in critically ill patients. J Crit Care. 2008; 23: 11-7.

[16]   Haron E, Vartivarian S, Anaissie E, Dekmezian R, Bodey GP. Primary *Candida* pneumonia. Experience at a large cancer center and review of the literature. Medicine (Baltimore) 1993; 72: 137-42.

[17]   Masur H, Rosen PP, Armstrong D. Pulmonary disease caused by *Candida* species. Am J Med 1977; 63: 914-25.

[18]   el-Ebiary M, Torres A, Fabregas N *et al.* Significance of the isolation of *Candida* species from respiratory samples in critically ill, non-neutropenic patients. An immediate postmortem histologic study. Am J Respir Crit Care Med 1997; 156: 583-90.

[19]   Sheng WH, Wang JT, Lin MS, Chang SC. Risk factors affecting in-hospital mortality in patients with nosocomial infections. J Formos Med Assoc 2007; 106: 110-8.

[20]   Sobieraj DM, White CM, Coleman CI. Benefits and risks of adjunctive inhaled corticosteroids in chronic obstructive pulmonary disease: a meta-analysis. Clin Ther 2008; 30: 1416-25.

[21]   Li S, An YZ. [Retrospective analysis of invasive fungal infection in surgical intensive care unit]. Zhonghua Yi Xue Za Zhi 2010; 90: 382-5.

[22]   Navarro J, Rainisio M, Harms HK *et al.* Factors associated with poor pulmonary function: cross-sectional analysis of data from the ERCF. European Epidemiologic Registry of Cystic Fibrosis. Eur Respir J 2001; 18: 298-305.

[23]   Chotirmall SH, O'Donoghue E, Bennett K, Gunaratnam C, O'Neill SJ, McElvaney NG. Sputum *Candida albicans* Presages FEV1 Decline and Hospital-Treated Exacerbations in Cystic Fibrosis. Chest 2010; 138: 1186-95.

[24]   Roux D, Gaudry S, Dreyfuss D *et al. Candida albicans* impairs macrophage function and facilitates *Pseudomonas aeruginosa* pneumonia in rat. Crit Care Med 2009; 37: 1062-7.

[25]   Muthig M, Hebestreit A, Ziegler U, Seidler M, Muller FM. Persistence of *Candida* species in the respiratory tract of cystic fibrosis patients. Med Mycol 2010; 48: 56-63.

[26]   Kullberg BJ, Sobel JD, Ruhnke M *et al.* Voriconazole versus a regimen of amphotericin B followed by fluconazole for candidaemia in non-neutropenic patients: a randomised non-inferiority trial. Lancet 2005; 366: 1435-42.

[27]   DiNubile MJ, Hille D, Sable CA, Kartsonis NA. Invasive candidiasis in cancer patients: observations from a randomized clinical trial. J Infect 2005; 50: 443-9.

[28]   Fanci R, Guidi S, Bonolis M, Bosi A. *Candida krusei* fungemia in an unrelated allogeneic hematopoietic stem cell transplant patient successfully treated with Caspofungin. Bone Marrow Transplant 2005; 35: 1215-6.

[29]   Ostrosky-Zeichner L, Rex JH, Pappas PG *et al.* Antifungal susceptibility survey of 2,000 bloodstream *Candida* isolates in the United States. Antimicrob Agents Chemother 2003; 47: 3149-54.

[30]   Pfaller MA, Messer SA, Boyken L *et al. In vitro* activities of voriconazole, posaconazole, and fluconazole against 4,169 clinical isolates of *Candida spp.* and *Cryptococcus neoformans* collected during 2001 and 2002 in the ARTEMIS global antifungal surveillance program. Diagn Microbiol Infect Dis 2004; 48: 201-5.

[31]   Pfaller MA, Messer SA, Hollis RJ, Jones RN, Diekema DJ. *In vitro* activities of ravuconazole and voriconazole compared with those of four approved systemic antifungal agents against 6,970 clinical isolates of *Candida spp.* Antimicrob Agents Chemother 2002; 46: 1723-7.

[32]   Denning DW. Invasive aspergillosis. Clin Infect Dis 1998;2 6: 781-803.

[33]   Chotirmall SH, Branagan P, Gunaratnam C, McElvaney NG. *Aspergillus*/allergic bronchopulmonary aspergillosis in an Irish cystic fibrosis population: a diagnostically challenging entity. Respir Care 2008; 53: 1035-41.

[34]   Rankin NE. Disseminated aspergillosis and moniliasis associated with agranulocytosis and antibiotic therapy. Br Med J 1953; 1: 918-9.

[35]   Marr KA, Carter RA, Crippa F, Wald A, Corey L. Epidemiology and outcome of mould infections in hematopoietic stem cell transplant recipients. Clin Infect Dis 2002; 34: 909-17.

[36]   Marty FM, Lee SJ, Fahey MM *et al.* Infliximab use in patients with severe graft-versus-host disease and other emerging risk factors of non-*Candida* invasive fungal infections in allogeneic hematopoietic stem cell transplant recipients: a cohort study. Blood 2003; 102: 2768-76.

[37]   Patterson TF, Kirkpatrick WR, White M *et al.* Invasive aspergillosis. Disease spectrum, treatment practices, and outcomes. I3 *Aspergillus* Study Group. Medicine (Baltimore). 2000; 79: 250-60.

[38]   Perfect JR, Cox GM, Lee JY *et al.* The impact of culture isolation of *Aspergillus* species: a hospital-based survey of aspergillosis. Clin Infect Dis 2001; 33: 1824-33.

[39]   Bulpa P, Dive A, Sibille Y. Invasive pulmonary aspergillosis in patients with chronic obstructive pulmonary disease. Eur Respir J 2007; 30: 782-800.

[40]   Samarakoon P, Soubani AO. Invasive pulmonary aspergillosis in patients with COPD: a report of five cases and systematic review of the literature. Chron Respir Dis 2008; 5: 19-27.

[41]   Clark H, Reid K. The potential of recombinant surfactant protein D therapy to reduce inflammation in neonatal chronic lung disease, cystic fibrosis, and emphysema. Arch Dis Child 2003; 88: 981-4.

[42]   Wert SE, Yoshida M, LeVine AM *et al.* Increased metalloproteinase activity, oxidant production, and emphysema in surfactant protein D gene-inactivated mice. Proc Natl Acad Sci U S A 2000; 97: 5972-7.

[43]   Ader F, Nseir S, Le Berre R *et al.* Invasive pulmonary aspergillosis in chronic obstructive pulmonary disease: an emerging fungal pathogen. Clin Microbiol Infect 2005; 11: 427-9.

[44]   Balloy V, Huerre M, Latge JP, Chignard M. Differences in patterns of infection and inflammation for corticosteroid treatment and chemotherapy in experimental invasive pulmonary aspergillosis. Infect Immun 2005; 73: 494-503.

[45]   Musher B, Fredricks D, Leisenring W, Balajee SA, Smith C, Marr KA. *Aspergillus* galactomannan enzyme immunoassay and quantitative PCR for diagnosis of invasive aspergillosis with bronchoalveolar lavage fluid. J Clin Microbiol 2004; 42: 5517-22.

[46]   Althoff Souza C, Muller NL, Marchiori E, Escuissato DL, Franquet T. Pulmonary invasive aspergillosis and candidiasis in immunocompromised patients: a comparative study of the high-resolution CT findings. J Thorac Imaging. 2006; 21: 184-9.

[47]   Millar FA, Simmonds NJ, Hodson ME. Trends in pathogens colonising the respiratory tract of adult patients with cystic fibrosis, 1985-2005. J Cyst Fibros 2009; 8: 386-91.

[48]   Baddley JW, Pappas PG, Smith AC, Moser SA. Epidemiology of *Aspergillus terreus* at a university hospital. J Clin Microbiol 2003; 41: 5525-9.

[49]   Hagerty JA, Ortiz J, Reich D, Manzarbeitia C. Fungal infections in solid organ transplant patients. Surg Infect (Larchmt) 2003; 4: 263-71.

[50]   Perkhofer S, Lass-Florl C, Hell M *et al.* The Nationwide Austrian *Aspergillus* Registry: a prospective data collection on epidemiology, therapy and outcome of invasive mould infections in immunocompromised and/or immunosuppressed patients. Int J Antimicrob Agents 2010; 36: 531-6.

[51]   Mastella G, Rainisio M, Harms HK *et al.* Allergic bronchopulmonary aspergillosis in cystic fibrosis. A European epidemiological study. Epidemiologic Registry of Cystic Fibrosis. Eur Respir J 2000; 16: 464-71.

[52]   Rapaka RR, Kolls JK. Pathogenesis of allergic bronchopulmonary aspergillosis in cystic fibrosis: current understanding and future directions. Med Mycol 2009; 47: S331-7.

[53]   Allard JB, Poynter ME, Marr KA, Cohn L, Rincon M, Whittaker LA. *Aspergillus fumigatus* generates an enhanced Th2-biased immune response in mice with defective cystic fibrosis transmembrane conductance regulator. J Immunol 2006; 177: 5186-94.

[54]   Chauhan B, Santiago L, Hutcheson PS *et al.* Evidence for the involvement of two different MHC class II regions in susceptibility or protection in allergic bronchopulmonary aspergillosis. J Allergy Clin Immunol 2000; 106: 723-9.

[55]   Brouard J, Knauer N, Boelle PY *et al.* Influence of interleukin-10 on *Aspergillus fumigatus* infection in patients with cystic fibrosis. J Infect Dis 2005; 191: 1988-91.

[56]   Knutsen AP, Kariuki B, Consolino JD, Warrier MR. IL-4 alpha chain receptor (IL-4Ralpha) polymorphisms in allergic bronchopulmonary aspergillosis. Clin Mol Allergy 2006; 4: 3.

[57]   Saraceno JL, Phelps DT, Ferro TJ, Futerfas R, Schwartz DB. Chronic necrotizing pulmonary aspergillosis: approach to management. Chest. 1997; 112: 541-8.

[58]   Soubani AO, Chandrasekar PH. The clinical spectrum of pulmonary aspergillosis. Chest. 2002; 121: 1988-99.

[59]   Denning DW, Riniotis K, Dobrashian R, Sambatakou H. Chronic cavitary and fibrosing pulmonary and pleural aspergillosis: case series, proposed nomenclature change, and review. Clin Infect Dis 2003; 37: S265-80.

[60]   Smith NL, Denning DW. Underlying conditions in chronic pulmonary aspergillosis, including simple aspergilloma. Eur Respir J 2010 ePub

[61]   Diekema DJ, Messer SA, Hollis RJ, Jones RN, Pfaller MA. Activities of caspofungin, itraconazole, posaconazole, ravuconazole, voriconazole, and amphotericin B against 448 recent clinical isolates of filamentous fungi. J Clin Microbiol 2003; 41: 3623-6.

[62]   Johnson LB, Kauffman CA. Voriconazole: a new triazole antifungal agent. Clin Infect Dis 2003; 36: 630-7.

[63]   Manavathu EK, Cutright JL, Chandrasekar PH. Organism-dependent fungicidal activities of azoles. Antimicrob Agents Chemother 1998; 42: 3018-21.

[64]   Torres HA, Hachem RY, Chemaly RF, Kontoyiannis DP, Raad, II. Posaconazole: a broad-spectrum triazole antifungal. Lancet Infect Dis 2005; 5: 775-85.

[65]   Chiou CC, Mavrogiorgos N, Tillem E, Hector R, Walsh TJ. Synergy, pharmacodynamics, and time-sequenced ultrastructural changes of the interaction between nikkomycin Z and the echinocandin FK463 against *Aspergillus fumigatus*. Antimicrob Agents Chemother 2001; 45: 3310-21.

[66]   Groll AH, Kolve H. Antifungal agents: *in vitro* susceptibility testing, pharmacodynamics, and prospects for combination therapy. Eur J Clin Microbiol Infect Dis 2004; 23: 256-70.

[67]   Summerbell RC, Krajden S, Kane J. Potted plants in hospitals as reservoirs of pathogenic fungi. Mycopathologia 1989; 106: 13-22.

[68]   Lake FR, Tribe AE, McAleer R, Froudist J, Thompson PJ. Mixed allergic bronchopulmonary fungal disease due to *Pseudallescheria boydii* and *Aspergillus*. Thorax 1990; 45: 489-91.

[69]   Blyth CC, Middleton PG, Harun A, Sorrell TC, Meyer W, Chen SC. Clinical associations and prevalence of *Scedosporium* spp. in Australian cystic fibrosis patients: identification of novel risk factors? Med Mycol 2010; 48: S37-S44.

[70]   Husain S, Munoz P, Forrest G *et al.* Infections due to *Scedosporium apiospermum* and *Scedosporium prolificans* in transplant recipients: clinical characteristics and impact of antifungal agent therapy on outcome. Clin Infect Dis 2005; 40: 89-99.

[71]   Symoens F, Knoop C, Schrooyen M *et al.* Disseminated *Scedosporium apiospermum* infection in a cystic fibrosis patient after double-lung transplantation. J Heart Lung Transplant 2006; 25: 603-7.

[72]   Troke P, Aguirrebengoa K, Arteaga C *et al.* Treatment of scedosporiosis with voriconazole: clinical experience with 107 patients. Antimicrob Agents Chemother 2008; 52: 1743-50.

[73]   Latge JP. *Aspergillus fumigatus* and aspergillosis. Clin Microbiol Rev. 1999; 12: 310-50.

[74]   Rementeria A, Lopez-Molina N, Ludwig A *et al.* Genes and molecules involved in *Aspergillus fumigatus* virulence. Rev Iberoam Micol 2005; 22: 1-23.

[75]   Levitz SM. Interactions of Toll-like receptors with fungi. Microbes Infect 2004; 6: 1351-5.

[76]   Clark IA, Gray KM, Rockett EJ *et al.* Increased lymphotoxin in human malarial serum, and the ability of this cytokine to increase plasma interleukin-6 and cause hypoglycaemia in mice: implications for malarial pathology. Trans R Soc Trop Med Hyg 1992; 86: 602-7.

[77]   Akira S, Uematsu S, Takeuchi O. Pathogen recognition and innate immunity. Cell 2006; 124: 783-801.

[78]   Braedel S, Radsak M, Einsele H *et al. Aspergillus fumigatus* antigens activate innate immune cells *via* toll-like receptors 2 and 4. Br J Haematol 2004; 125: 392-9.

[79]   Netea MG, Warris A, Van der Meer JW *et al. Aspergillus fumigatus* evades immune recognition during germination through loss of toll-like receptor-4-mediated signal transduction. J Infect Dis 2003; 188: 320-6.

[80]   Chai LY, Vonk AG, Kullberg BJ *et al. Aspergillus fumigatus* cell wall components differentially modulate host TLR2 and TLR4 responses. Microbes Infect 2010 ePub.

[81]   Shoham S, Levitz SM. The immune response to fungal infections. Br J Haematol 2005; 129: 569-82.

[82]   Wang JE, Warris A, Ellingsen EA *et al.* Involvement of CD14 and toll-like receptors in activation of human monocytes by *Aspergillus fumigatus* hyphae. Infect Immun 2001; 69: 2402-6.

[83]   Bochud PY, Chien JW, Marr KA *et al.* Toll-like receptor 4 polymorphisms and aspergillosis in stem-cell transplantation. N Engl J Med 2008; 359: 1766-77.

[84]   Meier A, Kirschning CJ, Nikolaus T, Wagner H, Heesemann J, Ebel F. Toll-like receptor (TLR) 2 and TLR4 are essential for *Aspergillus*-induced activation of murine macrophages. Cell Microbiol 2003; 5: 561-70.

[85]   Ramaprakash H, Ito T, Standiford TJ, Kunkel SL, Hogaboam CM. Toll-like receptor 9 modulates immune responses to *Aspergillus fumigatus* conidia in immunodeficient and allergic mice. Infect Immun 2009; 77: 108-19.

[86]   Ramirez-Ortiz ZG, Specht CA, Wang JP *et al.* Toll-like receptor 9-dependent immune activation by unmethylated CpG motifs in *Aspergillus fumigatus* DNA. Infect Immun 2008; 76: 2123-9.

[87]   Carvalho A, Pasqualotto AC, Pitzurra L, Romani L, Denning DW, Rodrigues F. Polymorphisms in toll-like receptor genes and susceptibility to pulmonary aspergillosis. J Infect Dis. 2008; 197: 618-21.

[88]   Novak N, Yu CF, Bussmann C *et al.* Putative association of a TLR9 promoter polymorphism with atopic eczema. Allergy. 2007; 62: 766-72.

[89]   Salvenmoser S, Seidler MJ, Dalpke A, Muller FM. Effects of caspofungin, *Candida albicans* and *Aspergillus fumigatus* on toll-like receptor 9 of GM-CSF-stimulated PMNs. FEMS Immunol Med Microbiol. 2010; 60: 74-7.

[90]   Balloy V, Chignard M. The innate immune response to *Aspergillus fumigatus*. Microbes Infect 2009; 11: 919-27.

[91]   Steele C, Rapaka RR, Metz A *et al.* The beta-glucan receptor dectin-1 recognizes specific morphologies of *Aspergillus fumigatus*. PLoS Pathog 2005; 1: e42.

[92]   Latge JP. Tasting the fungal cell wall. Cell Microbiol 2010; 12: 863-72.

[93]   Brown GD, Gordon S. Immune recognition. A new receptor for beta-glucans. Nature 2001; 413: 36-7.

[94]   Lanier LL. On guard--activating NK cell receptors. Nat Immunol 2001; 2: 23-7.

[95]   Ravetch JV, Bolland S. IgG Fc receptors. Annu Rev Immunol 2001; 19: 275-90.

[96]   Gantner BN, Simmons RM, Canavera SJ, Akira S, Underhill DM. Collaborative induction of inflammatory responses by dectin-1 and Toll-like receptor 2. J Exp Med 2003; 197: 1107-17.

[97]   Christin L, Wysong DR, Meshulam T, Hastey R, Simons ER, Diamond RD. Human platelets damage *Aspergillus fumigatus* hyphae and may supplement killing by neutrophils. Infect Immun 1998; 66: 1181-9.

[98]   Werner JL, Metz AE, Horn D *et al.* Requisite role for the dectin-1 beta-glucan receptor in pulmonary defense against *Aspergillus fumigatus*. J Immunol 2009; 182: 4938-46.

[99]   Kozel TR, Wilson MA, Farrell TP, Levitz SM. Activation of C3 and binding to *Aspergillus fumigatus* conidia and hyphae. Infect Immun. 1989; 57: 3412-7.

[100]   Behnsen J, Hartmann A, Schmaler J, Gehrke A, Brakhage AA, Zipfel PF. The opportunistic human pathogenic fungus *Aspergillus fumigatus* evades the host complement system. Infect Immun 2008; 76: 820-7.

[101]   Garlanda C, Hirsch E, Bozza S, Salustri A *et al.* Non-redundant role of the long pentraxin PTX3 in anti-fungal innate immune response. Nature 2002; 420: 182-6.

[102]   Bellocchio S, Bozza S, Montagnoli C *et al.* Immunity to *Aspergillus fumigatus*: the basis for immunotherapy and vaccination. Med Mycol 2005;43: S181-8.

[103]   Mehrad B, Strieter RM, Standiford TJ. Role of TNF-alpha in pulmonary host defense in murine invasive aspergillosis. J Immunol 1999; 162: 1633-40.

[104]   Mehrad B, Wiekowski M, Morrison BE *et al.* Transient lung-specific expression of the chemokine KC improves outcome in invasive aspergillosis. Am J Respir Crit Care Med 2002; 166: 1263-8.

[105]   Rivera A, Van Epps HL, Hohl TM, Rizzuto G, Pamer EG. Distinct CD4+-T-cell responses to live and heat-inactivated *Aspergillus fumigatus* conidia. Infect Immun 2005; 73: 7170-9.

[106]   Bellocchio S, Montagnoli C, Bozza S *et al.* The contribution of the Toll-like/IL-1 receptor superfamily to innate and adaptive immunity to fungal pathogens *in vivo*. J Immunol 2004; 172: 3059-69.

[107]   Zelante T, De Luca A, Bonifazi P *et al.* IL-23 and the Th17 pathway promote inflammation and impair antifungal immune resistance. Eur J Immunol 2007; 37: 2695-706.

[108]   Balloy V, Si-Tahar M, Takeuchi O *et al.* Involvement of toll-like receptor 2 in experimental invasive pulmonary aspergillosis. Infect Immun 2005; 73: 5420-5.

[109] Leonard EJ, Yoshimura T. Neutrophil attractant/activation protein-1 (NAP-1 [interleukin-8]). Am J Respir Cell Mol Biol 1990; 2: 479-86.

[110] Gibson PG, Wark PA, Simpson JL *et al.* Induced sputum IL-8 gene expression, neutrophil influx and MMP-9 in allergic bronchopulmonary aspergillosis. Eur Respir J 2003; 21: 582-8.

[111] Kelly E, Greene CM, McElvaney NG. Targeting neutrophil elastase in cystic fibrosis. Expert Opin Ther Targets 2008; 12: 145-57.

[112] Bozza S, Gaziano R, Spreca A *et al.* Dendritic cells transport conidia and hyphae of *Aspergillus fumigatus* from the airways to the draining lymph nodes and initiate disparate Th responses to the fungus. J Immunol 2002; 168: 1362-71.

[113] Funk MO, Isaac R, Porter NA. Letter: Free radical cyclization of unsaturated hydroperoxides. J Am Chem Soc 1975;9 7: 1281-2.

[114] Bulawa CE, Miller DW, Henry LK, Becker JM. Attenuated virulence of chitin-deficient mutants of *Candida albicans*. Proc Natl Acad Sci U S A 1995; 92: 10570-4.

[115] Buurman ET, Westwater C, Hube B, Brown AJ, Odds FC, Gow NA. Molecular analysis of CaMnt1p, a mannosyl transferase important for adhesion and virulence of *Candida albicans*. Proc Natl Acad Sci U S A 1998 ; 95: 7670-5.

[116] Lussier M, Sdicu AM, Shahinian S, Bussey H. The *Candida albicans* KRE9 gene is required for cell wall beta-1, 6-glucan synthesis and is essential for growth on glucose. Proc Natl Acad Sci U S A 1998; 95: 9825-30.

[117] Csank C, Schroppel K, Leberer E *et al.* Roles of the *Candida albicans* mitogen-activated protein kinase homolog, Cek1p, in hyphal development and systemic candidiasis. Infect Immun 1998; 66: 2713-21.

[118] Masuoka J. Surface glycans of *Candida albicans* and other pathogenic fungi: physiological roles, clinical uses, and experimental challenges. Clin Microbiol Rev 2004; 17: 281-310.

[119] Timpel C, Strahl-Bolsinger S, Ziegelbauer K, Ernst JF. Multiple functions of Pmt1p-mediated protein O-mannosylation in the fungal pathogen *Candida albicans*. J Biol Chem 1998; 273: 20837-46.

[120] Cutler JE. N-glycosylation of yeast, with emphasis on *Candida albicans*. Med Mycol 2001; 39: 75-86.

[121] Ernst JF, Prill SK. O-glycosylation. Med Mycol 2001; 39: 67-74.

[122] Underhill DM, Ozinsky A. Phagocytosis of microbes: complexity in action. Annu Rev Immunol 2002; 20: 825-52.

[123] Marr KA, Balajee SA, Hawn TR *et al.* Differential role of MyD88 in macrophage-mediated responses to opportunistic fungal pathogens. Infect Immun 2003; 71: 5280-6.

[124] Underhill DM, Gantner B. Integration of Toll-like receptor and phagocytic signaling for tailored immunity. Microbes Infect 2004; 6: 1368-73.

[125] Underhill DM, Ozinsky A. Toll-like receptors: key mediators of microbe detection. Curr Opin Immunol 2002; 14: 103-10.

[126] Underhill DM, Ozinsky A, Hajjar AM *et al.* The Toll-like receptor 2 is recruited to macrophage phagosomes and discriminates between pathogens. Nature 1999; 401: 811-5.

[127] Kilpatrick DC. Mannan-binding lectin: clinical significance and applications. Biochim Biophys Acta 2002; 1572: 401-13.

[128] Brouwer N, Dolman KM, van Houdt M, Sta M, Roos D, Kuijpers TW. Mannose-binding lectin (MBL) facilitates opsonophagocytosis of yeasts but not of bacteria despite MBL binding. J Immunol 2008; 180: 4124-32.

[129] Lee SJ, Gonzalez-Aseguinolaza G, Nussenzweig MC. Disseminated candidiasis and hepatic malarial infection in mannose-binding-lectin-A-deficient mice. Mol Cell Biol 2002; 22: 8199-203.

[130] Brown GD. Dectin-1: a signaling non-TLR pattern-recognition receptor. Nat Rev Immunol 2006; 6: 33-43.

[131] Brown GD, Herre J, Williams DL, Willment JA, Marshall AS, Gordon S. Dectin-1 mediates the biological effects of beta-glucans. J Exp Med 2003; 197: 1119-24.

[132] Ghosh S, Howe N, Volk K, Tati S, Nickerson KW, Petro TM. *Candida albicans* cell wall components and farnesol stimulate the expression of both inflammatory and regulatory cytokines in the murine RAW264.7 macrophage cell line. FEMS Immunol Med Microbiol 2010; 60: 63-73.

[133] McGreal EP, Rosas M, Brown GD *et al.* The carbohydrate-recognition domain of Dectin-2 is a C-type lectin with specificity for high mannose. Glycobiology 2006; 16: 422-30.

[134] Sato K, Yang XL, Yudate T *et al.* Dectin-2 is a pattern recognition receptor for fungi that couples with the Fc receptor gamma chain to induce innate immune responses. J Biol Chem 2006; 281: 38854-66.

[135] Jouault T, El Abed-El Behi M, Martinez-Esparza M *et al.* Specific recognition of *Candida albicans* by macrophages requires galectin-3 to discriminate Saccharomyces cerevisiae and needs association with TLR2 for signaling. J Immunol 2006; 177: 4679-87.

[136] Cambi A, Gijzen K, de Vries JM *et al.* The C-type lectin DC-SIGN (CD209) is an antigen-uptake receptor for *Candida albicans* on dendritic cells. Eur J Immunol 2003; 33: 532-8.

[137] Kery V, Krepinsky JJ, Warren CD, Capek P, Stahl PD. Ligand recognition by purified human mannose receptor. Arch Biochem Biophys 1992; 298: 49-55.

[138] Lemaitre B, Nicolas E, Michaut L, Reichhart JM, Hoffmann JA. The dorsoventral regulatory gene cassette spatzle/Toll/cactus controls the potent antifungal response in *Drosophila* adults. Cell. 1996; 86: 973-83.

[139] Simon A, Kullberg BJ, Tripet B *et al.* Drosomycin-like defensin, a human homologue of *Drosophila melanogaster* drosomycin with antifungal activity. Antimicrob Agents Chemother 2008; 52: 1407-12.

[140] Ozinsky A, Underhill DM, Fontenot JD *et al.* The repertoire for pattern recognition of pathogens by the innate immune system is defined by cooperation between toll-like receptors. Proc Natl Acad Sci U S A 2000; 97: 13766-71.

[141] Netea MG, Van Der Graaf CA, Vonk AG, Verschueren I, Van Der Meer JW, Kullberg BJ. The role of toll-like receptor (TLR) 2 and TLR4 in the host defense against disseminated candidiasis. J Infect Dis 2002; 185: 1483-9.

[142] Villamon E, Gozalbo D, Roig P, O'Connor JE, Fradelizi D, Gil ML. Toll-like receptor-2 is essential in murine defenses against *Candida albicans* infections. Microbes Infect 2004; 6: 1-7.

[143] Netea MG, van de Veerdonk F, Verschueren I, van der Meer JW, Kullberg BJ. Role of TLR1 and TLR6 in the host defense against disseminated candidiasis. FEMS Immunol Med Microbiol 2008; 52: 118-23.

[144] Blasi E, Mucci A, Neglia R *et al.* Biological importance of the two Toll-like receptors, TLR2 and TLR4, in macrophage response to infection with *Candida albicans*. FEMS Immunol Med Microbiol 2005; 44: 69-79.

[145] Netea MG, Sutmuller R, Hermann C *et al.* Toll-like receptor 2 suppresses immunity against *Candida albicans* through induction of IL-10 and regulatory T cells. J Immunol 2004; 172: 3712-8.

[146] Sutmuller RP, den Brok MH, Kramer M *et al.* Toll-like receptor 2 controls expansion and function of regulatory T cells. J Clin Invest 2006; 116: 485-94.

[147] van de Veerdonk FL, Netea MG, Jansen TJ *et al.* Redundant role of TLR9 for anti-Candida host defense. Immunobiology 2008; 213: 613-20.

[148] Tessarolli V, Gasparoto TH, Lima HR *et al.* Absence of TLR2 influences survival of neutrophils after infection with *Candida albicans*. Med Mycol 2010 ;48: 129-40.

[149] Romani L. Immunity to fungal infections. Nat Rev Immunol 2004; 4: 1-23.

[150] Villamon E, Gozalbo D, Roig P *et al.* Myeloid differentiation factor 88 (MyD88) is required for murine resistance to *Candida albicans* and is critically involved in Candida -induced production of cytokines. Eur Cytokine Netw 2004; 15: 263-71.

[151] Cenci E, Romani L, Vecchiarelli A, Puccetti P, Bistoni F. T cell subsets and IFN-gamma production in resistance to systemic candidosis in immunized mice. J Immunol 1990; 144: 4333-9.

[152] Romani L, Mocci S, Bietta C, Lanfaloni L, Puccetti P, Bistoni F. Th1 and Th2 cytokine secretion patterns in murine candidiasis: association of Th1 responses with acquired resistance. Infect Immun 1991; 59: 4647-54.

[153] Belkaid Y, Rouse BT. Natural regulatory T cells in infectious disease. Nat Immunol 2005; 6: 353-60.

[154] Montagnoli C, Bacci A, Bozza S *et al.* B7/CD28-dependent CD4+CD25+ regulatory T cells are essential components of the memory-protective immunity to *Candida albicans*. J Immunol 2002; 169: 6298-308.

[155] Sakaguchi S. Naturally arising CD4+ regulatory T cells for immunologic self-tolerance and negative control of immune responses. Annu Rev Immunol 2004; 22: 531-62.

[156] Lee HK, Iwasaki A. Innate control of adaptive immunity: dendritic cells and beyond. Semin Immunol 2007; 19: 48-55.

[157] d'Ostiani CF, Del Sero G, Bacci A *et al.* Dendritic cells discriminate between yeasts and hyphae of the fungus *Candida albicans*. Implications for initiation of T helper cell immunity *in vitro* and *in vivo*. J Exp Med 2000; 191:1661-74.

[158] Pasare C, Medzhitov R. Toll-dependent control mechanisms of CD4 T cell activation. Immunity 2004; 21: 733-41.

[159] Pasare C, Medzhitov R. Toll-like receptors: linking innate and adaptive immunity. Adv Exp Med Biol 2005; 560: 11-8.

[160] Yang Y, Huang CT, Huang X, Pardoll DM. Persistent Toll-like receptor signals are required for reversal of regulatory T cell-mediated CD8 tolerance. Nat Immunol 2004; 5: 508-15.

[161] Netea MG, Van der Meer JW, Kullberg BJ. Toll-like receptors as an escape mechanism from the host defense. Trends Microbiol 2004; 12: 484-8.

[162] Huang W, Na L, Fidel PL, Schwarzenberger P. Requirement of interleukin-17A for systemic anti-Candida albicans host defense in mice. J Infect Dis 2004; 190: 624-31.

[163] Bourgeois C, Majer O, Frohner IE, Tierney L, Kuchler K. Fungal attacks on mammalian hosts: pathogen elimination requires sensing and tasting. Curr Opin Microbiol 2010; 13: 401-8.

[164] Ferwerda G, Netea MG, Joosten LA, van der Meer JW, Romani L, Kullberg BJ. The role of Toll-like receptors and C-type lectins for vaccination against *Candida albicans*. Vaccine 2010; 28: 614-22.

[165] Stevens DA, Clemons KV, Liu M. Developing a vaccine against aspergillosis. Med Mycol 2010 ePub.

[166] Wells CA, Salvage-Jones JA, Li X *et al.* The macrophage-inducible C-type lectin, mincle, is an essential component of the innate immune response to *Candida albicans.* J Immunol 2008; 180: 7404-13.

[167] Kabelitz D, Medzhitov R. Innate immunity--cross-talk with adaptive immunity through pattern recognition receptors and cytokines. Curr Opin Immunol 2007; 19:1-3.

[168] Miyake K. Innate immune sensing of pathogens and danger signals by cell surface Toll-like receptors. Semin Immunol 2007; 19: 3-10.

[169] Poulain D, Jouault T. *Candida albicans* cell wall glycans, host receptors and responses: elements for a decisive crosstalk. Curr Opin Microbiol 2004; 7: 342-9.

[170] West AP, Koblansky AA, Ghosh S. Recognition and signaling by toll-like receptors. Annu Rev Cell Dev Biol 2006; 22: 409-37.

CHAPTER 10

The Role of Toll-Like Receptors in Lung Transplantation

Jonathan C. Yeung, Shaf Keshavjee and Mingyao Liu[*]

The Latner Thoracic Surgery Research Laboratories, Toronto General Research Institute, University Health Network, Department of Surgery, Faculty of Medicine, University of Toronto, Canada

Abstract: Lung transplantation is now a mainstream therapy for end-stage lung disease. However, long-term survival remains diminished by antigen-independent ischemia-reperfusion injury and antigen-dependent acute and chronic rejection. While rejection has traditionally been considered an adaptive immune response, the innate immune response, and events mediated by Toll-like receptors in particular, have recently been shown to be important to the priming and modulation of this adaptive immune response. Unlike other solid organ transplants, the lung is in constant communication with the outside environment and innate immunity likely plays a more significant role in lung transplantation. In this chapter, we will review Toll-like receptor responses in the context of lung transplantation.

Keywords: Lung transplantation, TLRs, ischemia reperfusion injury, chronic rejection, transplantation tolerance.

1. INTRODUCTION

Following the first successful clinical lung transplant in Toronto in 1983 [1], lung transplantation now represents a mainstream therapy for end-stage lung disease globally. Between 1988 and 2008, the number of lung transplants performed worldwide increased dramatically from 83 to approximately 2200 procedures annually [2]. Today, the indications for lung transplant span the spectrum of lung diseases, the most common being: chronic obstructive pulmonary disease, emphysema, idiopathic pulmonary fibrosis, cystic fibrosis, idiopathic pulmonary arterial hypertension, and Eisenmenger's syndrome.

Barriers to successful lung transplantation continue to exist in the modern era. The 5-year survival for lung transplant recipients (about 50%) remains the lowest among solid organ transplant recipients [2]. Primary Graft Dysfunction (PGD) is largely caused by ischemia-reperfusion injury (IRI), an acute inflammatory multi-factorial and antigen-independent acute lung injury characterized clinically by pulmonary edema and impaired gas exchange immediately or in the early period following lung transplantation [3]. The clinical presentation has many similarities to the adult respiratory distress syndrome caused by an over-exuberant inflammatory response. Injury to the donor lung during donor brain death, complications from intensive care, mechanical ventilation and the lung preservation strategy can all contribute towards this inflammatory injury. Recent improvements in donor selection and management along with improved lung preservation strategies have lowered but not eliminated the risk for PGD. Late graft failure is likely related more to antigen-dependent factors, and improvements in surgical technique and lung preservation have not resulted in significant improvements in long-term outcomes. The immunosuppression protocols used for lung transplantation today remain primarily focused on impairing the T-cell response, yet episodes of acute rejection occur on a regular basis [4]. Moreover, bronchiolitis obliterans (BOS), the progressive fibrosis and obliteration of the small airway lumens, remains the major cause of late mortality, and is seen in the majority of lung transplant recipients despite adequate immunosuppression [2, 5].

The innate immune system has been largely overlooked during the development of lung transplantation and there is now increasing evidence for the critical role of the innate immune response in influencing both antigen-independent early graft dysfunction and antigen-dependent adaptive immunity [6-8]. Toll-like

---

*Address correspondence to Mingyao Liu:** Professor of Surgery, Faculty of Medicine, University of Toronto, 101 College Street, Toronto Medical Discovery Tower, Room 2-814,Toronto, Ontario, M5G 1L7 Canada; Tel: 416-581-7500; E-mail: mingyao.liu@utoronto.ca

receptors (TLR) and other pattern recognition receptors appear to be vital to the innate immune response to transplantation and a better understanding of this response may lead to better immunosuppression strategies and improved long term outcomes [9, 10].

2. PROCESS OF LUNG TRANSPLANTATION

The procedure of lung transplantation proceeds through several distinct steps (Fig. **1**) [11]. First, the lung retrieval operation is performed, usually at a distant hospital, during which the donor lung is assessed clinically and then removed from the donor after the pulmonary vasculature is flushed anterograde and retrograde with a cold low-potassium dextran solution. The lungs are stored inflated with 50% oxygen following removal and cooled on ice for transport back to the transplant hospital and for the anesthetic and surgical preparation of the lung recipient. Altogether, this time on ice is known as the *cold ischemic time* and generally does not exceed 12 hours [12].

Following the removal of the recipient's native lungs, a donor lung is removed from the ice for implantation into the recipient. As the lung is no longer chilled on ice, the lung is now considered to be "warm", and this time is considered the *warm ischemic time*. In practice, a cooling jacket is placed around the lung to slow the warming of the lung. Warm ischemic time ends with the completion of the surgical anastamoses and the start of reperfusion of the lung. Following reperfusion, the chest is closed and the patient is brought to the intensive care unit for postoperative care and assessment of the early function of the lung.

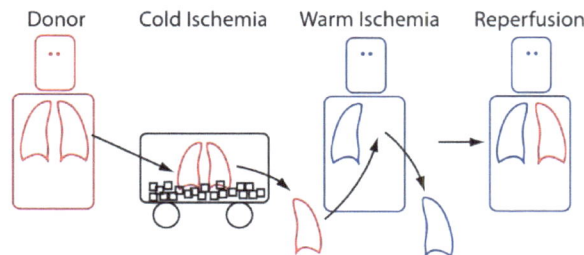

Figure 1: Schematic for the process of lung transplantation. A single lung transplant is depicted; double lung transplantation is performed as sequential single lung transplants [11].

3. TOLL-LIKE RECEPTORS

A brief overview of the Toll-like receptor will be discussed in this chapter with an emphasis on mechanisms important to understanding current animal models of transplantation. More detailed discussion can be found elsewhere in this book or in the following reviews [13, 14]. Following the discovery of Toll as an important receptor to fight fungal infection in *Drosophila*, a mammalian Toll-like receptor, TLR4, was identified as an important inducer of pro-inflammatory genes [9, 10]. TLRs are now known to be receptors encoded by the genome which are involved in recognizing highly conserved molecular patterns on both pathogenic microorganisms and endogenous injury molecules. These patterns have been named pathogen associated molecular patterns (PAMPs) and damage-associated molecular patterns (DAMPs), respectively [15]. Thus, TLRs can act as sensors of microbial infection and cellular injury. PAMPs include distinctly non-self molecules such as lipopolysaccharide (LPS), peptidoglycan, flagellin, unmethylated CpG DNA, dsRNA, and ssRNA. In comparison, DAMPs are endogenous proteins and include high mobility group box 1 protein (HMGB1), oxidized phospholipids, fibrinogen, hyaluronic acid, and heat shock proteins. TLRs are a family of at least 12 members and are expressed on many cell types, including professional antigen-presenting cells (APC), T-cells, endothelial cells, and lung epithelial cells [6]. Currently, 10 TLRs have been identified in humans. TLRs 1, 2, 4, 5, 6, and 10 are expressed at the cellular membrane, while the remaining TLRs are expressed within endosomes for the recognition of bacterial and viral RNA and DNA.

TLRs are type 1 integral membrane proteins [13]. The extracellular N-terminal consists of leucine rich repeating regions and the C-terminal consists of an IL-1 receptor homology region known as the Toll/IL-1 receptor (TIR) domain. This domain is required for downstream signal transduction. Following ligand recognition, TIR domain adaptor proteins are recruited to the TLR. These adaptors include MyD88, TIRAP, TRIF, and TRAM. The majority of TLRs link either directly or indirectly to the adaptor protein MyD88, and use of the MyD88 knockout mouse has greatly increased our understanding of innate immunity in transplantation. An alternative pathway is the TRIF pathway of TLR4 and TLR3. TLR3 utilizes the TRIF pathway exclusively, while TLR4 can activate both MyD88 and TRIF pathways. TLR activation can result in NF-κB activation, MAPK activation, and type 1 interferon expression.

4. TLR INVOLVEMENT IN ISCHEMIA-REPERFUSION INJURY

Contribution of the innate immune response to inflammation post-transplantation is increasingly being recognized and TLRs are being implicated as the sensors and effectors of this response [16]. One early report of innate immunity and TLRs in lung transplantation was by Andrade and colleagues. They studied gene expression of TLRs in human lung tissues collected during clinical transplantation. Lung biopsies from 14 patients who received double lung transplantation were studied pre- and post- reperfusion and expression levels of multiple TLRs were highly correlated with that of cytokine mRNAs [17]. A correlation was found between the cytokine IL-8 and TLR4 levels both before and after reperfusion. Higher donor lung IL-8 has been shown to be associated with poorer post-transplant lung function [18], thus higher expression of TLR4 may also reflect the inflammatory status of donor lungs. Andrade and colleagues also noted that HSP70 was significantly induced by reperfusion and may represent an important DAMP in lung transplantation.

The initial donor lung condition, lung preservation strategy and the process of transplantation can cause a certain degree of unavoidable cellular injury with the subsequent release of endogenous DAMPs. TLR4 is the mammalian sensor of LPS, but it has also been shown to be activated by DAMPs such as HMGB1, hyaluronans, surfactant protein A, and others [16]. The contribution of TLR4 to ischemia-reperfusion has been modeled in TLR4 knockout mice by Shimamoto and colleagues using a 60 minute hilar-clamp model of lung ischemia-reperfusion injury (IRI) [19]. By comparing the TLR4 knockout mice to wildtype mice, they were able to show that TLR4 deficiency results in significantly reduced (but not completely absent) IRI using permeability index, MPO activity, and BAL cell count readouts. They also demonstrated that TLR4 activity during IRI was associated with activation of MAPK and JNK, and nuclear translocation of NF-κB and AP-1, known downstream mediators of TLR4. One can argue that this model of warm ischemia/reperfusion without the cold ischemia (hypothermic preservation) of the donor lung does not accurately model the lung transplant process. However, activation of MAPK and JNK have been noted from samples collected from human [20] as well as from rat lung transplantation [21], which is associated with alteration of protein tyrosine phosphorylation and other signaling events [22].

Recently, Zanotti and colleagues studied the role of TLR4 in ischemia-reperfusion injury and found that TLR4 activation may cause pulmonary edema by regulation of the endothelial cell cytoskeleton rather than by alterations in gene expression and inflammation [23]. First, they confirmed the Shimamoto results using a 60-minute warm ischemia model of lung IRI in a TLR4-defective mouse strain and showed that TLR4-deficiency resulted in less edema formation and faster resolution of edema. They then extended the work by showing that TLR4 blockade by the inhibitor CRX-526 also prevented edema formation. In an attempt to identify the downstream signaling of this response, they examined a strain of MyD88 deficient mice but found that these mice developed the same level of edema as the wild type mice. This implies that although TLR4 may be involved in IRI-induced pulmonary edema formation, the downstream signal from TLR4 may be not be the MyD88-dependent pathway. TRIF is a well known alternative signal pathway by which TLR4 can transmit signals; however, TRIF is not expressed on murine endothelial cells [24]. The development of edema may thus be due to other unknown signaling pathways, or due to TLR4 activity on non-endothelial cells, such as the alveolar macrophages or the pulmonary epithelium. Previous studies have shown the importance of the epithelial side of the epithelial-endothelial border in the development of lung edema [25] and of the role of alveolar macrophages in the development of lung ischemia-reperfusion injury [26, 27]. In order to distinguish between TLR activation on alveolar macrophages and TLR activation on parenchymal (*i.e.* lung epithelial) cells, chimeric mice with either TLR4 function only in parenchymal cells or only in myeloid cells were generated [23]. Lung edema formation only occurred when TLR4 function was present on parenchymal cells, suggesting that the role of alveolar macrophage TLR is not important to the development of IRI. With regards to downstream MAPK and NF-κB activation, they found that while TLR4 deficiency delays and reduces both MAPK and NF-κB activation, it is not completely abrogated and NF-κB activation also occurs in the presumed normal contralateral lung. Thus, a direct correlation between reduced NF-κB activation and lung edema formation was not found [23].

To better understand the mechanism of TLR4 activation, Zanotti and his colleagues used an *in vitro* model of warm IRI [23]. By replacing culture media with Ringer's Lactate from a confluent monolayer of human microvascular endothelial cells (HMVEC) for one hour and culturing cells in a 100% oxygen environment, they simulated warm ischemia and ventilation with 100% oxygen as in their *in vivo* hilar clamp model. Reperfusion was simulated by replenishing the cells with normal media and culturing in the normal 5% CO_2 environment. Gap junction and actin rearrangements in the monolayers occurred following "reperfusion" in this cellular model and was blocked by the TLR4 inhibitor CRX-526. Interestingly, conditioned Ringer's Lactate from HMVECs after 1 hour of warm ischemia was not able to create the same actin rearrangements nor activate NF-κB suggesting that a soluble DAMP was not present within the medium. However, further studies will need to confirm this finding. Cardella and colleagues have used human lung epithelial (A549) cells to simulate a cold ischemia-reperfusion process of lung transplantation [28]. Although these model systems can only reflect certain features of lung preservation and transplantation, they may help to delineate the contribution of TLRs in different cell types in IRI. Selection of the appropriate cell types and culture conditions are important for the experimental design and interpretation of results.

The importance of TLR4 to IRI has been reflected in similar studies using liver and kidney models of ischemia-reperfusion or transplantation. While all of these studies implicate TLR4 in ischemia-reperfusion injury, the proposed mechanism is not as clear. Again, all these studies used a warm IRI model. In contrast to the Zanotti study, Tsung and colleagues showed that TLR4-mediated hepatic IRI requires TLR4-expression on non-parenchymal cells, in particular the Kupffer cell which is analogous to the alveolar macrophage in the lung [29]. Similar to the Zanotti study, Zhai and colleagues also found that TLR4 mediated liver IRI was not MyD88 dependent [30]. In a study by Wu and colleagues where a warm kidney ischemia-reperfusion injury model was used, again, TLR4 was found to be important to the development of kidney IRI [31]. However, it appears that in kidneys, TLR4-mediated IRI proceeds through a MyD88-dependent pathway, but like the lung, is dependent on parenchymal TLR4 expression. Thus, a unified mechanism to explain TLR-mediated IRI in all organs has not been found and organ specific differences may exist. Lungs, which communicate with the environment, may ultimately have different mechanisms of injury than that of the "sterile" solid organs.

Given the evidence for the importance of TLR4 activation in the development of IRI, the actual ligand has not yet been identified. Ischemia-reperfusion injury is seen in many organs, thus the ligand is more likely to be an endogenous DAMP rather than a PAMP. A recently studied DAMP is HMGB1. This protein is one of the most conserved proteins in the eukaryokic kingdom and works in the nucleus to bind and bend DNA [32]. When released from necrotic or damaged cells, however, HMGB1 acts as a potent danger signal and proinflammatory mediator and appears to signal through TLR4 [33]. In the liver, inhibition of HMGB1 by a neutralizing antibody was shown to be protective of IRI and administration of exogenous recombinant HMGB1 was shown to worsen IRI [34].

The process of brain death has been associated with an adrenergic and cytokine storm which can injure organs while in the donor body and has also been shown to promote IRI in rat models of lung transplantation [35, 36]. While it is unclear in the lung transplant literature whether this effect is related to TLR activation during brain death, there is some evidence of brain death-induced DAMP formation in the kidney transplant literature due to the prevalent use of living-donor kidneys. Kruger and colleagues recently compared human donor kidneys from living-donors to those from brain-dead donors in clinical kidney transplantation [37]. They observed that HMGB1 expression was increased in tubular cells of brain-dead donor kidneys when compared to living donor kidneys. They also looked at two loss-of-function single nucleotide polymorphisms in TLR4, Asp299Gly and Thr399Ile [38]. In the 30 recipients of kidneys from

TLR4 mutant donors, immediate graft function was superior and there was lower intra-graft pro-inflammatory gene expression.

Overall, there is now convincing evidence that TLRs play a role in the development of IRI. This should provide the rationale for further work in the context of lung transplantation. In particular, a study on the role of brain death in TLR activation would be valued. One limitation of the data in the lung is the reliance on warm IRI models. Utilization of a lung cold ischemia model typically necessitates the orthotopic transplantation of the lung. In order to take advantage of knockout mice, this represents the need for a murine orthotopic lung transplant model. Such a model has recently been developed using a cuff technique for transplantation [39]. While highly technically demanding, use of this model would open up not just a cold ischemic model, but could be combined with models of brain death, pneumonia, or aspiration to assess these clinically relevant problems on TLR mediated IRI. Ultimately, this may lead to new insights into the role of the lung's contact with the environment on activation of TLRs.

5. TLR INVOLVEMENT IN ACUTE REJECTION

For many decades, acute allograft rejection has been thought of as a primarily T-cell mediated phenomenon and current clinically used immunosuppressive agents remain largely targeted against this response [4]. However, it is now known that activation of T-cells requires more than just a foreign peptide-MHC interaction, but also requires T-cell co-stimulation by antigen presenting cells (APCs). Janeway first proposed that APCs were quiescent, *i.e.* no costimulatory molecule expression, until activated by a PAMP [40]. Toll-like receptors were subsequently implicated as a key PAMP sensor and TLR activation in APCs has now been shown to cause the upregulation of costimulatory molecules leading to activation of the adaptive immune response [41]. The Matzinger danger hypothesis has built upon this model and suggests that the immune system is more concerned with damage than with foreignness [42]. In addition to PAMPs, Matzinger postulated that endogenous "danger" or "alarm" signals secreted or released by injured cells could also activate APCs. The recent discovery of TLR binding endogenous molecules (DAMPs) lends support to this hypothesis. All organ grafts undergo sequential injuries during brain death, surgical organ retrieval and storage, and ischemia-reperfusion all of which can lead to DAMP molecule presentation. Organs such as the lung, but also skin and bowel, are exposed to the outside environment and thus process a variety of commensal and pathogenic bacteria which may translocate during the transplantation process. It has been shown that lung and bowel transplants have higher rates of acute rejection when compared to other solid organs. Alegre, Chong, and others have advanced the hypothesis that these organs reject more frequently because of the combination of DAMP and PAMP molecules priming the adaptive immune response [43, 44].

Currently, there has been no study utilizing a model of lung transplantation to study TLR ligation in acute rejection. However, experimental skin transplantation models have been utilized and, given that skin is also continuously exposed to the environment, these models could be considered a prelude to experiments with lung transplantation. Using a minor mismatch (male to female) model of skin transplantation, Goldstein and colleagues showed that recipient mice would accept a donor skin graft permanently if both donor and recipient were MyD88$^{-/-}$; however, MyD88 expression in either the donor graft or recipient mouse would lead to the rejection of the skin graft [45]. Consistent with the hypothesis that reduced APC activation by TLR signaling leads to a reduction in T-cell activation, the investigators found that mature dendritic cells (DC) within the lymph nodes of the recipients was reduced. Reconstitution with delivery of either wild type DCs or primed wild type spleen cells led to rejection. It must be noted, however, that this could also be due to decreased migration of DCs rather than just decreased activation. In an attempt to identify the specific TLR needed for this effect, the investigators attempted to replicate the MyD88$^{-/-}$ results in TLR4$^{-/-}$ and TLR2$^{-/-}$ mice. While TLR2$^{-/-}$ mice appeared to slow rejection, TLR4$^{-/-}$ mice rejected at the same rates as wild type. Thus, multiple TLRs *via* multiple PAMPs/DAMPs may be important in signaling to MyD88 for the acute rejection response. Overall, in this model, MyD88 appears to be important in DC maturation or migration and subsequent T-cell activation.

It was subsequently shown by the same group that knockout of MyD88 in both donor and recipient was unable to prolong the survival of a fully allogeneic skin graft [46]. In the analysis of DCs within the draining lymph nodes of these recipients, DCs were found and could present co-stimulatory molecules, but the absolute numbers of DCs were reduced. Furthermore, these DCs were found to be able to stimulate allo-primed T-cells, but were impaired at priming naïve T-cells. Thus, while MyD88 appears to be involved in acute rejection in a minor-mismatch model of skin transplantation, it is not the sole pathway towards the development of acute rejection in a major mismatch model. The logical hypothesis arising from this study would be that the MyD88 independent pathway of TLR signaling, the TRIF pathway, becomes vital in the absence of MyD88. Thus, McKay and colleagues used donor mice with double-knockouts of MyD88 and TRIF [47]. Again, a major mismatch skin model was utilized, but the double knockout skin grafts were transplanted into wild type recipients. In this model, there was slightly prolonged graft survival. As the recipient was wild type, this may represent blunting of the early donor derived DC activation of T-cells (direct allorecognition). In addition, they showed that there was reduced migration of donor DCs to the draining lymph nodes, thus TLRs may affect DC migration rather than maturation. A study of MyD88 and TRIF knockout in both the donor and recipient was not performed.

TLR signaling has been shown to increase Th1 immune responses but not Th2. Correspondingly, in the above studies, TLR signaling blockade appeared to impair Th1 but not Th2 immune responses. In the case of a minor-antigen mismatch model, IFN-γ and IL-4 levels, classic Th1 and Th2 cytokines, respectively, were measured by RT-PCR in draining nodes [45]. There was a significant drop in IFN-γ but not IL-4 following MyD88$^{-/-}$ blockade. In a subsequent study, Tesar and colleagues used an ELISPOT-effector assay to assess spleen cells following transplantation of fully MHC-mismatched skin grafts between MyD88$^{-/-}$ donors and recipients [46]. They found that rejection occurred at the same rate as wild type skin transplants; however, the MyD88$^{-/-}$ transplant recipients' spleen cells had a reduced number of IL-2 and IFN-γ producing cells compared to IL-4 producing cells. There was still an increase of IL-2 and IFN-γ production compared to responder only controls, thus this represents an impaired not an abrogated Th1 response. Moreover, given that the speed of rejection remained the same, Th2-mediated rejection may be possible in the setting of reduced Th1 responses.

A relatively newly discovered subset of T helper cells, Th17 cells, have been implicated in driving autoimmune disease and in playing a role in the anti-microbial function of the epithelial/mucosal barrier, of which the lung has plenty [48]. Chen and colleagues have recently studied the role of CpG, a TLR9 agonist, in the driving of acute rejection in a murine cardiac transplant model [49]. CpG administration resulted in the systemic production of IL-6 and IL-12. Subsequently, alloreactive T-cells secreted not only IFN-γ, but also IL-17, implying that both Th1 and Th17 differentiation of alloreactive T cells is involved in TLR induced acute rejection. Using chimeric mice, they were able to show that this response is mediated by TLRs of recipient cells of hematopoietic origin.

Further experimental evidence demonstrating local innate immunity triggering of acute allograft rejection was provided by Garantziotis and colleagues using a murine bone marrow transplant (BMT) model [50]. In their model, fully mismatched BMT was performed with careful donor cell titration to avoid post-BMT systemic graft-*versus*-host-disease (GVHD). In essence, due to the exchange of immune systems, an immunologic "lung transplant" had been performed without surgical injury, ischemia-reperfusion injury, and release of DAMPs. Following aerosolized LPS administration intra-tracheally, the "new" immune system was primed by TLR activation and led to a pronounced T-cell mediated rejection of the lung. In addition, by using different combinations of TLR4-deficient mice as recipient or as donor, they showed that it was the TLR expressed on the donor leukocyte which was important. As GVHD can be considered the mirror of acute rejection, this appears to support the data by Chen and colleagues that it is recipient cells of hematopoietic origin that are important to TLR mediated acute rejection.

Thus, while TLRs play a role in the initiation of T-cell mediated rejection, much like the role of TLR in IRI, the actual ligand or ligands important for this effect remain unclear. HMGB1 is again implicated in TLR-mediated acute rejection. It can strongly affect DC maturation and polarize towards the Th1 response [51]. In a murine model of heart transplantation, Huang and colleagues showed that HMGB1 is released by damaged cells in both syngeneic and allogeneic hearts, as well as actively secreted by graft-infiltrated DCs and macrophages [52]. There was an immediate but transient increase of HMGB1 in syngeneic grafts which likely reflects injury surrounding retrieval and ischemia-reperfusion. On the contrary, allogeneic grafts maintained a high HMGB1 level following transplantation. Blockade of HMGB1 led to decreased TNF-α and IFN-γ levels. Other DAMPs have also been shown to be involved in alloimmunity *via* TLR signaling. Tesar and colleagues studied the putative DAMP, hyaluronan [53]. Fragmented hyaluronan was shown to induce dendritic cell maturation *in vitro* and to be dependent on TLRs 2 and 4 and the adaptor protein TIRAP, but surprisingly independent of MyD88 or TRIF. These DCs could also prime allogeneic T-cells *in vitro* in a largely TLR4-dependent fashion. Using a minor-mismatch skin transplantation model, they showed that rejecting skin grafts expressed higher levels of hyaluronan. They subsequently analyzed the amount of hyaluronan in the BAL of human lung transplant recipients. Patients with BOS had higher levels of hyaluronan than patients who did not. While they did not correlate levels of hyaluronan release with acute lung rejection, a relationship between hyaluronan and acute clinical kidney rejection has been shown [54]. Other DAMPs have been studied in the context of acute rejection. HSP60 and 70 were shown to be endogenous ligands for TLRs by Vabulas and colleagues [55] and Ohashi and colleagues [56], respectively, but this could not be replicated by Tesar and colleagues [53]. Much like in TLR activation in IRI, it is unlikely that during the global insults of transplantation, only one specific DAMP would be critical for IRI and priming of the acute allograft response.

TLRs have also been studied in the context of susceptibility to infection and TLR polymorphisms found to render a person susceptible to infection have been described. In particular, patients with either the Asp299Gly or Thr399Ile polymorphisms demonstrated lower responses to LPS. Thus, perhaps recipients with these polymorphisms would also be less susceptible to DAMPs and PAMPs during transplantation. Palmer and colleagues analyzed the fate of lung transplant recipients who had these polymorphisms compared to wild type recipients and found a lower rate of acute rejection at 6 months and also at 3 years post-transplant [57, 58]. They also noted a reduced severity of BOS at the 3 year time point. Interestingly, TLR4 polymorphisms in the recipient, but not in the donor, were associated with the reduced rates of acute rejection. This implies that it is the recipient cells, not the donor cells, which are important to this effect and corroborates the above animal studies. This same group further looked at the 159TT promoter polymorphism in CD14, a molecule which can assist with the binding of LPS to TLR4 [59]. This polymorphism results in increased transcription of CD14 and patients with this polymorphism had earlier acute rejection, BOS, and graft loss with increased CD14, TNF-α, and IFN-γ.

6. TLR SIGNALING AND TRANSPLANTATION TOLERANCE

Modern immunosuppressive regimens have been the key to the success of organ transplantation in recent decades. However, such life-long regimens have significant morbidities such as increased risks of infection, malignancy and kidney disease. Induction of immunological tolerance towards the graft is the elusive "holy grail" of transplantation. Costimulation blockade for the induction of tolerance has led to the long-term acceptance of skin and cardiac allografts in mouse [60]. Unfortunately, translation to non-human primate models has been met with little success [61]. Given that TLR activation can activate APCs and lead to increased costimulatory signals, TLR signaling may prime the immune response and interfere with costimulation blockade tolerance strategies. Thornley and colleagues have worked on a skin transplantation model [62]. In one costimulation protocol, donor-specific transfusion and anti-CD154 antibody, has been shown to significantly prolong major-mismatch skin transplantation in mouse by the deletion of alloreactive T-cells. However, lymphocytic choriomeningitis virus infection at the time of donor specific transfusion abrogates this survival benefit [63]. Likely, the virus acted as a PAMP for TLR activation. To test this theory, they administered TLR agonists, LPS (TLR4 agonist), Pam3Cys (TLR2 agonist), poly I:C (TLR3 agonist), and CpG DNA (TLR9 agonist) during costimulation blockade and replicated the abrogation of survival benefit by the prevention of apoptosis of graft-specific T-cells [62]. Subsequently, this same group has shown that LPS abrogates tolerance in skin grafts *via* TLR4 and MyD88 and that poly I:C does so in a TLR3-independent fashion. The end result of both pathways is the upregulation of type 1 interferons and signaling through IFN-R1 [64].

TLR abrogation of transplantation tolerance can also occur in "sterile" organs such as the heart. In fully allogeneic cardiac allografts, Chen and colleagues showed that B6 recipients could accept a BALB/c heart in the long-term if anti-CD154 therapy was given [43]. This is less stringent than the skin model where MyD88 knockout in both donor and recipient is required for anti-CD154 therapy to work and may represent the additional immunogenicity of environmentally exposed organs. When CpG or Pam3Cys was administered, anti-CD154 induced cardiac tolerance was abrogated [43]. They showed that intra-graft CCR4-expressing Treg chemokines CCL17 and CCL22 were reduced with a corresponding decrease in the recruitment of FoxP3+ Tregs. The same group subsequently showed that CpG administration could result in decreased conversion of graft-reactive T-cells into inducible regulatory T-cells. The cytokine profile also changed following CpG administration. A rapid systemic production of IL-12 and IL-6 led to the expression of IFN-γ and IL-17 by graft infiltrating CD4+ T-cells despite anti-CD154 therapy, suggesting that TLR stimulation promotes Th1 and Th17 differentiation [49]. CpG mediated prevention of anti-CD154-mediated allograft acceptance was halted in anti-IL-17 mAb treated IL-6 knockout mice suggesting that IL-6 and IL-17 cytokines were vital for this effect. Interestingly, blockade of IL-17 and IL-6 in the absence of anti-CD154 resulted in rapid rejection suggesting that acute rejection and CpG-mediated rejection of anti-CD154 treated recipients operates by different mechanisms. Thus, ligation of TLR at the time of transplantation can alter proinflammatory events and stimulate rejection. The actual mechanisms, whether through changes in cytokine production, Th differentiation, Treg recruitment, or others, remain to be fully elucidated. It is likely that redundant pathways lead to the same clinical phenotype of rejection.

The above studies on rejection have centered on skin transplantation models and heterotopic heart models of transplantation and no studies have yet been performed using lung transplant models. The technically demanding nature of orthotopic lung transplantation in mice coupled with the graft-dependent survival of the recipient animal complicates the study of acute rejection using lungs. Skin is thus a reasonable substitute for the lung as it is also exposed to the environment and can also develop lymphoid neogenesis. However, there are likely to be organ-specific differences that will ultimately need to be addressed with a lung model.

One of the most pressing concerns in lung transplantation is that of bronchiolitis obliterans syndrome. This is the major factor contributing to the low 5 year survival of lung transplant recipients and is currently poorly understood. BOS continues to occur despite adequate immunosuppression and increased rates of BOS are associated with episodes of IRI and acute rejection, thus the immune process likely plays a role [65]. A variety of animal models have been developed for BOS research, each with advantages and limitations [66]. Recently, a murine intrapulmonary tracheal transplant model has been developed as a model for BOS [67]. It represents many pathological and molecular features of BOS, it is relatively easy to perform, and animals do not rely on the function of the transplanted grafts for survival. Perhaps utilization of this and other similar models with knockout mice will help to elucidate the role of TLRs in BOS.

7. CONCLUSIONS AND PERSPECTIVES

After decades of focus on T-cell responses to lung (and organ) transplantation, the role of the innate immune system and in particular, the role of TLRs, is now being studied and elucidated (Fig. **2**). The innate immune system is a phylogenetically ancient mechanism representing the first line of defense against foreign invasion and damage response. Lung transplantation is a highly un-natural event and ischemic injury during organ storage and surgical trauma during implantation may lead to the release of DAMPs and the activation of TLRs. In an organ constantly exposed to the environment such as the lung, increased exposure to PAMPs may occur leading to increased TLR activation. TLR activation has been shown to influence ischemia-reperfusion injury as well as promote rejection and break current tolerance protocols. TLR blockade and/or blockade of downstream signals may eventually be useful in clinical practice, but current knowledge of these signals is too incomplete for the safe development of such a strategy. Like the modern immunosuppression strategies of today, strategic targeting in TLR blockade will be essential to minimize the theoretical potential for increased risk of infection and malignancy.

Detailed knowledge regarding the ligands important to the innate immune response and the signaling events which occur following TLR ligation are still lacking. Models studying the TLR response in transplantation have included a variety of TLR ligands and span DAMPs and PAMPs. Clinical studies have implicated HMGB1, HSPs, and hyaluronans, but it is unlikely that these are the sole culprits. It is also unlikely that

TLRs are the only PRRs important to the innate immune response. Other PRRs exist such as NOD, RAGE, or DC-Sign which could signal an adaptive immune response through common and/or distinct pathways.

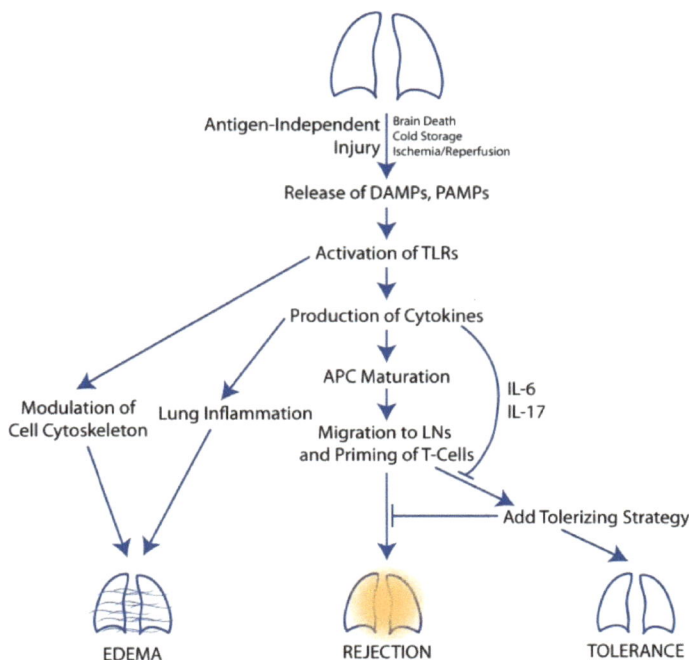

Figure 2: Antigen-independent injury of the lung can cause release of TLR ligands which can promote edema *via* cell cytoskeleton modulation [23] and/or lung inflammation [26, 27]. Release of cytokines can promote the maturation of APCs and prime the adaptive immune response [44]. Moreover, certain cytokines released can block currently known tolerance strategies in animal models [49].

The lack of appropriate models of lung transplantation for the use of transgenic mice has limited the study of TLRs in lung transplantation. However, recent developments in murine orthotopic lung transplant and murine intrapulmonary tracheal transplant models should hopefully stimulate the study of TLRs in lung-specific models. Studies focused on BOS will be of particular value given the significant clinical relevance.

In summary, a role for TLRs and the innate immune response in the development of ischemia-reperfusion injury and the promotion of graft rejection has been established. Specific mechanisms of this response remain to be fully elucidated and further studies, particularly in the lung, need to be done in order to develop strategies to control the innate immune contribution to acute and chronic lung allograft dysfunction

REFERENCES

[1] Cooper JD, Pearson FG, Patterson GA *et al.* Technique of successful lung transplantation in humans. J Thorac Cardiovasc Surg 1987; 93: 173-81.

[2] Taylor DO, Stehlik J, Edwards LB *et al.* Registry of the international society for heart and lung transplantation: twenty-sixth official adult heart transplant report-2009. J Heart Lung Transplant 2009; 28: 1007-22.

[3] de Perrot M, Liu M, Waddell TK, Keshavjee S. Ischemia-reperfusion-induced lung injury. Am J Respir Crit Care Med 2003; 167: 490-511.

[4] Bhorade SM, Stern E. Immunosuppression for lung transplantation. Proc Am Thorac Soc 2009; 6: 47-53.

[5] Sato M, Keshavjee S. Bronchiolitis obliterans syndrome: alloimmune-dependent and -independent injury with aberrant tissue remodeling. Semin Thorac Cardiovasc Surg 2008; 20: 173-82.

[6] Manicassamy S, Pulendran B. Modulation of adaptive immunity with Toll-like receptors. Semin Immunol 2009; 21: 185-93.

[7] Andrade CF, Waddell TK, Keshavjee S, Liu M. Innate immunity and organ transplantation: the potential role of toll-like receptors. Am J Transplant 2005; 5: 969-75.

[8]   Liu M. Innate immunity and lung transplantation. In: Society CT, Ed. Contributions in Transplantation: Innate Immunity in Organ Transplantation. Barcelona: Prous Science 2006; pp. 3-13.

[9]   Lemaitre B, Nicolas E, Michaut L, Reichhart JM, Hoffmann JA. The dorsoventral regulatory gene cassette spatzle/Toll/cactus controls the potent antifungal response in *Drosophila* adults. Cell 1996; 86: 973-83.

[10]   Medzhitov R, Preston-Hurlburt P, Janeway CA, Jr. A human homologue of the *Drosophila* Toll protein signals activation of adaptive immunity. Nature 1997; 388: 394-7.

[11]   Boasquevisque CH, Yildirim E, Waddel TK, Keshavjee S. Surgical techniques: lung transplant and lung volume reduction. Proc Am Thorac Soc 2009; 6: 66-78.

[12]   Fischer S, Matte-Martyn A, De Perrot M *et al.* Low-potassium dextran preservation solution improves lung function after human lung transplantation. J Thorac Cardiovasc Surg 2001; 121: 594-6.

[13]   Takeda K, Kaisho T, Akira S. Toll-like receptors. Annu Rev Immunol 2003; 21: 335-76.

[14].   O'Neill LA, Bowie AG. The family of five: TIR-domain-containing adaptors in Toll-like receptor signaling. Nat Rev Immunol 2007; 7: 353-64.

[15]   Bianchi ME. DAMPs, PAMPs and alarmins: all we need to know about danger. J Leukoc Biol 2007; 81: 1-5.

[16]   Mollen KP, Anand RJ, Tsung A, Prince JM, Levy RM, Billiar TR. Emerging paradigm: toll-like receptor 4-sentinel for the detection of tissue damage. Shock 2006; 26: 430-7.

[17]   Andrade CF, Kaneda H, Der S *et al.* Toll-like receptor and cytokine gene expression in the early phase of human lung transplantation. J Heart Lung Transplant 2006; 25: 1317-23.

[18]   Fisher AJ, Donnelly SC, Hirani N *et al.* Elevated levels of interleukin-8 in donor lungs is associated with early graft failure after lung transplantation. Am J Respir Crit Care Med 2001; 163: 259-65.

[19]   Shimamoto A, Pohlman TH, Shomura S, Tarukawa T, Takao M, Shimpo H. Toll-like receptor 4 mediates lung ischemia-reperfusion injury. Ann Thorac Surg 2006; 82: 2017-23.

[20]   Sakiyama S, Hamilton J, Han B *et al.* Activation of mitogen-activated protein kinases during human lung transplantation. J Heart Lung Transplant 2005; 24: 2079-85.

[21]   Sakiyama S, dePerrot M, Han B, Waddell TK, Keshavjee S, Liu M. Ischemia-reperfusion decreases protein tyrosine phosphorylation and p38 mitogen-activated protein kinase phosphorylation in rat lung transplants. J Heart Lung Transplant 2003; 22: 338-46.

[22]   Keshavjee S, Zhang XM, Fischer S, Liu M. Ischemia reperfusion-induced dynamic changes of protein tyrosine phosphorylation during human lung transplantation. Transplantation 2000; 70: 525-31.

[23]   Zanotti G, Casiraghi M, Abano JB *et al.* Novel critical role of Toll-like receptor 4 in lung ischemia-reperfusion injury and edema. Am J Physiol Lung Cell Mol Physiol 2009; 297: L52-63.

[24]   Harari OA, Alcaide P, Ahl D, Luscinskas FW, Liao JK. Absence of TRAM restricts Toll-like receptor 4 signaling in vascular endothelial cells to the MyD88 pathway. Circ Res 2006; 98: 1134-40.

[25]   Pierre AF, DeCampos KN, Liu M *et al.* Rapid reperfusion causes stress failure in ischemic rat lungs. J Thorac Cardiovasc Surg 1998; 116: 932-42.

[26]   Naidu BV, Krishnadasan B, Farivar AS *et al.* Early activation of the alveolar macrophage is critical to the development of lung ischemia-reperfusion injury. J Thorac Cardiovasc Surg 2003; 126: 200-7.

[27]   Zhao M, Fernandez LG, Doctor A *et al.* Alveolar macrophage activation is a key initiation signal for acute lung ischemia-reperfusion injury. Am J Physiol Lung Cell Mol Physiol 2006; 291: L1018-26.

[28]   Cardella JA, Keshavjee S, Mourgeon E *et al.* A novel cell culture model for studying ischemia-reperfusion injury in lung transplantation. J Appl Physiol 2000; 89: 1553-60.

[29]   Tsung A, Hoffman RA, Izuishi K *et al.* Hepatic ischemia/reperfusion injury involves functional TLR4 signaling in nonparenchymal cells. J Immunol 2005; 175:7661-8.

[30]   Zhai Y, Shen XD, O'Connell R, Gao F *et al.* Cutting edge: TLR4 activation mediates liver ischemia/reperfusion inflammatory response *via* IFN regulatory factor 3-dependent MyD88-independent pathway. J Immunol 2004;173(12):7115-9.

[31]   Wu H, Chen G, Wyburn KR, Yin J *et al.* TLR4 activation mediates kidney ischemia/reperfusion injury. J Clin Invest 2007; 117: 2847-59.

[32]   Lotze MT, Tracey KJ. High-mobility group box 1 protein (HMGB1): nuclear weapon in the immune arsenal. Nat Rev Immunol 2005; 5: 331-42.

[33]   Scaffidi P, Misteli T, Bianchi ME. Release of chromatin protein HMGB1 by necrotic cells triggers inflammation. Nature 2002; 418: 191-5.

[34]   Tsung A, Sahai R, Tanaka H *et al.* The nuclear factor HMGB1 mediates hepatic injury after murine liver ischemia-reperfusion. J Exp Med 2005; 201: 1135-43.

[35]   Avlonitis VS, Fisher AJ, Kirby JA, Dark JH. Pulmonary transplantation: the role of brain death in donor lung injury. Transplantation 2003; 75: 1928-33.

[36]   Avlonitis VS, Wigfield CH, Golledge HD, Kirby JA, Dark JH. Early hemodynamic injury during donor brain death determines the severity of primary graft dysfunction after lung transplantation. Am J Transplant 2007; 7: 83-90.

[37]   Kruger B, Krick S, Dhillon N *et al.* Donor Toll-like receptor 4 contributes to ischemia and reperfusion injury following human kidney transplantation. Proc Natl Acad Sci U S A 2009; 106: 3390-5.

[38]   Arbour NC, Lorenz E, Schutte BC *et al.* TLR4 mutations are associated with endotoxin hyporesponsiveness in humans. Nat Genet 2000; 25: 187-91.

[39]   Okazaki M, Krupnick AS, Kornfeld CG *et al.* A mouse model of orthotopic vascularized aerated lung transplantation. Am J Transplant 2007; 7: 1672-9.

[40]   Janeway CA. Approaching the asymptote? Evolution and revolution in immunology. Cold Spring Harbor Symposia on Quantitative Biology 1989; 54(1).

[41]   Akira S, Uematsu S, Takeuchi O. Pathogen recognition and innate immunity. Cell 2006; 124: 783-801.

[42 Matzinger P. The danger model: a renewed sense of self. Science 2002; 296: 301-5.

[43]   Chen L, Wang T, Zhou P *et al.* TLR engagement prevents transplantation tolerance. Am J Transplant 2006; 6: 2282-91.

[44]   Obhrai J, Goldstein DR. The role of toll-like receptors in solid organ transplantation. Transplantation 2006; 81: 497-502.

[45]   Goldstein DR, Tesar BM, Akira S, Lakkis FG. Critical role of the Toll-like receptor signal adaptor protein MyD88 in acute allograft rejection. J Clin Invest 2003; 111: 1571-8.

[46]   Tesar BM, Zhang J, Li Q, Goldstein DR. TH1 immune responses to fully MHC mismatched allografts are diminished in the absence of MyD88, a toll-like receptor signal adaptor protein. Am J Transplant 2004; 4: 1429-39.

[47]   McKay D, Shigeoka A, Rubinstein M, Surh C, Sprent J. Simultaneous deletion of MyD88 and Trif delays major histocompatibility and minor antigen mismatch allograft rejection. Eur J Immunol 2006; 36: 1994-2002.

[48]   Korn T, Bettelli E, Oukka M, Kuchroo VK. IL-17 and Th17 Cells. Annu Rev Immunol 2009; 27: 485-517.

[49]   Chen L, Ahmed E, Wang T *et al.* TLR signals promote IL-6/IL-17-dependent transplant rejection. J Immunol 2009; 182: 6217-25.

[50]   Garantziotis S, Palmer SM, Snyder LD *et al.* Alloimmune lung injury induced by local innate immune activation through inhaled lipopolysaccharide. Transplantation 2007; 84: 1012-9.

[51]   Messmer D, Yang H, Telusma G *et al.* High mobility group box protein 1: an endogenous signal for dendritic cell maturation and Th1 polarization. J Immunol 2004; 173: 307-13.

[52]   Huang Y, Yin H, Han J *et al.* Extracellular hmgb1 functions as an innate immune-mediator implicated in murine cardiac allograft acute rejection. Am J Transplant. 2007; : 799-808.

[53]   Tesar BM, Jiang D, Liang J, Palmer SM, Noble PW, Goldstein DR. The role of hyaluronan degradation products as innate alloimmune agonists. Am J Transplant 2006; 6: 2622-35.

[54]   Wells A, Larsson E, Fellstrom B, Tufveson G, Klareskog L, Laurent T. Role of hyaluronan in chronic and acutely rejecting kidneys. Transplant Proc 1993; 25: 2048-9.

[55]   Vabulas RM, Wagner H, Schild H. Heat shock proteins as ligands of toll-like receptors. Curr Top Microbiol Immunol 2002; 270: 169-84.

[56]   Ohashi K, Burkart V, Flohe S, Kolb H. Cutting edge: heat shock protein 60 is a putative endogenous ligand of the toll-like receptor-4 complex. J Immunol 2000; 164: 558-61.

[57]   Palmer SM, Burch LH, Trindade AJ *et al.* Innate immunity influences long-term outcomes after human lung transplant. Am J Respir Crit Care Med 2005; 171: 780-5.

[58]   Goldstein DR, Palmer SM. Role of Toll-like receptor-driven innate immunity in thoracic organ transplantation. J Heart Lung Transplant 2005; 24: 1721-9.

[59]   Palmer SM, Klimecki W, Yu L *et al.* Genetic regulation of rejection and survival following human lung transplantation by the innate immune receptor CD14. Am J Transplan. 2007; 7:693-9.

[60]   Larsen CP, Elwood ET, Alexander DZ *et al.* Long-term acceptance of skin and cardiac allografts after blocking CD40 and CD28 pathways. Nature 1996;381: 434-8.

[61]   Kean LS, Gangappa S, Pearson TC, Larsen CP. Transplant tolerance in non-human primates: progress, current challenges and unmet needs. Am J Transplant 2006; 6: 884-93.

[62]   Thornley TB, Brehm MA, Markees TG *et al.* TLR agonists abrogate costimulation blockade-induced prolongation of skin allografts. J Immunol 2006; 176: 1561-70.

[63]   Turgeon NA, Iwakoshi NN, Meyers WC *et al.* Virus infection abrogates cd8(+) t cell deletion induced by donor-specific transfusion and anti-cd154 monoclonal antibody. Curr Surg 2000; 57: 505-6.

[64]   Miller DM, Thornley TB, Pearson T *et al.* TLR agonists prevent the establishment of allogeneic hematopoietic chimerism in mice treated with costimulation blockade. J Immunol 2009; 182: 5547-59.

[65]   Estenne M, Maurer JR, Boehler A *et al.* Bronchiolitis obliterans syndrome 2001: an update of the diagnostic criteria. J Heart Lung Transplant 2002; 21: 297-310.

[66]   Sato M, Keshavjee S, Liu M. Translational research: animal models of obliterative bronchiolitis after lung transplantation. Am J Transplant 2009; 9: 1981-7.

[67]   Wagnetz D, Sato M, Hirayama S *et al.* The mouse intrapulmonary tracheal transplant model of obliterative bronchiolitis: a novel tool to investigate lymphoid neogenesis in the lung after ransplantation. J Heart Lung Transplant 2009; 28: S247.

INDEX

A